UPDATED GUIDELINES FOR SURVIVING PROSTATE CANCER

UPDATED GUIDELINES FOR SURVIVING PROSTATE CANCER

E. Roy Berger, M.D., F.A.C.P. and James Lewis, Jr., Ph.D.

Health Education Literary Publisher

ISBN: 1-4107-9128-9 (e-book)
ISBN: 1-4107-9127-0 (Paperback)
ISBN: 1-4107-9129-7 (Dust Jacket)

For information, contact:
Health Education Literary Publisher
380 North Broadway – Suite 304
Jericho, New York 11753
Phone: 516-942-5000
Fax: 516-942-5025
Email: ecpcp@aol.com

1stBooks-rev 12/09/03

DEDICATION

To all of the prostate cancer patients and their families that we have learned so much from in our efforts to help them in every way possible. Each and every one has touched us and added to our ability to give to others as we seek better answers for those who follow in their footsteps.

CONTRIBUTORS

We are grateful to the following physicians, researchers, scientists, and other individuals who contributed their expertise, making Updated Guidelines a reality.

Rebecca Carley, M.D.
Specialist in Vaccine-Induced
Diseases
9 Sutherland Rd.
Hicksville, NY 11801
Tel/Fax: 516-433-0774
www.drcarley.com

Frank A. Critz, M.D.
Radiation Oncologist
Radiotherapy Clinics of Georgia
2349 Lawrenceville Highway
Decatur, GA 30033
Tel: 404-320-1550

Bruce Curran
Vice President
NOMOS Corporation
2591 Wexford Bayne Rd., Ste 400
Sewickley, PA 15143
Tel: 724-934-8200

Jeffrey Demanes, M.D.
Radiation Oncologist
California Endocurietherapy
3012 Summit St., Ste. 2675
Oakland, CA 94609
Tel: 510-986-0690

Winston Dyer
Patient Advocate/Advisor
115-70 202nd St.
St. Albans, NY 11412
Tel: 718-712-3997

Steven Evans
President & Senior Research
Scientist
Genetic Services Mgmt., Inc.
418 N. 38th St.
Omaha, NE 68131
Tel: 402-551-1020
Fax: 402-556-5743
sevans@gsm-usa.com

Edward Goldman, M.D.
Vice President of Medical Affairs
Intl. Urology Network, LLC
World Trade Center
401 E. Pratt St., 11th Floor
Baltimore, MD 21202
Tel: 410-659-7488

Llewellyn Hyacinthe, M.D.
Urologist
Urology Associates
60 Plaza St. East
Brooklyn, NY 11238
Tel: 718-638-9222

Michael N. Kattan, Ph.D.
Outcomes Research Scientist
Dept. of Urology
Epidemiology @ Biostatistics
Memorial Sloan-Kettering
Cancer Center
1275 York Ave.
New York, NY 10021
Tel: 646-422-4386

Charles Knouse, D.O.
Medical Oncologist
Aidan Clinic
621 South 48th St., Ste. 111
Tempe, AZ 85281
Tel: 480-446-8181
Toll-free: 1-877-585-7684
aidan@aidan-az.com

John Kurhanewitz, Ph.D.
Asst. Professor Radiology,
Bioengineering, Pharmaceutical
Chemistry
U.C.S.F. Comprehensive Cancer
Center
Dept. of Radiology
Box 1290, USCF
San Francisco, CA 94143
Tel: 415-476-0312

Fred Lee, M.D.
Cryosurgeon, Radiologist
Rochester Urology
1135 W. University Dr., Ste. 420
Rochester Hills, MI 48307
Tel: 248-650-4699

Arlene J. Lennox, M.D.
Clinical Physicist
Fermi National Accelerator
Laboratory
PO Box 500, MS 301
Batavia, IL 60510-0500
Tel: 630-840-3865

Sonny Levinbook, A.C.S.W.
Oncology Social
Worker/Psychotherapist
3771 Nesconset Hwy
Ste. 101-B
South Setauket, NY 11720
Tel: 631-689-1854

Mario Menelly
Advisor/Patient Advocate
Education Center for
Prostate Cancer Patients
380 North Broadway, Ste. 304
Jericho, NY 11753
Tel: 516-942-5000

Charles Myers, M.D.
Medical Oncologist
American Institute for Disease of
the Prostate
690 Bent Oaks Drive
Earlysville, VA 22936
Tel: 434-964-0212

Ed Van Overloop
Nutritional Advisor
Nature's Market Place
One West Ridgewood Ave.
Ridgewood, NJ 07450
Tel: 201-455-9210

John S. Pellerito, M.D.
Radiologist
Radiology/Ultrasound Dept.
North Shore Hospital
300 Community Drive
Manhasset, NY 11030
Tel: 516-562-2796

Julie Ann Plantamura, R.N.,
M.S.N., F.N.P.
Nurse Practitioner
North Shore
Hematology/Oncology Associates
235 North Belle Mead Rd.
East Setauket, NY 11733
Tel: 631-751-0506

Rodney R. Rodriguez, M.D.,
Ph.D.
Radiation Oncologist
California Endocurietherapy
3012 Summit St., Ste. 2675
Oakland, CA 94609
Tel: 510-986-0690

Edward T. Samuel M.D., Ph.D.
Medical Oncologist
Sub-Specialty Pain and
Neurologic Oncology
North Shore
Hematology/Oncology Assoc.
235 North Belle Mead Rd.
East Setauket, NY 11733
Tel: 631-751-3000

Jeffrey Scott, M.D.
National Medical Director
Intl. Oncology Network
World Trade Center
410 E. Pratt St.
Baltimore, MD 21201
Tel: 410-385-2900

Katsuto Shinohara, M.D.
Urologist
Subspecialty in Oncology
U.C.S.F.
Box 0711
San Francisco, CA 94143-0711
Tel: 415-476-1611

Martin Silverstein, M.D.
Radiation Oncologist
North Shore Radiation/Oncology
181 North Belle Mead Rd.
East Setauket, NY 11733
Tel: 631-689-6776

Richard Stock, M.D.
Radiation Oncologist
Professor and Chairman of
Radiation Oncology
Mt. Sinai Medical Center
11854 5th Ave., 1st floor
Mt. Sinai, NY 11766
Tel: 212-241-7502

Stephen B. Strum, M.D.
Medical Oncologist
538 Granite Street
Ashland, OR 97520
Tel: 541-482-5884

Robert Walshon
V.P. Managed Care
Intl. Urology Network
World Trade Center
401 East Pratt Street
Baltimore, MD 21202
Tel: 877-223-2400

Harold Wodinsky, MA, MHSC.
Chief Operating Officer
Intl. Urology Network
World Trade Center
401 E. Pratt Street
Baltimore, MD 21202
Tel: 877-223-2400

*We would also like to thank those
who assisted us with the
production of this book:*

Ann Favilla, ECPCP,
Administrative Assistant

Maria Marino, ECPCP,
Executive Assistant

Bettye Rainwater, ECPCP,
Director of Communication

Patricia Mansfield Phelan,
Glanville Enterprises, Ltd., Copy
Editor.

Michael Cochran, Cochran
Designs

William Britton, EditText

CONTENTS

PART IV PROSTATE CANCER INFORMATION

QUALIFYING STATEMENT

INTRODUCTION

New Guidelines for Surviving Prostate Cancer, our first book, was highly acclaimed as one of the finest, most easy-to-read, and most comprehensive books on the many facets of prostate cancer. At that time, Dr. Berger stated, "Research is continually ongoing, and as more information is collected, treatment options may change." He continued, "I expect many sequels to this book, or books like it, to be necessary to keep the public up-to-date on the state-of-the-art diagnosis and treatment of prostate cancer." Dr. Berger's words ring true. We knew there would be changes in the diagnosis and treatment of the second leading cause of death in men in the United States. We just didn't know how many changes there would be or how rapidly they would take place. In fact, it was difficult for us to complete Updated Guidelines because as soon as we incorporated the latest treatment into the text, another one would appear on the scene. For instance, two new treatments, which we had to leave out due to reasons of space, are two promising alternative therapies: an herb called Artemisinin and a protein known as Azurin. We just compared the number of chapters in the first edition, which was 26, to the 44 chapters in this updated version, a nearly 69 percent increase. Updated Guidelines is divided into four parts: Diagnosing Prostate Cancer, Imaging the Prostate, Treating Prostate Cancer, and Important Prostate Cancer Information. It also includes an appendix of resources and a glossary.

PART I: DIAGNOSING PROSTATE CANCER

Part I begins with the normal diagnostic sequence urologists use to screen men for prostate cancer. The exact sequence is important because if any step is performed out of order or omitted, it may delay diagnosis or treatment. For example, if you have a PSA level of 4.0 to 10 ng/ml "the gray area" and the free/total PSA ratio is not checked, you may end up being biopsied unnecessarily. This ratio helps determine whether the PSA level is elevated due to prostate cancer or to benign causes such as prostatitis or an enlarged prostate. Another example: if your urologist fails to conduct a transrectal ultrasound of your prostate, he or she may miss a suspicious area that should have been biopsied, possibly delaying a diagnosis of prostate cancer. Chapter 1 begins with the need for all men age 50 years and older to get a blood test known as a prostatic specific antigen (PSA) test. Men at higher risk should have the test beginning at age 40. The PSA test is the first step in a sequence of four to detect whether a man has prostate cancer. The PSA test is divided into two forms — the complex and the free — to separate men with cancer from those who do not have it. Some attention is given to the PSA range according to age, race, and nationality. A probability table — the Partin Tables — is also included to help understand the pathologic stage of the tumor based upon PSA, Gleason score, and clinical stage. Other blood markers are also discussed. Chapter 2 discusses the need for the doctor to perform the second step in the sequential diagnostic procedure, a digital rectal examination. It explains how the DRE is performed and presents some of its limitations. This step, along with the PSA test, is essential for the initial detection of prostate cancer. If one of these tests is omitted or not performed in the proper manner, the patient's disease may go undetected. Chapter 3, Transrectal Ultrasound, is devoted to the third step in the diagnostic sequence: the visualization of the prostate on a transrectal ultrasound in order to look for suspicious areas and target them for biopsy. Some attention is also given to the pros and cons of the ultrasound as a screening device. The fourth step in the diagnostic sequence, the extraction of tissue known as a biopsy, is presented in Chapter 4. The pathologist conducts tests on the extracted tissue to determine if malignant cells are visible and, if so, to determine the Gleason score. Until recently, if the result of the biopsy was inconclusive, the patient would eventually need to undergo a second biopsy. However, an alternative procedure has evolved in which laboratories in at least three hospitals take the "inconclusive" tissues to look for certain overexpressing genes. These genes may give enough evidence of prostate cancer that a repeat biopsy can be avoided. Chapter 5 presents information on a gene for metastatic prostate cancer. Not only does the presence of the gene determine if a patient has prostate cancer, but it also determines how aggressive the cancer is — and whether or not it is metastasized.

PART II: IMAGING THE PROSTATE

Currently, hundreds of millions of dollars are spent on two tests that are not necessary. If a man's PSA level is less than 10 ng/ml, it is highly unlikely that a CT scan or bone scan will add useful information to the staging procedure. It is probably more prudent for the patient to avoid these two tests and to save the money for an image modality known as an MRSI, which has an excellent record in determining localized prostate cancer. Chapters 6 and 7 highlight this imaging technique. As of this writing, however, it is generally not available to most prostate cancer patients. The sequence chapters discuss improved ways to image either the areas around the prostate or the gland itself. In Part II, information is presented on imaging modalities for the detection of metastatic disease using either the PET scan or ProstaScint scan.

PART III: TREATING PROSTATE CANCER

Part III discusses the need to detoxify the body to establish a fertile environment for using both conventional and complementary treatments for prostate cancer. Maintaining a healthy body demands an effort to balance the pH level. Although watchful waiting is not a treatment, it is offered to readers so they will understand when it should be used — and when it should not. The typical conventional treatments are reviewed. Some attention is given to IMRT, the latest and best technology for applying external beam radiation. Because several of the chapters are somewhat technical, they have been reviewed by experts in their respective fields and, in some cases, revised by them. Because a number of patients have asked why certain radiation topics were omitted from the first edition, we have included them in the updated version. Innovations produced by NASA have enabled the medical community to develop additional treatment modalities and more effective treatment for defeating prostate cancer. A treatment using light, referred to as CLT, is also covered in this section. PCLT, a modified form of CLT, is also discussed, detailing the advantages of the latter over the former treatment. All of the approaches to radiation, such as neutron beam, proton beam, photon beam, and high-dose, are tackled in individual chapters. The two major patterns of brachytherapy are discussed, sometimes referred to as combination radiation when seed implants and external beam radiation are combined. Each of the authors discusses why he prefers one or the other. Most patients are familiar with hormonal therapy being used as a palliative treatment. Some attention is given to whether it can also be used as a definitive treatment. New revelations and the uses of hormone blockade are included. How patients can live longer with hormonal-refractory disease is discussed in detail. A new hormonal-refractory treatment using a vitamin and drug is also included in Part III. An herbal product called PC SPES was discussed in our last book, but unfortunately the form that was known to be effective is no longer available. A new herb, an extract of ginseng, shows excellent promise. Soon after our first book was published, Viagra became popular. Now we have Befar, a new treatment for erectile dysfunction that challenges Viagra. This treatment is not only safer than Viagra, but it also works faster and is more effective for more patients. Part III also includes a treatment for multiple bone sites as well as a promising vaccine.

PART IV: IMPORTANT PROSTATE CANCER INFORMATION

Part IV provides pertinent information about your health insurance plans, second opinions, and how to appeal an HMO's negative decision. Attention is given to nutrition and colon-stimulating agents in the fight against prostate cancer and injections, which may result from some of the treatments. The benefits of joining a support group may lengthen a patient's life due to the information and experience gained from other group members. Part IV ends with an assortment of questions from inquiring prostate cancer patients – and our answers.

APPENDIX: RESOURCES

The appendix lists medical doctors according to treatments, the locations of IMRT sites, combination radiation sites, neutron radiation centers, Provenge clinical study centers, and MRSI hospitals.

GLOSSARY

The glossary presents terms commonly used in the prostate cancer field, including many used throughout Updated Guidelines.

James Lewis Jr., Ph.D.
E. Roy Berger, M.D., F.A.C.P.

PART I DIAGNOSING PROSTATE CANCER

Chapter 1

THE PSA TEST

Prostate cancer is the second-leading cause of cancer death among men in the United States. During 2002, approximately 189,000 new cases of prostate cancer were diagnosed in the United States, and over 32,000 American men died of this terrible disease. A man has a one in six chance (15.4%) of developing invasive prostate cancer during his lifetime, though it is clear that the risk increases with age. From birth to age 30, the chances are 1:10,000; from age 40 to 59, the chances are 1:103; from age 60 to 79, the chances are 1:8. At the age of 50, a man has a 42 percent chance of developing prostate cancer, a 2.9 percent chance of dying from the disease. The incidence of prostate cancer has increased dramatically worldwide over the past ten years. In the United States for example, the age-adjusted incidence has increased from 84.4/100,000 in 1984 to 163/100,000 in 1991. Most of this increase may be attributed to the increase of early detection programs based on the prostate specific antigen (PSA). As a result of new screening techniques, an increased incidence of disease is to be expected. A subsequent decrease in the incidence is also to be expected as prevalent cases of a disease process are removed from the population.

What is Prostate-Specific Antigen (PSA)?

Prostate specific antigen (PSA) is a glycoprotein produced primarily by cells in the prostate gland. Men who have prostate cancer frequently have high or abnormal PSA levels due to the enhanced production of PSA and various changes in the size and shape of the prostate that allow the PSA greater access to the circulatory system. Therefore, the amount of PSA in the blood can serve as a marker for prostate cancer. In addition, an elevated PSA level can indicate such conditions or events as biopsy of the prostate, transrectal prostatectomy, acute urinary retention, acute and chronic prostatitis, ejaculation, and benign prostatic hyperplasia. The test measures total PSA, and the results are reported in nanograms per milliliter (ng/ml). Despite the wide use of the PSA test in the detection and monitoring of prostate cancer, its sensitivity and specificity are quite low. The ideal blood test would be 100 percent sensitive — that is, it would detect all cancer in a group of men with no false negatives. It would also be 100 percent specific — that is, it would not diagnose cancer when none exists. Unfortunately, the PSA test sometimes produces false negatives and false positives.

E. Roy Berger, M.D., F.A.C.P. and James Lewis, Jr., Ph.D

Identifying the PSA Origin

In 1970, Ablin et al. were the first to identify the prostate specific antigen. Shortly thereafter, Hara et al. identified and confirmed PSA in the seminal fluid. In 1973, Li and Beling purified the PSA in seminal fluid. Eight years after the identification of PSA by Ablin et al., Sensabaugh and Crim confirmed that seminal fluid and the prostate gland had common antigens and that the origin was the prostate. It didn't take long for Wang et al. to isolate and purify the PSA from tissue of the prostate gland. Finally, in 1980, Papsidero et al. located PSA in the blood. In 1986, the U.S. Food and Drug Administration (FDA) approved two uses for the PSA test: (1) determining if treatment for prostate cancer had eliminated all of the diseased tissue and (2) monitoring a patient for a recurrence of the disease. In 1994, the FDA approved the use of the PSA test for detecting prostate cancer. Today the PSA test is used for:

- estimating the time to clinical failure after treatment
- calculating the rate of change in a patient's cancer cell load
- estimating a patient's pathological stage and lymph-node involvement
- monitoring for a recurrence of prostate cancer
- separating patients with benign prostatic hyperplasia (BPH) from those with prostate cancer.

Free and Complex

There are two forms of PSA: free and complex. Free PSA, sometimes referred to as PSA II, is a protein that circulates unbound through the blood. Complex PSA is attached to a protein that circulates within the blood. A PSA level of 4 to 10 ng/ml is considered the gray area in which it is difficult to determine if the elevated PSA is due to prostate cancer, prostatitis, or an enlarged prostate gland. If free PSA is 25 percent or more of total PSA, then an elevated PSA is most likely due to prostatitis or an enlarged prostate. However, if free PSA is less than 25 percent, there is a likelihood of prostate cancer. Not all physicians test for the free PSA, but a patient should insist on it if his PSA is in the 4 to 10 range. For example, a patient had an elevated PSA of 6.8 ng/ml. His urologist did not believe in the free PSA, so he asked his primary doctor to do the test. It showed his free PSA was 24 percent and the total PSA was 3.8 ng/ml. Thus a physician should not depend on the initial PSA level, but should perform another test within a week or two to confirm that the initial PSA was abnormal.

Race- and Age-Specific PSA

The race- and age-specific PSA is a method that compares a man's PSA level with those of men of the same race and age group. Higher PSA levels are more common in black men and in older men compared to younger men. If a man's PSA level is higher than the upper limit of normal for his race and age group, there is a greater probability he has prostate cancer. Table 1-1 illustrates the race and age-specific PSA levels.

Table 1-1 Race- and Age-Specific PSA Reference Range

PSA Level (ng/ml)

Age	Asian	Black	White
40-49	0-2.0	0-2.5	0-2.5
50-59	0-3.0	0-4.0	0-3.5
60-69	0-4.0	0-4.5	0-4.5
70-79	0-5.0	0-5.5	0-6.5

A study of the National Institute on Aging at Johns Hopkins University found that while the PSA blood test alone detects 20 to 25 percent of men with prostate cancer, both tests used together can detect prostate cancer in 53 to 70 percent of men.

Some Facts about PSA

- When free and total PSA were normal, prostate cancer was detected in only 2.3 percent of those tested (Drago 1994).
- Patients with a PSA level below 100 ng/ml do better than those with a PSA exceeding 100 ng/ml (Buck 1995).
- The PSA test has a lower probability of error (36 percent) in detecting prostate cancer than does a digital rectal examination or a transrectal ultrasound (TRUS).
- A PSA test is combined with a digital rectal examination (DRE) has the lowest probability of error (50 percent) among various double combinations of the PSA, DRE, and TRUS (Catalona et al. 1994).
- After radical prostatectomy, patients with residual cancer are most likely to have elevated PSA levels within the first two years.

- A PSA level above 0.2 ng/ml after radical prostatectomy or 0.5-1.0 ng/ml after external beam radiation indicates that the prostate cancer may have recurred.
- No treatment decision should be made based on a low PSA reading alone.
- The PSA level alone can identify between 24 and 25 percent of patients with prostate cancer. With the digital rectal examination, it can identify from 50 to 60 percent of such patients.
- Whenever a patient undergoes a bilateral orchiectomy (that is, castration) or combination hormone therapy, the PSA level almost always decreases.
- Ten percent of men with BPH will be found to have prostate cancer (Nash 1994).

How the PSA Level Can Be Influenced

The PSA level can be influenced by such factors as:

- age
- prostate size
- benign prostatic hyperplasia
- prostate cancer
- Proscar, a drug sometimes used in hormone therapy
- prostatitis
- ischemia
- infarction (tissue death)

Ways the PSA Test Can Be Used

Age-specific PSA

- If you do not have prostate cancer but would like to monitor your PSA level, the age-specific PSA can determine the upper limits of your PSA level. For example, if you are a 72-year-old Caucasian man, the upper limit of the PSA for your age group would be 6.5 ng/ml (instead of the old limit of 4.0). However, the age-specific PSA level for African-American men is lower, with the upper limit being 5.5.

PSA II

- Let's say your PSA is 7.5 ng/ml, and your doctor is not certain whether you have BPH or prostate cancer. He or she could order a PSA II to determine whether free or complex PSA is more dominant. If the lab reports that you have a higher percentage of free PSA, you probably have BPH.

PSA-DT

- If you have undergone either radical prostatectomy or external beam radiation, your doctor can determine if your prostate cancer has recurred by observing the doubling time of your PSA within 4 months. If your baseline PSA level at 6 months was 0.8 ng/ml and 4 months later it rose to 2.3, there is a high probability your prostate cancer has recurred.

PSA velocity

- If your PSA level rises more than 0.75 ng/ml on three consecutive occasions following your treatment or if it rises continuously, there is a possibility the disease has recurred.

PSA-T

- For the PSA-T test, the doctor measures the volume of the transitional zone of your prostate using a TRUS and then divides it by the PSA level. If your PSA-T is greater than 0.01, you are likely to have prostate cancer.

Predictive-value PSA

- Let's say your PSA is 11 ng/ml, your stage is T2b, and your Gleason score is 3. Using these data, the doctor can predict fairly accurately if your prostate cancer has spread to the lymph nodes or seminal vesicles, or has penetrated the prostatic capsule.

As a Diagnostic Tool

- The PSA test is prostate-specific, not cancer-specific.
- The PSA test has limited accuracy.

- It is assumed, but not yet proven, that men should get a PSA test because it may save lives.
- As of this writing, PSA is the best biomarker for diagnosing prostate cancer.
- You can have prostate cancer and still have a low PSA level.
- Twenty-five percent of men with a low PSA have prostate cancer.
- Many men with high or stable PSA levels do not have prostate cancer.
- There is no reason for most men over 75, or any man with a life expectancy of less than 10 years, to have a PSA test (Walsh 1995).
- Depending on age and general medical condition, a man should have a biopsy if a nodule is detected on the prostate, regardless of his PSA level.
- Patients with low PSA levels can have prostate cancer that has spread to the bones (Walsh 1995).
- An abnormal PSA level should be verified by repeating the test.
- A high prostatic acid phosphatase (PAP) level means that the cancer has probably metastasized, frequently to the pelvic lymph nodes.
- A high alkaline phosphatase (AP) indicates a likelihood of metastases to the bones.
- When both the digital rectal examination and PSA were abnormal, prostate cancer was detected in 50 to 60 percent of patients.

As a Monitoring Tool

- The PSA level is the most sensitive marker available for monitoring the progression of prostate cancer.
- The drug finasteride (Proscar) can mask the PSA level by artificially lowering it.

To Establish Prognosis

- A PSA level of 0.3 ng/ml or less after radical prostatectomy usually means the disease is in remission. A number greater than this usually indicates a recurrence. For example, if a patients PSA is 0.1 ng/ml following a radical prostatectomy, but his PSA rises every 3 months by 0.2 ng/ml, his PSA level will be 0.7 ng/ml, which signals a recurrence of his disease.
- A PSA level greater than 100 usually means the cancer has metastasized to the bones.
- Prostate cancer patients whose PSA level decreases to the normal range (below 2.5 ng/ml) or becomes undetectable within 6 months after

hormonal therapy will usually enjoy a prolonged response to hormonal treatment (Stamey et al. 1989).

To Signal a Disease Recurrence

- A continuous rise in PSA level after treatment usually means a recurrence of prostate cancer.
- A recurrence of prostate cancer will usually lag behind PSA elevation by up to 48 months.
- A PSA level exceeding 30 ng/ml indicates a high probability of metastasis in the lymph nodes, soft tissue, or bones.

Which PSA Assay Is Best?

An <u>assay</u> is a biochemical analysis of the purity or effectiveness of drugs and other biologic substances. Researchers at Emory University School of Medicine in Atlanta, Georgia, studied four PSA assays – the Abbott Imx, the Tosoh, the Chiron ACS PSA, and the Chiron ACS PSA2 – to see which was best able to detect the recurrence of prostate cancer after radical prostatectomy. The results of each PSA assay were compared using linear regression. Blood was drawn from all men who had undergone a radical prostatectomy who were seen in the Emory urology clinic in March 1995. Twenty-two patients had an undetectable PSA level by the Imx PSA assay. The PSA level was over the residual cancer detection limit (RCDL) of the Tosoh assay in five of these patients. The PSA levels exceeded the RCDL of the ACS PSA in 15 patients, and was over the RCDL of the PSA2 in two patients. No patients whose PSA level was measurable by any of the other assays had a PSA level less than the RCDL of the ACS PSA assay.[1]

Determining Clinical Stage

Bluestein Table

With a combination of local clinical stage (indicates the size of the tumor and extent of the spread of cancer) and Gleason score (the degree of aggressiveness of prostate cancer), determined at biopsy, Bluestein and colleagues used PSA level to predict whether prostate cancer had spread to the lymph nodes (see Table 1-2). They reviewed the records of 1,632 patients who had undergone lymph-node dissection for staging purposes. Using logistic regression analysis, the PSA level was determined to be the best predictor for calculating whether prostate cancer had spread to the lymph nodes. However, to enhance the predictive value of PSA, they also used a combination of PSA, Gleason score, and stage to determine if the disease had spread to the lymph nodes. By incorporating a statistical model with all three variables, a probability chart was developed that could help determine the probability that a patient's cancer had spread to the lymph nodes. The predictive value of PSA, using the PSA in combination with Gleason score and stage, is not only important in terms of sparing a patient an unnecessary radical prostatectomy, but also in terms of sparing him a costly staging procedure (both in terms of dollars and morbidity).

Table 1-2

The Bluestein Table

Combinations of local clinical stage, primary Gleason grade, and serum PSA* to yield a false-negative rate of 3 percent for positive lymph nodes.		
Local Clinical Stage	Primary Gleason Grade	Serum PSA (ng/ml)
T1a-T2b (A1-B1)	1, 2	17.1
T1c	3	8.0
	4, 5	4.2
T2c (B2)	1, 2	4.1
	3	H2.0
	4, 5	1.0
T3a (C1)	1, 2	1.4
	3	0.7
	4, 5	0.3

* Patients with lower serum PSA values have a false-negative rate of less than 3 percent.

Partin Table

Men with prostate cancer have a much better chance of cure if the cancer is confined to the prostate at the time of radical prostatectomy. Therefore, this surgery typically is performed only on men who are thought to have organ-confined disease by clinical exam. However, men with T1-T2 prostate cancer are found to have extracapsular disease about half the time. As a result, about 50 percent of men with clinically localized cancer who undergo prostatectomy have RP will have a significantly lower potential cure rate than would otherwise be predicted. Therefore, it is important to know how the factors of pretreatment PSA, stage, and grade can influence the likelihood of extracapsular disease and thus the chance of cure by surgery alone. The Partin tables contain such information as the patient's clinical stage based on the DRE, the Gleason score on the pathology report of the biopsy, and the PSA. The Partin tables correlate these factors with the pathological findings on the specimens removed during prostatectomy. The outcomes for the Partin tables shown in tables 1-3 through 1-7 indicate:

1. organ-confined disease
2. established capsular penetration
3. seminal-vesicle involvementI
4. lymph-node involvement

In 1993, the Partin tables were developed based upon 1,058 prostate cancer patients who underwent a retropubic radical prostatectomy during 1982-1991 at the Johns Hopkins Hospital in Baltimore, Maryland. The surgeon was Patrick Walsh, M.D. In 1997, the Partin tables were updated and published based upon 4,133 prostate cancer patients undergoing surgery at three medical centers: Johns Hopkins, Baylor College of Medicine, and the University of Michigan. Again in 2001, the Partin tables were updated and published this time based on 5,071 prostate cancer patients from one hospital, namely, Johns Hopkins, with the operations being performed by Dr. Patrick Walsh between 1994 and 2000.To use these tables, find the one for the range in which your PSA level falls. Then go to the left of the table and find your Gleason score. Now, move across the columns until you locate your clinical stage and then read the probabilities for organ-confined disease (OC), capsular penetration (CP), seminal-vesicle involvement (SV+), and lymph-node involvement (LN+). Any number represents a 95 percent probability (that is, you have a 95 percent chance of having the condition within the range indicated).

Table 1-3

Gleason Score	Path Stage	PSA 0 – 2.5 ng/ml							
		Clinical Stage							
		T1c		T2a		T2b		T2c	
2-4	OC	95	89-99	91	79-98	88	79-97	86	71-97
	CP	5	1-11	9	2-21	12	3-27	14	3-29
	SV+	0	0-0	0	0-0	0	0-0	0	0-0
	LN+	0	0-0	0	0-0	0	0-0	0	0-0
5-6	OC	90	88-93	81	77-85	75	69-81	73	63-81
	CP	9	7-12	17	13-21	22	17-28	24	17-33
	SV+	0	0-1	1	0-2	2	0-3	1	0-4
	LN+	0	0-0	0	0-1	1	0-2	1	0-4
3+4=7	OC	79	74-85	64	56-71	54	46-63	51	38-63
	CP	17	13-23	29	23-26	35	28-43	36	26-48
	SV+	2	1-5	5	1-9	6	2-12	5	1-13
	LN+	1	0-2	2	0-5	4	0-10	6	0-18
4+3=7	OC	71	62-79	53	43-63	43	33-54	39	26-54
	CP	25	18-34	40	30-49	45	35-56	45	32-59
	SV+	2	1-5	4	1-9	5	1-11	5	1-12
	LN+	1	0-4	3	0-8	6	0-14	9	0-26
8-10	OC	66	54-76	47	35-59	37	26-49	34	21-48
	CP	28	20-38	42	32-53	46	35-58	47	33-61
	SV+	4	1-10	7	2-16	9	2-20	8	2-19
	LN+	1	0-4	3	0-9	6	0-16	10	0-27

PSA 2.6 – 4.0 ng/ml								
Gleason Score	**Path Stage**	**Clinical Stage**						
		T1c		**T2a**		**T2b**		**T2c**
2-4	OC	92	82-98	85	69-96	80	61-95	78	58-94
	CP	8	2-18	15	4-31	20	5-39	22	6-42
	SV+	0	0-0	0	0-0	0	0-0	0	0-0
	LN+	0	0-0	0	0-0	0	0-0	0	0-0
5-6	OC	84	81-86	71	66-75	63	57-59	61	50-70
	CP	15	13-18	27	23-31	34	28-40	36	27-45
	SV+	1	0-1	2	1-3	2	1-4	2	1-5
	LN+	0	0-0	0	0-1	1	0-2	1	0-4
3+4=7	OC	68	62-74	50	43-57	41	33-48	38	27-50
	CP	27	22-33	41	35-48	47	40-55	48	37-59
	SV+	4	2-7	7	3-12	9	4-15	8	2-17
	LN+	1	0-2	2	0-4	3	0-8	5	0-15
4+3=7	OC	58	48-67	39	30-48	30	22-39	27	18-40
	CP	37	29-46	52	43-61	57	47-67	57	44-70
	SV+	4	1-7	6	2-12	7	3-14	6	2-16
	LN+	1	0-3	2	0-6	4	0-12	7	0-21
8-10	OC	52	41-63	33	24-44	25	17-34	23	14-34
	CP	40	31-50	53	44-63	57	46-68	57	44-70
	SV+	6	3-12	10	4-18	12	5-22	10	3-22
	LN+	1	0-4	3	0-8	5	0-14	8	0-22

Table 1-5

PSA 4.1 – 6.0 ng/ml								
Gleason Score	Path Stage	Clinical Stage						
		T1c		T2a		T2b		T2c	
2-4	OC	90	78-98	81	63-95	75	55-93	73	52-93
	CP	10	2-22	19	5-37	25	7-45	27	7-48
	SV+	0	0-0	0	0-0	0	0-0	0	0-0
	LN+	0	0-0	0	0-0	0	0-0	0	0-0
5-6	OC	80	78-83	66	62-70	57	52-63	55	44-64
	CP	19	16-21	32	28-36	39	33-44	40	32-50
	SV+	1	0-1	1	1-2	2	1-3	2	1-4
	LN+	0	0-1	1	0-2	2	1-3	3	1-7
3+4=7	OC	63	58-68	44	39-50	35	29-40	31	23-41
	CP	32	27-36	46	40-52	51	44-57	50	40-60
	SV+	3	2-5	5	3-8	7	4-11	6	2-11
	LN+	2	1-3	4	2-7	7	4-13	12	5-23
4+3=7	OC	52	43-60	33	254-41	25	18-32	21	14-31
	CP	42	35-50	56	48-64	60	50-68	57	43-68
	SV+	3	1-6	5	2-8	5	3-9	4	1-10
	LN+	3	1-5	6	3-11	10	5-18	16	6-32
8-10	OC	46	36-56	28	20-37	21	14-29	18	11-28
	CP	45	36-54	58	49-66	59	49-69	57	43-70
	SV+	5	3-9	8	4-13	9	4-16	7	2-15
	LN+	3	1-6	6	2-12	10	4-20	16	6-33

Table 1-6

Gleason Score	Path Stage	PSA 6.1 – 10.0							
		Clinical Stage							
		T1c		T2a		T2b		T2c	
2-4	OC	87	73-97	76	56-94	69	47-91	67	45-91
	CP	13	3-27	24	6-44	31	9-53	33	9-55
	SV+	0	0-0	0	0-0	0	0-0	0	0-0
	LN+	0	0-0	0	0-0	0	0-0	0	0-0
5-6	OC	75	72-77	58	54-61	49	43-55	46	36-56
	CP	23	21-25	37	34-41	44	39-49	46	37-55
	SV+	2	2-3	4	3-5	5	3-8	5	2-9
	LN+	0	0-1	1	0-2	2	1-3	3	1-6
3+4=7	OC	54	49-59	35	30-40	26	22-31	24	17-32
	CP	36	32-40	49	43-54	52	46-58	52	42-61
	SV+	8	6-11	13	9-18	16	10-22	13	6-23
	LN+	2	1-3	3	2-6	6	4-10	10	5-18
4+3=7	OC	43	35-51	25	19-32	19	14-25	16	10-24
	CP	47	40-54	58	51-66	60	52-68	58	46-69
	SV+	88	4-12	11	6-17	13	7-20	11	4-21
	LN+	2	1-4	5	2-8	8	5-14	13	6-25
8-10	OC	37	28-46	21	15-28	15	10-21	13	8-20
	CP	48	39-57	57	48-65	57	48-67	56	43-69
	SV+	13	8-19	17	11-26	19	11-29	16	6-29
	LN+	3	1-5	5	2-10	8	4-16	13	5-26

Table 1-7

Gleason Score	Path Stage	PSA > 10							
		Clinical Stage							
		T1c		T2a		T2b		T2c	
2-4	OC	80	61-95	65	43-89	57	35-86	54	32-85
	CP	20	5-39	35	11-57	43	14-65	46	15-68
	SV+	0	0-0	0	0-0	0	0-0	0	0-0
	LN+	0	0-0	0	0-0	0	0-0	0	0-0
5-6	OC	62	58-64	42	38-46	33	28-38	30	21-38
	CP	33	30-36	47	43-52	52	46-56	51	42-60
	SV+	4	3-5	6	4-8	8	5-11	6	2-12
	LN+	2	1-3	4	3-7	8	5-12	13	6-22
3+4=7	OC	37	32-42	20	17-24	14	11-17	11	7-17
	CP	43	38-48	49	43-55	47	40-53	42	30-55
	SV+	12	9-17	16	11-22	17	12-24	13	6-24
	LN+	8	5-11	14	9-21	22	15-30	33	18-49
4+3=7	OC	27	21-34	14	10-18	9	6-13	7	4-12
	CP	51	44-59	55	46-64	50	40-60	43	29-59
	SV+	11	6-17	13	7-20	13	8-21	10	3-20
	LN+	10	5-17	18	10-27	27	16-39	38	20-58
8-10	OC	22	16-30	11	7-15	7	4-10	6	3-10
	CP	50	42-59	52	41-62	46	36-59	41	27-57
	SV+	17	10-25	19	12-29	19	12-29	15	5-28
	LN+	11	5-18	17	9-29	27	14-40	38	20-59

Improving on the PSA

A number of organizations have attempted to improve on the PSA. Some of them are cited below.

Ultrasensitive Tests

The first-generation PSA test had a sensitivity of 0.3 (up to 50 ng/ml). The second-generation test has a sensitivity of 0.1 ng/ml. Now the third-generation, or ultrasensitive, PSA test, can detect a recurrence of prostate cancer much earlier than could the previous two tests. Thomas Stamey, M.D. and colleagues estimate that after surgery, the average time for the PSA level to increase from 0.1 to 0.3 ng/ml in a patient with early metastatic prostate cancer is about 12 months. However, an ultrasensitive PSA test can determine a recurrence several months earlier. Nichols Institute has introduced a third-generation PSA test with a sensitivity of 0.02 ng/ml. This test has several advantages over the earlier tests:

- It can detect a recurrence of prostate cancer 15 to 30 months earlier than any other PSA test.
- It is a more accurate assessment of the efficiency of adjuvant therapy.
- It is a more sensitive indicator of residual prostate cancer after a radical prostatectomy.

The benefit of monitoring prostate cancer patients using ultrasensitive measurements of PSA is frequently discussed. Usually, the analytic lower detection limit of an ultrasensitive assay is determined by the manufacturer. As the analytic lower detection limit does not take into account interfering factors of human blood, the biologic lower detection limit, which is defined as PSA concentration detected in PSA-free human blood, plus 3 standard deviations, is of greater interest. The researchers investigated the biologic lower detection limit of six ultrasensitive PSA assays. Blood from 15 patients with bladder cancer after radical cystoprostatectomy and blood from 30 healthy patients were investigated. Hence, the investigator expected no PSA of prostatic origin.

NMP48

A blood test known as NMP48 and developed by Matritech of Newton, Massachusetts, using mass spectrometry to detect specific proteins that are markers for prostate cancer, is currently under study. In preclinical research, Matritech's scientists found that the NMP48 test had greater sensitivity in diagnosing prostate cancer than did the PSA test. The NMP48 test identified 92 percent of the cancers that the PSA test failed to detect. The typical PSA test misses almost one-third of patients with prostate cancer. Matritech's research also showed that NMP48 could correctly rule out men with benign prostate disease. Patients with benign disease often have elevated PSA levels because the PSA test is not cancer-specific. As a result, patients with false positives must undergo invasive testing, including biopsy, to rule out prostate cancer. Matritech intends to offer the NMP48 in the future for laboratory testing service in conjunction with a national clinical laboratory. The company plans to do this immediately following a positive clinical trial, although FDA approval is not required for laboratory testing.

TGF-Beta

Researchers at Houston's Baylor College of Medicine have discovered that all men diagnosed with prostate cancer are more likely to need aggressive treatment because their cancer is more likely to spread. This revelation is important because prostate cancer is more easily treated when it is confined to the prostate gland; however, it is much more difficult to control after it spreads. Kevin Slawin, M.D., associate professor of urology and director of the Baylor Prostate Center, and his team analyzed blood samples from 120 patients who underwent prostatectomy removal for localized cancer at the Methodist Hospital. Levels of the growth factor TGF-beta were measured before surgery and at intervals after surgery. The blood samples taken were then compared with those of (1) healthy men and (2) men whose cancerous cells had already spread. "This marker, measured through a simple blood test, indicates at a very early stage which patients may have prostate cancer that has already begun to spread to other areas of the body," said Dr. Slawin. "It can give us an early warning for who will need more aggressive therapy." Screening for prostate cancer with the PSA test has become widespread in the United States in the last decade or so. But, while the PSA test has had the enormous benefit of allowing earlier detection of prostate cancer, unlike the TGF-beta levels, it does not predict cancer progression. "The PSA test is not as effective at predicting the aggressive behavior of prostate cancer, especially when the PSA is low," explained Dr. Slawin. "What's most important in managing patients with prostate cancer is both an early diagnosis and the ability to determine which patients have more aggressive forms of cancer, those likely to recur and spread." A study by S.F. Shariat and colleagues concluded that plasma TGF-beta level were markedly elevated in men with prostate cancer that had metastasized to lymph nodes and bone. In patients without evidence of metastases, the preoperative plasma TGF-beta level was a strong predictor of biochemical progression after surgery, presumably because of an association with occult metastatic disease present at the time of radical prostatectomy.

Prostate-Specific Membrane Antigen

Researchers at Memorial Sloan-Kettering Cancer Center in New York City have devised a test for detecting prostate cancer that measures the level of prostatic-specific membrane antigen in the blood. This test, which can detect one prostate cancer cell among 10 million blood cells, may be able to give doctors a much earlier warning of cancer than the does PSA test. It is currently not available commercially.

ProstAsure Test

The ProstAsure test works by combining PSA, prostatic acid phosphatase (PAP), and three isoenzymes of creatinine kinase (CK-BB, CK-MB, CK-MM), along with the patient's age in the SMARTDiagnostics system to create a diagnostic interpretation. It has been shown in clinical trials involving more than 800 patients to have a positive predictive value of 90 percent. This is about twice as effective as the PSA test and digital rectal examination combined. This superior accuracy comes from the ability of ProstAsure to recognize and differentiate patterns in biomarker variation for normal prostate tissue, BPH, and palpable prostate tumors, thereby demonstrating a unique profile for each clinical condition. The FDA is expected to approve ProstAsure in the very near future. Like most diagnostic procedures, ProstAsure has both advantages and disadvantages, as indicated below:

Advantages

- ProstAsure can help detect clinically significant prostate cancer in older patients.
- It can help identify potentially curable prostate cancer cases in younger patients.
- It can help differentiate between high-risk and low-risk BPH patients.
- It can help determine if a patient's prostate cancer is confined to the capsule.
- The ProstAsure report also includes an age-specific reference range.

Disadvantage

- ProstAsure has not yet demonstrated its ability to identify early-stage, nonpalpable prostate cancer. (Clinical trials are currently being planned for this study.)

How to Use This Information

1. If your PSA level is between 4 and 10 ng/ml, ask your doctor to do a "free PSA" test. If your free PSA is 25 percent of your total PSA, you probably don't have prostate cancer.
2. If your PSA is 20 ng/ml or greater, there is a high probability that you have prostate cancer. Have another PSA test in a week to confirm your initial PSA.
3. Remember, you can have a low PSA level with metastatic disease. See Chapter 5, A Gene for Metastatic Prostate Cancer.

Chapter 2

THE DIGITAL RECTAL EXAM

The second step in the sequence for detecting prostate cancer is the digital rectal exam (DRE). Of the several tests used to detect prostate cancer, the DRE is the most widely used. Initially, detection was based on the results of the DRE. However, in a review of the DRE as a detection test, it was concluded that the detection rate is low in several reported studies with a variation between 0.13 percent and 1.65 percent. In 1989, Chodak et al. reported a detection rate of 1.45 percent and a positive predictive value of 25 percent. Others reported positive predictive values between 6 and 39 percent. As a result of several studies, it can be concluded that the DRE has a low sensitivity and specificity for the detection of prostate cancer. The DRE has the tendency to detect the larger cancerous tumors, and the risk or probability of detecting clinically insignificant tumors with the DRE is quite low. On the other hand, small multi-focal lesions with an aggressive biologic potential are not detected with the DRE alone. The general belief by most physicians and researchers is that the DRE is highly subjective. These limitations of the DRE is the salient reason why the PSA and DRE should be used in combination to detect a larger percentage of men with prostate cancer.

How the DRE is Performed?

During a digital rectal exam, the doctor's gloved index finger is carefully inserted into the patient's rectum to feel for any hardness on the surface of the prostate gland. The rectum is thin and flexible enough so that the prostate can be felt through it. A normal prostate feels firm but pliable, much like the tip of the nose. An infected gland feels swollen or mushy — what some doctors call "boggy." A small, hard lump or nodule sometimes indicates cancer. Before performing the DRE, your doctor will ask you to either take down your pants or put on a hospital gown. Next, he or she will ask you to assume a position that will allow him to examine you. The doctor may ask you to stand next to the examination table and bend forward a little, to kneel on the table, or to lie on the table in a fetal position.

Sometimes the DRE yields a false positive result. This may be due to:

- nodule(s) caused by BPH
- prostate stones

- prostatitis
- anomaly of the ejaculation duct
- anomaly of the seminal vesicles
- phlebolith of the rectal wall
- polyp or tumor of the rectal wall

Some Facts about the DRE

- The DRE takes only three to five seconds to perform.
- The DRE should not be painful. If it is painful, you may have prostatitis, an inflammation of the prostate.
- The DRE is safe. It does not cause rectal bleeding or any other injury.
- The DRE is inexpensive.
- Men aged 50 or more should have a DRE and a PSA test at least once a year.
- The DRE should be the first test performed during a genitourinary examination.

Why Men Fail to Have a DRE

Many men avoid having a DRE for the following reasons:
- The doctor is rude, gruff, disrespectful, or uncommunicative.
- The physician performing the DRE is a woman, which causes some men to feel especially embarrassed.
- Some men are fearful, particularly on their first visit.

Limitations of the DRE

A DRE is not without its limitations. Prostate cancer patients should be aware of these limitations and avoid them if possible.

1. The DRE identifies only 15 to 20 percent of patients with prostate cancer. Therefore, it should not be used as a sole diagnostic test for the disease.
2. The DRE's ability of the DRE to detect localized prostate cancer is limited. Dr. Chodak and colleagues performed the DRE on 2,131 men and had a detection rate of 15 percent. However, after surgery, 50 percent of the patients with stage B disease were upgraded to stage C or D1. Other studies revealed similar results.

3. The average detection rate using the DRE alone was 1.4 percent for men between 57 and 70 years of age.
4. DRE alone is a poor diagnostic tool because some prostate cancers detected by this method are advanced and thus incurable.
5. Studies indicate that the DRE lacks specificity and that it has a false negative rate as high as 36 percent.
6. The subjectivity of the DRE varies among doctors, resulting in great variability in the yield of prostate cancer in men with an abnormality using this test.
7. Using the DRE to assess the size of the prostate is known to be notoriously inaccurate.
8. The overall detection rate is estimated at about 15 to 20 percent.

- The percentage of cancers detected has been approximately 1 to 2 percent in most reported screening series in the United States. The European screening studies have markedly lower percentages. Waaler and associates screened 480 men 45 to 67 years old and had a detection rate of 0.2 percent. Only 16 patients had an abnormal examination that warranted a biopsy. Similarly, Vihko and associates screened 771 men with DRE and PAP, and their detection rate was 1.2 percent, but they performed only 66 biopsies. The rate of biopsies was higher in the American studies in which the detection rate was higher. The detection rate obviously varies depending on age, patient symptoms, rate of biopsy, and prevalence of the disease in each country.

How to Use This Information

Although the digital rectal examination by itself only detects a small percentage of patients with prostate cancer, this rate increases substantially when other diagnostic tests follow. To capitalize on this diagnostic step, consider the following:

- If your doctor fails to do a DRE, insist that one be performed.
- If a nodule is detected, ask the doctor how it feels.
- Don't be fooled into believing you don't have prostate cancer just because the doctor does not feel a suspicious area on your prostate.
- When considering the unpleasant aspect of a DRE, forget about your macho image; your life may be at stake.

Chapter 3

TRANSRECTAL ULTRASOUND

The transrectal ultrasound (TRUS) test is the third sequential diagnostic test that should be performed to detect prostate cancer. Unfortunately, many urologists and oncologists skip the TRUS and perform a biopsy. Nevertheless, TRUS should be done — before any biopsy is ordered — to determine the percentage of free PSA compared to complex PSA. Depending on the results of the TRUS, a biopsy may be unnecessary. The TRUS is important in prostate cancer not only in detection of the disease, but also in staging the disease. It is particularly relevant to determine if there is any evidence of extracapsular extension (ECE). ECE is also useful for determining prostate cancer that has invaded the seminal vesicles. Although TRUS alone is reasonably accurate in determining the presence of ECE, it is apparent at this time that the DRE in combination with the TRUS is more effective in the detection of extracapsular extension.

Advantages

There are many advantages to the transrectal ultrasound:

1. TRUS is easily performed with a handheld endorectal probe.
2. TRUS can be used to estimate the total prostate volume and the volume of tumors within the prostate.
3. TRUS is important not only in the diagnosis of prostate cancer, but also in staging the disease.
4. TRUS sometimes shows evidence of extracapsular penetration.
5. TRUS can determine seminal-vesicle invasion.
6. TRUS tends to be more accurate with a color Doppler.
7. The color Doppler has improved the accuracy of scanning of prostate gland.
8. TRUS permits reasonably accurate measurements of both the total gland volume and the transition-zone volume.
9. TRUS can reveal hypoechoic foci in the peripheral zone of the prostate.
10. TRUS provides the most convenient and accurate way of obtaining a biopsy.
11. Complications from the TRUS are minimal.

12. Although more uncomfortable and intrusive then transabdominal scanning, TRUS provides greater accuracy because the probe is so close to the prostate.
13. Many investigators have found that TRUS is preferable to transabdominal, transperineal, and transurethral techniques for viewing the prostate because it is more consistent and reproducible.

Limitations

Transrectal ultrasound is not without its limitations. For example:

1. TRUS results may be informative, but scans providing more anatomical details are necessary to determine if the tumor is confined to the prostate or has metastasized.
2. TRUS is not suitable as a first-line screening test for prostate cancer because of its limited sensitivity and specificity.

Technology Used to Perform the TRUS

TRUS is performed with a handheld probe, which is inserted into the rectum. If air gets between the probe and the prostate gland, the image will deteriorate. Thus some probes incorporate a surrounding condom fixed with degassed water. Most probes have 7.5-MHz transducers that provide a spatial resolution down to 0.2 mm. Therefore, a biplanar scanning in the sagittal and transverse axial planes permits a more complete scanning of the prostate. In addition, a color Doppler allows blood flow within the prostate to be assessed, thus helping to distinguish between malignancy and inflammation.

Understanding the TRUS

Prior to your undergoing a TRUS, your doctor will ask you to have an enema so that the area between the probe and the anterior rectal wall is clear. You will be positioned on a table in a left lateral knee-to-chest position or in a knee-to-chest position. The tip of the probe is well lubricated to facilitate insertion into the rectum. Then, the doctor usually scans the prostate in the transverse axial plane in a step-wide fashion, from the base of the bladder down to the apex of the prostate gland. Abnormalities within the prostate and seminal vesicles may be observed. Next, step-wide scanning is performed in the longitudinal plane to identify any abnormalities that are not apparent on transverse scanning and to estimate the three-dimensional features of abnormalities that are apparent.

Most scanning now incorporates a feature that can be used to estimate the total prostate volume and the volume of the tumors within the prostate. Some transrectal ultrasounds also include software that allows the technician to calculate prostate volume by drawing around the periphery of the prostate gland with a cursor on both longitudinal and transverse scans.

Power Doppler versus the TRUS

Although the transrectal ultrasound is effective for performing a biopsy, the power Doppler is a much better instrument.

- Most TRUS technology shows images in black-and-white. However, most power Dopplers display images in color, and, so, more can be seen.

How to Use This Information

If you undergo a TRUS, pay attention to each stage of the procedure and ask your doctor to describe the condition of your prostate. Can he or she see your seminal vesicles? Are there any suspicious areas? How large is the prostate gland and tumor?

Chapter 4

BIOPSYING THE PROSTATE

The fourth step in the sequence for detecting prostate cancer is the biopsy, which involves extracting prostate tissue for examination under a microscope. Only by retrieving actual tissue samples can the urologist determine whether prostate cancer is present. Usually, a pattern of samples are extracted from the prostate to represent each section of the gland. Microscopic examination of the tissue by a pathologist allows for an analysis of the nature and virulence of the cancer. After the biopsy, cancerous tissue is given a Gleason score to denote the loss of normal gland formation according to the size, shape, and differentiation of the specimen in order to classify the aggressiveness of the cancer. In most cancers, histological confirmation is an important prerequisite before determining a treatment for prostate cancer. A number of different biopsy techniques have been used. At one time, the digital guidance has been used to direct the biopsy of palpable lesions via the transrectal or transperineal routes. However, the TRUS guidance has been shown to be superior to digital guidance in directing the biopsy of both palpable and impalpable prostate cancers. Because TRUS is also beneficial in staging prostate cancer, it is only natural to perform all prostate cancer biopsies using the TRUS guidance.

What Is a Biopsy?

A biopsy is usually performed by a urologist who uses a thin needle attached to a biopsy gun, guided by a transrectal ultrasound or the doctor's finger. The needle is inserted through the rectum to extract prostatic tissue. A sextant biopsy – one that takes six samples — is usually performed. Some physicians have modified the sextant biopsy to extract additional cores from the prostate. Although some researchers claim that the sextant biopsy has better than a 90 percent accuracy rate, more biopsies usually increase the accuracy. Another biopsy method, which is probably an improvement over the sextant biopsy, is the 5-region biopsy developed by several doctors in Wake Forest, North Carolina. They maintain that the 5-region biopsy detects 37 percent more cancers than does the sextant biopsy, thereby minimizing the number of false negatives.

E. Roy Berger, M.D., F.A.C.P. and James Lewis, Jr., Ph.D

Why Have a Biopsy?

Biopsies are performed for several reasons:

1. The biopsy is used to determine if a man has prostate cancer or a precancerous condition and to obtain information about pathologic stage and Gleason score, critical elements in predicting the aggressiveness of the cancer.

2. It can be used to perform a DNA ploidy analysis – that is, to determine if the tumor is <u>diploid</u> (has the normal 46 chromosomes per cell), <u>tetraploid</u> (has four times the normal number of chromosomes per cell), or <u>aneuploid</u> (has an uneven number of chromosomes – more or less than the 46 per cell).

3. A biopsy is sometimes necessary to rule out progression of cancer to the seminal vesicles. This is often beneficial for men with bulky, higher-grade tumors, PSA levels over 10, or both.

   Among 67 men who underwent radical prostatectomy for clinically localized prostate cancer, Vallancien andv coworkers determined that seminal-vesicle biopsy detected 61 percent of those men with seminal-vesicle invasion with no false-positive biopsies. They recommended seminal-vesicle biopsy for all men with localized prostate cancer and a PSA level over 10 ng/ml.

4. Branches of the neurovascular bundles – two groups of nerves and blood vessels — enter the prostate on the posterior lateral surface. Prostate cancer frequently penetrates the capsule of the prostate, invading the perineural spaces.
   Bastacky and colleagues examined whether perineural invasion found on needle biopsies was a predictor of extracapsular penetration in 302 men with stage 2 prostate cancer who underwent surgery. Perineural invasion was seen in 20 percent of needle biopsies taken before treatment.

5. A 5-region biopsy is taken from several different areas of the prostate to get a representative sampling of the entire gland. It includes a sextant biopsy as described by Hodge and colleagues, two samples from each lateral aspect of the gland, and three from the middle of the prostate, for a total of at least 13 samples per patient.

Preparing for a Biopsy

The first step in preparing for a needle biopsy is to stop taking medication that can interfere with the ability of the blood to clot 10 to 14 days before the procedure. If you take aspirin regularly, stop it one to two weeks before the biopsy. However, if you have had a stroke or transient ischemic attack (TIA), it is not always safe to stop taking aspirin. In this case, alternative arrangements need to be made. Similarly, if you take Ticlid or Plavix, discontinue it two weeks before to the biopsy. Persantine (dipyridamole) should be stopped for two days, and Coumadin (warfarin) for five days. For some patients, it will be necessary to receive intravenous heparin shortly after stopping the Coumadin. It is important that before discontinuing Coumadin, you speak with the doctor who prescribed it. Finally, any nonsteroidal anti-inflammatory drugs that you take – such as Motrin, Advil, Nuprin, Aleve, and Naprosyn – should be stopped several days prior to the biopsy. However, it is all right to take Tylenol, Tylenol with codeine, or Percocet before the biopsy. Two days before the biopsy, begin taking the antibiotic that your doctor has prescribed. (Generally, Cipro, Floxin, or Levaquin is prescribed.) If you have a pacemaker, an artificial joint, such as an artificial hip, or other implanted device, additional antibiotics might be required. If you have a heart murmur or an abnormality of a heart valve, your doctor might arrange for you to receive intravenous antibiotics.

On the day of the biopsy, eat breakfast. Eat lunch, too, if the procedure is in the afternoon.

If the biopsy is scheduled for early morning, use a Fleet enema the night before. Otherwise, have the enema in the morning.

During the Biopsy

Generally, patients are prescribed Percocet (basically, Tylenol with an opiate called oxycodone) and Valium (diazepam) before the biopsy. After arriving in the urologist's office and checking that the biopsy will proceed on schedule, take whatever medication has been prescribed.

A caveat here: We know a man who underwent a biopsy without any sedation or painkillers. Oh, he asked for some, but his urologist (who soon became his former urologist) said he wouldn't need it. Well, when our friend left the treatment room and went out to meet his wife, she took one look at him and knew he had basically been tortured. He was then sent home without any painkillers, but he was in so much pain he could not even sit. Luckily, he had some codeine in the house, which gave him relief.

During the biopsy, you may feel pressure as if you have to urinate. Some patients feel pressure as if they have to move their bowels.

In situations where many samples are going to be extracted, the biopsy is sometimes done in the hospital and the patient is put under anesthesia.

Transrectal ultrasound with an ultrasound-guided biopsy of the prostate is done in the urologist's office. You will be asked to lie on your left side on an exam table. An ultrasound probe, shaped like a finger, is covered with a latex condom lubricated with water-soluble jelly and is inserted into the rectum. Using the probe, pictures of the prostate are obtained. The pictures show the size and dimensions of the prostate, the size and shape of the seminal vesicles, the condition of the capsule around the prostate, and any areas of abnormality within the prostate. If, in the tissue near the rectal surface or on the lateral sides of the prostate, there is an area that transmits more sound than the surrounding tissue, it will appear darker. Such an area has a greater possibility of having prostate cancer than does the adjacent tissue.

To obtain the best views of the prostate, two ultrasound probes are generally used. The biopsy is performed with guidance from a third ultrasound probe, which has more maneuverability for guiding the placement of the needle. This spring-loaded needle is placed within a guide pathway along the side of the ultrasound probe. The needle traverses the rectal wall and enters the prostate, driven by a spring, which makes the procedure very quick.

To thoroughly sample the prostate, the doctor will perform a sextant biopsy and then may extract tissues from the right lateral, middle, and left lateral regions, for a total of 13 samples. The tissues are sent to a pathologist to determine whether prostate cancer is present.

Aspirin and Biopsies

Aspirin is widely used for pain control, as an antiinflammatory, and at low doses to prevent cardiovascular disease. A group of surgeons in Denmark conducted a study to determine whether aspirin use causes complications for prostate patients after either biopsy or radical surgery. Some doctors maintained that aspirin was a significant cause of postprostatectomy hemorrhage, but no controlled studies had ever been done.

The Danish researchers found that after prostate biopsy, "aspirin-induced hemorrhagic complications have been reported." They recommended stopping aspirin "one week prior to invasive urologic procedures." They also explained how to correct bleeding complications with desmopressin, platelet concentrates, or fresh frozen plasma.

Do U.S. doctors follow a consistent standard on stopping aspirin and Coumadin? No study has been done. Do American physicians follow a standard for preparing men for biopsy? In 1998, a team in Hawaii asked 900 randomly selected American urologists how they prepared men for a prostate biopsy.

"Approximately 63 percent (568 of 900) of the surveys were returned," they report, "and showed considerable differences among those urologists." A total of 98.6 percent prescribed antibiotics to prevent infection, while a small percentage did not.

Reducing Biopsy Pain

Transrectal ultrasound-guided prostate biopsy causes pain in some patients. It has been suggested that local anesthesia may be of value in such cases, but the most effective technique has not been determined.

Injection of local anesthetic into the prostate capsule reduces the pain associated with biopsy more effectively than do alternative techniques, German researchers report.

M. Schostak, M.D., and colleagues from the Free University of Berlin compared anesthetic block of the prostatic plexus, apex infiltration of the capsule, a combination of these two, and no anesthesia in patients undergoing 10-core prostate biopsies.

A total of 170 men took part in the study and were randomized to one of the four groups. The subjects reported pain or discomfort using a visual analogue scale and a numeric analogue scale.

No pain was reported by 4.5 percent of men in the no-anesthesia group, while mild pain was reported by 86.4 percent, moderate pain by 6.8 percent, and severe pain by 2.3 percent. In this group, average pain scores were 2.33 (on a scale of 1 to 10).

In contrast, pain scores reported by the other groups were 1.68 in patients who received anesthetic block of the prostatic plexus, 1.07 in those who received anesthesia of the capsule of the apex, and 1.23 in the combination group.

In these three groups, pain scores associated with actual delivery of the local anesthesia were 1.52, 1.05, and 1.79, respectively. Greater pain was reported at the apex, in the area adjacent to the urethra, and in the transitional zone than in the proximal peripheral zone during biopsy.

The researchers conclude that local anesthesia of the capsule is easier to perform than anesthetic block of the prostatic plexus, and it is also associated with lower pain levels. There is no additional benefit of combining the two.

Dr. Schostak and colleagues conclude, "Apex infiltration is recommended, especially for 10-core prostate biopsy, in view of its high efficacy and minimal invasiveness and morbidity."

How the Pathologist Identifies Cancer

The pathologist looks for unusual cells, especially ones where the nucleus becomes relatively large compared with the cytoplasm (the rest of the cell). (The nucleus is where DNA, the cell's blueprint, is kept.) Cancer cells generally reproduce at a higher rate than normal cells, and so the nucleus is busy turning out lots of copies of the DNA. If the nucleus were an egg yolk, it would become very large compared to the white (the cytoplasm). This distortion is characteristic of cancer cells.

In addition, because prostate cells form glands, which are separated by muscle and supporting tissue layers, the pathologist looks for distortions in gland formation. Bizarre or disorganized glands, formation of "glands in glands" (cribriform gland formation), and back-to-back glands without intervening tissue are all signs of cancer. The diagnostic finding of cancer, however, is the presence of cells or groups of cells invading beyond their natural borders into other areas of the prostate.

After the Biopsy

After a biopsy, the patient should have someone drive him home. He should not drive for the rest of the day.

A small percentage of patients may have some difficulty urinating. If this happens, call your doctor. He or she may insert a Foley catheter, a tube that passes through the urinary passageway and drains the bladder. It can be connected to a bag that is worn on the leg underneath your trousers. Generally, after a few days of drainage, the catheter will be taken out, and normal urination will resume.

Although rectal bleeding sometimes occurs after a biopsy, it generally clears up after a few days.

There is usually some blood in the urine. The urine can be light red to pink for two or three days, and there may be a spot of blood at the start or finish of urination for a few weeks. A week after the biopsy, a small stringy clot may pass in the urinary stream.

Avoid any vigorous activity for the first couple of days after the biopsy, and avoid sexual activity for four or five days. Blood may be present in the ejaculate for up to two months. Do not be alarmed. If the blood is dark red, this means it is old, and you may continue with sexual activity. If the blood is very bright red, however, wait another week before engaging in sexual activity.

Occasionally, a biopsy stirs up an old prostate infection or creates a new urinary-tract or prostate infection. However, the likelihood of this happening is low.

Limitations of the Biopsy

Biopsies have certain limitations:

1. Sometimes cancer is present, but the biopsy needle misses it. Known as a *sampling error,* this occurs about 15 percent of the time. If a patient's biopsy is negative, but his DRE and PSA test indicate cancer, he should return to the physician's office in three months for a follow-up.
2. At times, the biopsy may not reveal the full extent of the cancer. The tissues extracted from the prostate may show only a small amount of the tumor when there is actually much more.
3. The biopsy may be uncomfortable or painful.
4. The biopsy may transfer germs from the rectum into the prostate. However, this is rare, as patients have an enema before the biopsy and take antibiotics before and after it.
5. The biopsy may cause the prostate to swell, leading to difficulty in urinating.
6. A patient with a grade III PIN (prostatic intraepithelial neoplasia) usually needs to undergo a second biopsy.

The Five-Region Biopsy

Since the 1980s, the ability to diagnose prostate cancer has been enhanced significantly by the advent of the PSA test. By taking a PSA level and performing a digital rectal exam on an annual basis, physicians are now able to detect prostate cancer at an early stage. Such early detection may offer the best chance for cure and for decreasing morbidity and death. The sextant biopsy, which is usually guided by the TRUS instrument, has detected a large number of cases of prostate cancer. However, one research study has indicated that the sextant biopsy misses about 22 percent of the cancers. Many physicians believe that six-tissue extractions are not enough, and they have increased this figure to seven, eight, and even higher. Depending on the number of suspicious areas, a doctor may take as many as 18 samples from a patient.

E. Roy Berger, M.D., F.A.C.P. and James Lewis, Jr., Ph.D

Urologists at the Bowman Gray School of Medicine of Wake Forest University at Winston-Salem, North Carolina, have developed a technique known as the 5-region prostate biopsy. It is probably superior to the sextant biopsy and may represent the best approach for conducting prostate biopsies.

A study was conducted to determine if additional biopsies performed in areas of the prostate beyond those sampled by the sextant biopsy increased the detection of prostate cancer. A total of 119 patients underwent TRUS-guided needle biopsy. In addition to sextant biopsies, cores were taken from the lateral and middle regions of the prostate. Pathological findings of the additional regions were analyzed and compared to those of the sextant biopsies. Of the 119 patients, 48 (40%) had prostate cancer. Of these 48 patients, 17 (35%) had cancer only in regions 1, 3, and 5 (right lateral, middle, and left lateral lobes). These tumors would have been missed had the sextant biopsy been used alone.

A study was conducted by Freedman et al. at Georgetown University, Walter Reed Army Medical Center, Armed Forces Institute of Pathology, entitled *Evaluation of Prostate Biopsy Protocols Based on 3D Simulation.*

Freedman and colleagues obtained digital images of over 200 step-sectioned, whole-mounted, radical prostatectomy specimens. Three-dimensional computer simulation software was developed to accurately depict the anatomy of the prostate and all individual tumor sites. Additional peripheral devices were incorporated in the system to perform interactive prostate biopsies. They also obtained 18 biopsies of each prostate model to determine the detection rates of various biopsy protocols.

The 10- and 12-pattern biopsies had a 99.0 percent detection rate, whereas the traditional sextant-biopsy rate was only 72.6 percent. The 14-pattern, which includes all the biopsies used in the 10- and 12-pattern protocols, added only one additional positive case (99.5%). The 5-region biopsy had a 90.5% detection rate. Transitional zone and seminal-vesicle biopsies did not result in a significantly increased detection rate when added to the patterns just mentioned. Only one positive model was obtained when transitional zone biopsies were added. The lateral sextant-biopsy revealed a detection rate of 95.5 percent, whereas the 4-pattern lateral biopsy had a 93.5 percent detection rate.

This study suggests that all protocols that use laterally placed biopsies based upon the five-region anatomical model are superior to the routinely used sextant-biopsy pattern. Lateral biopsies in the mid and apical zones of the gland are the most important. The three-dimensional models and biopsy simulation allowed the testing of multiple biopsy methods in more than 200 unique patients based on actual patterns of the location of cancer within the prostate.

What If Your Biopsy Is Inconclusive?

Research as well as personal observation have convinced us that there are far too many needle biopsies involving microscopic analysis of extracted prostatic tissue. Normally, 15 to 20 percent of these biopsies fail to detect prostate cancer. In fact, patients who undergo an initial biopsy are often reluctant to get a repeat biopsy because of a fear of seeding prostate cancer.

The JAMA (April 3, 2002) reported that a clinical trial was conducted to determine if a testing of biopsied prostatic tissue for a specific protein could help rule out or confirm prostate cancer without performing a repeat biopsy. This protein is found in a gene referred to as alpha-methylacyl coenzyme A racemase (AMACR).

The AMACR gene produces an enzyme important in fatty acid oxidation. It plays an important role in the breakdown of branched-chain fatty acid molecules such as those found in dairy products and beef.

It is not known whether an overexpression of the AMACR gene plays a role in the development of prostate cancer through increased oxidative stress that can damage cell components, such as the DNA. The link between consuming dairy products and beef and the increased expression of AMACR is unclear and is the focus of ongoing research. AMACR could be an invaluable early marker for prostate cancer and could possibly aid in identifying new dietary or chemical means for treating the disease.

Researchers have determined that more than 95 percent of prostate tumors show an overexpression of the AMACR gene, therefore making it one of the most consistent biological markers known for prostate cancer. It is an important improvement over the standard PSA test. Unlike the PSA, the AMACR is cancer-specific and is found almost exclusively in cancer cells. Because the PSA test cannot distinguish between cell changes caused by cancer and those caused by benign prostatic hyperplasia and prostatitis, it is limited in diagnosing prostate cancer.

Another AMACR study, conducted at the Brady Urological Institute of Johns Hopkins University using special genetic techniques, examined 94 prostate tissue samples for an overexpression of AMACR. When the results were compared to an analysis of prostate tissue removed through surgery, prostate cancer was identified in 97 percent of cases and was correctly ruled out in 100 percent of the cases.

Unfortunately, only a few medical laboratories in the United States conduct the AMACR test, although more are expected to offer it in the future. If your PSA test is inconclusive and or if your biopsy slides are available, you may not have to undergo a repeat biopsy. Instead, have your biopsy tissue submitted to one of the laboratories offering the AMACR.

Types of Cancer

Prostate cancer, or *prostatic adenocarcinoma*, is cancer of the cells that make up the prostate gland, which secretes fluid composing most of the semen.

Several types of cancer can occur in the body. *Sarcomas,* or cancer of muscles, bones, and supporting tissues, are very rare. Cancers of the blood and lymphatic systems are known as *leukemias* or *lymphomas*. Cancer of protective linings (such as the inside of the mouth) or of the skin are frequently *squamous* cancers. Cancers arising from glands that absorb or secrete fluids are called *adenocarcinomas*. These cancers frequently arise in the pancreas, colon, rectum, and lower esophagus and other digestive organs, as well as in the lung and prostate.

Types of Biopsies:

There are at least two types of biopsy: The most common is the sextant biopsy, which the urologist extracts a six-tissue sample from the prostate gland. However, it is not uncommon for a sextant biopsy to miss the tumor. Sextant biopsies are fairly good at detecting tumors greater than 2 cc and those in the peripheral zone; however, repeat biopsies should be strongly considered in patients with elevated PSA level and abnormal DREs but negative initial sextant biopsies.

Forty-three patients scheduled for prostatectomy had normal DRE findings. Immediately before surgery, all patients underwent sextant biopsies, and the location, amount, and Gleason grade of any cancer were recorded. After surgery, the prostate was serially sectioned, and the findings were compared with those of the biopsy specimens. There were 33 patients without prostate cancer in either the biopsies or the prostatectomy specimens. All patients who had cancer on the biopsies had cancer in the prostatectomy specimen. In six patients, cancer was found in both the biopsy and the prostatectomy specimen; these cancers ranged from 0.9 to 6.5 cc in volume. In the remaining four patients, there was no cancer on the biopsy, but the prostatectomy specimen revealed cancers of 0.05 to 2.5 cc. The overall sensitivity for sextant biopsies was 60 percent, with a specificity of 100 percent. When only cancers greater than 2 cc or cancers in the peripheral zone were considered, the sensitivity rose to 83.3 percent and 71.4 percent, respectively, with a minimal decrease in specificity (97.3% and 97.2%, respectively). In contrast, when transition zone cancers were evaluated, the sensitivity fell to 33.3 percent.

Ultrasound Power Doppler

Power Doppler imaging (known as PDI or power angio Doppler) can differentiate between cancer and benign prostatic hyperplasia. The sensitivity for malignancy diagnosis varies between 86 and 90 percent. Benign tumor vessels usually start from a single vascular pedicle and have regular caliber arterial vessels with regular course and regular vascular distribution. In contrast, malignant vessels have multiple vascular pedicles and irregular sizes and distributions.

Power Doppler imaging is five times more sensitive than traditional color Doppler imaging. The test is quick, painless, and uses sound waves, which are safe. Indeed, since the power Doppler finds out of 100 cases of cancer, some suggest that it be used to spare patients with elevated PSA levels from undergoing biopsies.

The areas to which cancer spreads may also be evaluated with the power Doppler. Areas of increased flow are 4.7 times more likely to contain cancer.

PIN

Some biopsies do not find prostate cancer but do show *prostatic intraepithelial neoplasia* (PIN), which many physicians believe to be the most likely precursor of prostate cancer. PIN is a proliferative lesion composed of prostatic epithelial cells that are dividing more rapidly than normal epithelium. However, these cells have not matured - that is, they have not yet become cancerous. PIN cells are classified as high-grade, medium-grade, and low-grade. Low-grade cells do not pose a problem unless, or until, they become high- or medium-grade. PIN cells do not elevate the PSA. They also do not invade the areas of the prostate outside the glandular structures.

DNA Ploidy Analysis

Sometimes a prostate cancer patient may have a biopsy in order to determine the prognosis of his disease. A study using needle biopsies indicated that a DNA ploidy analysis was more important than the Gleason grade. This study found a tenfold increase in risk for metastatic disease and a high risk for extracapsular spread if the needle biopsy showed nondiploid cells. A man who wants a DNA ploidy analysis should inform his urologist prior to the biopsy. We know several men who had biopsies and who later wanted the tissues to be assayed for DNA ploidy analysis, but they were unable to have it done due to the way the tissue was processed.

New Test Increases Accuracy of Diagnosis

Someday it may be possible to determine if a man has prostate cancer simply by testing a pattern of proteins found in a single drop of blood. David Ornstein, M.D., and his colleagues say they have found protein markers in a blood test that can be used to more accurately define those men at highest risk for prostate cancer. According to Dr. Ornstein, a prostate cancer specialist at the University of North Carolina in Chapel Hill, "This could help significantly reduce unnecessary biopsies."

In Ornstein's study, 95 percent of the cancer cases and 100 percent of those with a benign condition were diagnosed correctly by the computer-driven diagnostic.

PROSE Test

A new prostate cancer test called PROSE (*pro*state *s*pectroscopy and imaging *e*xamination) integrates spectroscopy technology with magnetic resonance imaging equipment. PROSE may be more effective as a screening test than is the PSA test, the sextant biopsy, or the standard MRI. For example, the PSA test must be used with the digital rectal exam and can detect only about 70 percent of patients with cancer. The sextant biopsy also has its limitations, and often the results are "inconclusive." The MRI often is unable to determine whether or not an abnormality appearing on the scan is cancerous. However, the PROSE exam is able to perform a chemical analysis of the prostate gland. Whenever PROSE is applied to the affected area, the spectroscopy displays a chemical analysis of the tumor, usually shown as an extended peak, which is characteristic of cancer.

The PROSE exam may eliminate multiple biopsies. If a patient has an elevated PSA and the biopsy comes back negative, he can undergo a PROSE exam to determine if cancer exists, where it is located, and how large it is. Based on the chemical makeup of the cancer, PROSE can also tell the physician how aggressive the cancer is, as well as its staging.

PROSE is more accurate in determining the size of the tumor and its location. Thus, if a patient opts for surgery, the surgeon may decide to take out surrounding tissue, along with the tumor, to ensure that all of the cancer has been removed. After surgery, PROSE can tell physicians if the surgery was successful in removing all the cancerous tissue. In addition, if a patient opts for other forms of treatment, such as radiation or seed implants, PROSE can be used to evaluate the progress of the therapy.

The PROSE system is available in approximately 20 hospitals nationwide and more than 70 hospitals worldwide. Leading medical centers offering PROSE in the United States are located in such cities as New York (tristate area), San Francisco, Baltimore, and Houston.

SELDI Process

SELDI (Surface-Enhanced Laser Desorption Ionization) is a process that involves the detection and quantitative mapping of protein biomarkers from trace quantities of biological fluids such as plasma, serum, urine, and saliva. LumiCyte's technology and the SELDI process do not require that the proteins be identified ahead of time, unlike other approaches using antibodies and aptamers. The seldiography provides for an analysis and comparison of multiple proteins that are increasing and decreasing relative to quantities of other proteins. LumiCyte technology and the SELDI process is an integrated procedure acting as a single solution to provide protein composition mapping discovery and validation with superior sensitivity, resolution, accuracy, throughput, and scalability. The combination of the superior sensitivity of SELDI and the efficiency and effectiveness of LumiCyte's technology will enable LumiCyte to provide new and better biomarkers, which are statistically more relevant improved biomarkers than the traditional ones such as the standard biopsy. However, clinical trials must be initiated before it becomes available.

How to Use This Information

1. If you are very anxious, ask your doctor to sedate you prior to a needle biopsy.
2. Be sure you are sedated before undergoing a 5-region biopsy for getting a DNA ploidy analysis.
3. Consider undergoing a biopsy using a power Doppler.
4. Before you undergo a biopsy, tell your doctor if you plan to get an AMACR. This will determine how the tissue is handled.

Chapter 5

A GENE FOR METASTATIC PROSTATE CANCER

Over the past 60 years, great strides have been made in treating localized prostate cancer. However, no significant changes or improvements have been made in the prognosis for men diagnosed with advanced prostate cancer. In addition, there was no way to tell at diagnosis which cancer would spread and which would not – at least not until Arul M. Chinnaiyan, M.D., and his research team at the University of Michigan's Comprehensive Cancer Center in Ann Arbor demonstrated that EZH2 was at "the top of the list" of 55 genes found to be more active in metastatic prostate cancer than in localized prostate cancer. When the gene EZH2 is active, the cell uses its coded instructions to produce EZH2 protein. The researchers believe that future diagnostic tests for high levels of this protein could serve as a marker for physicians and help save the lives of advanced prostate cancer patients.

Metastatic Prostate Cancer

Metastatic prostate cancer occurs when a secondary tumor forms as a result of a cancer cell or cells from the primary tumor site (in this case, the prostate), travel through the body, creates a new site, and then grows there.

The EZH2 Gene

EZH2 is one of several related proteins that control a cell's genetic memory and interfere with <u>transcription</u>, the process cells used to transcribe or copy their genetic code. The researchers indicated that an RNA nucleotides specifically targeted for the EZH2 gene and tested them on two different prostate cancer cell lines. Dr. Chinnaiyan says, "The first thing we noticed is the cells stopped growing. After 120 hours, 80 to 90 percent of the cultured cells containing the RNA nucleotides targeted for EZH2 had stopped dividing. When cells can't divide and grow, they die. This suggests that EZH2 could play an important role in the progression of prostate cancer."

To validate their findings, the researchers analyzed levels of EZH2 protein in more than a thousand prostate tissue samples. They included normal prostate tissue, tissue with nonmalignant cell changes, and tissue with localized and advanced cancer.

What the Research Concluded

Mark A. Rubin, M.D., one of the researchers, maintains that "one of the differences in our study is that we correlated EZH2 expression in prostate cells with clinical outcome." Dr. Rubin indicates that they analyzed "278 tissue samples from 64 men for EZH2 protein expression, as well as other common prognostic indicators used by pathologists such as Gleason score, tumor stage, or PSA level.... We found EZH2 protein expression to be significantly better at predicting clinical outcome than any other factor."

How to Use This Information

Have a blood test to determine if your EZH2 gene shows evidence of metastatic prostate cancer.

PART II IMAGING THE PROSTATE

Chapter 6

THE CT SCAN

The CT (computed tomography) scan of the pelvis and abdomen is used primarily for staging prostate cancer. The lymph nodes are evaluated for pathologic enlargement and the tissues surrounding the prostate for evidence of extracapsular penetration. The size, shape, and symmetry of the prostate can also be delineated by the CT scan. However, the zones of the prostate gland cannot be separated. As a result, it is not possible to distinguish normal tissue from that of benign prostatic hyperplasia and prostate cancer. The criteria for abnormalities are based on the size of the prostate and its symmetry, as well as the distortion of adjacent structures, such as the muscles, and bladder base and the fat of the pelvis. Soft-tissue densities, which are seen beyond the capsule, may indicate extracapsular disease.

What Is a CT Scan?

The CT scan combines images from multiple X-rays to produce three-dimensional pictures of the internal organs. It can be used to identify an enlargement of the prostate, but it is not always effective for determining the stage of prostate cancer. However, it is effective for evaluating metastases to the lymph nodes or more distant soft-tissue sites.

What Can the CT Scan Do?

The uses of the CT scan in diagnosing prostate cancer follow:

- The size of the prostate can be determined.
- Planning CT scans for radioactive seed implantation, external beam radiation, or both are easily performed. It requires minimal preparation and is not dependent on the skill of the person taking the scan. They are less subject to technical error in obtaining the scan.
- The PSA volumes shown by the CT are larger than the one shown by the TRUS.
- The pubic bones are well visualized on the CT scan, and thus their potential to interfere with implanting seed in the anterior portion of the prostate can be determined.
- Real-time CT imaging adds a degree of certainty that the seeds are placed as intended.

- Generally, only patients with PSA levels higher than 10 ng/ml are found to have metastases on the CT scan.
- The CT scan has proved moderately useful for staging prostate cancer patients when metastases exist.
- CT scanning can be useful in evaluating a patient with a high-grade or large tumor or a high PSA level who is likely to have nodal metastases.
- The CT scan can be used for accurate planning of the delivery of iodine-125 seed implants through the perineum.
- The CT scan is useful for evaluation of distant metastases from prostate cancer.
- The CT scan can sometimes be useful in distinguishing between stage B2 and C disease.
- The CT scan can be used to assess genitourinary disorders and is particularly helpful in imaging the kidneys, adrenal glands, and bladder.

Limitations of the CT Scan

Limitations of the CT scan follow:

- It cannot reliably image the presence or extent of intraprostatic cancers.
- It cannot produce well-defined images of the prostatic margins (that is, the outer edge of the prostate).
- It cannot distinguish between cancer and benign abnormalities of the prostate.
- It does not show microscopic extracapsular involvement.
- It cannot determine the cause of nodal enlargement.
- It usually cannot detect lymph-node metastases in patients with biochemical recurrence who have a PSA level under 10 ng/ml.
- It is unable to correlate CT findings with the PSA level. In patients who appear to have clinically localized prostate cancer with a PSA level of less than 20 ng/ml, the CT scan usually does not show lymph-node metastases, even if they are microscopically present.
- It is not useful in detecting local recurrences, unless they are larger.
- It includes restriction to the transaxial plane for direct imaging, tissue nonspecificity, low soft-tissue contrast resolution, and the need for contrast media, both oral and intravenous.
- It is generally not a modality for evaluation unless patients have a PSA level of at least 20 ng/ml and a Gleason score of 8.

- It cannot delineate the internal architecture of the prostate, and it often cannot separate normal parenchyma from the capsule.
- It is usually unable to determine if the cancer is in the bladder-base or seminal vesicles.
- It cannot detect microscopic metastases or the internal architecture of the lymph nodes.
- It is unable to definitively detect metastases based on lymph-node size. Nodes larger than 1.0 cm are considered suspicious, and those greater than 1.5 cm are considered abnormal.
- It lacks the resolution necessary to detect capsular penetration.

How to Use This Information

1. The CT scan is generally useful when the PSA level is greater than 20.
2. It has limited specificity, but can be helpful when there are gross metastases.
3. It may be helpful in diagnosing locally advanced disease.

Chapter 7

MONITORING PROSTATE CANCER WITH A BONE SCAN

Bone scanning is performed when prostate cancer has been diagnosed or is strongly suspected. A bone scan allows for staging, indicating if the cancer is confined to the prostate gland and therefore curable, or if it has spread outside the prostate gland and is probably not curable. One of the most common places to which prostate cancer is likely to spread is to the bones, particularly the spine, hips, pelvis, and the long bone of the upper legs. When prostate cancer does spread to the bones, it tends to debilitate the patient, damaging and even destroying the bone. As soon as this damage or destruction has occurred, the body's natural healing process begins to replace the damaged bone with new bone. A bone scan will reveal this.

What Is a Bone Scan?

A bone scan is an imaging of the entire skeleton - or a specific area - after the injection of technetium-99m, a radioactive isotope, into the blood, which transports it to the bones. Areas in the bone with prostate cancer, where cells are dividing rapidly, will pick up more of the radioactive substance, resulting in "hot spots." However, other conditions are also likely to show up as hot spots on a bone scan, thus making the bone scan difficult to interpret.

Why Have a Bone Scan?

Your physician may recommend you have a bone scan for the following reasons:

- Abdominal ultrasound.
- Intravenous urogram (showing abnormalities in the kidneys or urinary tract).
- You have a Gleason score of 8 or above.
- You have an extremely high PSA level, such as 100 ng/ml or more.
- You experience unusual bone pain.
- The bones are one of the most common areas for prostate cancer.
- Your PSA level is over 20 ng/ml.

- To assess systemic metastases.
- To detect a recurrence of prostate cancer.

How Is the Bone Scan Performed?

Prior to the Image Study

About three hours before the scanning procedure, you will receive an injection (usually in the arm) of a small amount of radioactive tracer that is "tagged" to a calcium-like material. Over the next few hours, the calcium will circulate in your body and be absorbed by your bones. After the injection, you can leave the nuclear medicine facility until it's time for your scan.

There are no dietary restrictions. You can eat before and after the injection and test. During the scanning procedure, you will be positioned on a scanning table, and a head-to-toe scan will be performed by a gamma camera. The entire procedure lasts 50 to 90 minutes.

Often an entire body scan is performed because the amount of radiation received is constant. Therefore, extra views of the skeleton can be taken if the radiologist so desires.

After the Scan

A normal bone scan will show symmetrical and uniform uptake of the tracer. An abnormal bone scan will show an increased uptake of the tracer where bone formation is occurring faster than the surrounding bone.

The Advantages of a Bone Scan

There are a host of benefits for getting a bone scan:

- False-negative scans occur in less than 1 percent of patients.
- Sensitivity approaches 100 percent in detecting metastases, compared to 18 percent for X-ray, 58 to 77 percent for the alkaline phosphatase test, and 50 to 60 percent for the acid phosphatase test.
- Used with combination hormonal therapy, it can determine if the patient has metastases.
- It is the gold standard for determining if there are skeletal metastases.
- It is useful for newly diagnosed patients with bone pain, a PSA level of under 10 ng/ml, or evidence of local or distant metastases.
- It can predict the duration of response to hormonal therapy.

45

- It can provide prognostic information.

The Disadvantages of Getting a Bone Scan

The disadvantages of a bone scan follow:

- Although many urologists prefer to have all prostate cancer patients undergo an initial baseline bone scan for staging purposes, it may not be necessary in all newly diagnosed patients. In a study that supports this concept, only 1 of 306 patients with a PSA level of 20 ng/ml or less had skeletal metastases, and none of 209 patients with a PSA level of 10 ng/ml or below had metastases. As a result, hundreds of millions of dollars are spent on unnecessary scans.
- A bone scan cannot distinguish between prostate cancer, arthritis, and Paget's disease.
- It has a high false-positive rate.
- It is unnecessary after prostatectomy in patients with a PSA level under 2.0 ng/ml.
- It may be too sensitive because it can also detect new and old fractures.

How to Use This Information

1. If you haven't had a bone scan in three years, do so now.
2. If your PSA is over 20 ng/ml and you have not had a bone scan in two years, do so now.
3. If you are experiencing any pain, get a bone scan immediately.

Chapter 8

THE PET SCAN AND LYMPH-NODE METASTASES

Metastases from prostate cancer usually begin in the lymph nodes, which are adjacent to the prostate in the pelvis near the iliac blood vessels. The most accurate markers for the presence of lymphatic metastases are the PSA level, the Gleason score, and the prostatic acid phosphatase (PAP) level. The incidence of lymphatic metastases in patients with clinically localized prostate cancer was reported in one study to be 7.5 percent (13 of 229). In another study, the rate reported was 2 percent. The detection of lymph-node involvement in prostate cancer is essential in planning treatment because aggressive local therapies such as radical prostatectomy, external beam radiation, radioactive seed implant, and cryosurgery are not likely to be effective in the long run when there is local or distant lymphatic spread.

In the past, lymphangiography was used in an attempt to detect lymphatic metastatic disease. In theory, it can detect metastases within the pelvic lymph nodes that are not enlarged; however, it is only 50 to 60 percent accurate. Lymphangiography has now been superseded by the CT and MRI scans, with which it is possible to see large-volume nodal metastases. Both scans can be used to determine the presence of metastatic disease; however, nodal metastases smaller than 5 mm in diameter are usually undetectable on CT and MRI scans.

What Is Positron Emission Tomography (PET)?

Positron emission tomography, or PET, scan, is a diagnostic examination that uses two radiotracer drugs to locate tumors and determine their activity.

What Is the PET Scan Used For?

A PET scan is used to:

- Identify and label a selected compound with a positron-emitting radionuclide.
- Administer this compound to the individual being studied.
- Image the distribution of the positron activity as a function of time by emission tomography.

- Elicit from the information acquired an understanding of the biological handling of the compound.

Specifically, PET scans are used to detect cancer and to examine the effects of cancer therapy by characterizing biochemical changes taking place within the cancer. These scans are performed on the whole body.

PET scans of prostate cancer patients are used to determine local and distant metastatic disease.

Functions of the PET Scan

The PET scan is useful for a variety of functions:

- It can assess biochemical changes in the body. Any region of the body that is experiencing an increase in glucose metabolism can be seen through PET.
- The PET scan is important in drug research and development, and it can be used to study how a drug is used and absorbed by the body and how the body reacts.
- The PET scan can be used to detect and locate lymphatic metastases, as well as lesions in other organs.
- The PET scan has the ability to model biological and physiological functions in the body by detection and modeling of regional concentrations of radioactivity tagged to glucose in a particular organ.
- The PET scan can be used to obtain improved localization of cancer activity by overlaying or imprinting the information from PET onto more detailed images of MRIs or CTs, or by employing a combined PET/CT device.

Preparing for a PET Scan

A PET scan is usually done on an outpatient basis. Wear comfortable, loose-fitting clothes. Do not eat anything for four hours before the scan, but water is allowed. Your doctor will instruct you about the use of medications before the test. Diabetic patients should ask the doctor for specific diet guidelines to control glucose levels on the day of the test.

Features of the PET Scan

The PET scanner is a machine that looks like a CT scanner; it has a hole in the middle and looks like a large, square-shaped doughnut. Within this machine are multiple rings of detectors that record the emission of energy from the radioactive substance in your body. The images are then displayed on the monitor of a nearby computer.

How Does the PET Scan Work?

Before the examination begins, a radioactive substance is produced in a machine called a Cyclotron. Then it is attached, or tagged, to a natural body compound, most commonly glucose.

This process is called *radiolabeling*.

Different colors or degrees of brightness on a PET image represent different levels of cellular function. For example, because healthy tissue uses glucose for energy, it accumulates some of the radiolabeled glucose; this will show up as background areas on the PET images.

Cancerous tissue will absorb more of the substance and appear brighter on the PET images.

Undergoing a PET Scan

While lying on an examination table you will be given the radioactive substance in an intravenous injection or through an intravenous line. It will take 30 to 60 minutes for the substance to travel through your body and be absorbed by the tissue under study. Then the scanning begins. It takes 30 to 45 minutes.

Some patients, in particular those with heart problems, may undergo a stress test in which PET scans are obtained while (1) they are at rest and (2) after a pharmaceutical is administered to alter the blood flow to the heart.

If given by intravenous injection, the administration of the radioactive substance will feel like a slight pinprick. You will then be made as comfortable as possible on the examination table before you are positioned into the hole of the PET scanner for the test. You will have to remain still throughout the examination. Patients who are claustrophobic may feel some anxiety while positioned in the scanner and may be given Valium. Also, some patients find it uncomfortable to hold one position for more than a few minutes. You will not feel the radioactive substance in your body.

Usually, there are no restrictions after the test, although you should drink plenty of fluids to flush the radioactive substance from your body.

A radiologist who has specialized training in PET will interpret the images and forward a report to the referring physician. This usually takes a couple of days.

Benefits of the PET Scan

The PET scan has several benefits:

- It allows for study of cellular function. As a result, it can help physicians detect alterations in biochemical processes that suggest disease before changes in anatomy are apparent.
- Its radioactivity is very short-lived; therefore, the patient's radiation exposure is extremely low. The amount of tracer is so small that it does not affect the normal processes of the body.
- It uses a noninvasive biochemical and/or physiologic reaction to detect prostate cancer.
- It can detect other cancers.
- It can identify metastases when other imaging studies are normal.
- It can show alterations in tumor metabolism before a CT or MRI can detect them.
- It may be more sensitive than CT for detecting lymph-node metastases.

Limitations of the PET Scan

PET can give false results if a patient's chemical balances are not normal. Specifically, test results of diabetics can be adversely affected because of blood sugar or insulin levels.

Also, because the radioactive substance decays quickly and is effective for only a short period of time, it must be produced in a laboratory near the PET scanner. It is important to receive the radioactive substance at the scheduled time. PET must be done by a radiologist who has specialized in nuclear medicine and has substantial experience with PET. Most large medical centers now have PET services available to their patients. Medicare and insurance companies cover many of the applications of PET, and coverage continues to increase; however, prostate cancer patients are not yet covered.

Finally, the PET scan should not be used alone as a diagnostic tool but should be part of a larger diagnostic workup. Unfortunately, the data have not yet supported the routine use of PET in prostate cancer.

How to Use This Information

If you have undergone a bone scan, ProstaScint scan, and an MRI and/or CT scan, you may verify the results by undergoing a PET scan for detection of metastatic lesions.

Chapter 9

THE PROSTASCINT SCAN

Approximately 40 to 60 percent of men with prostate cancer have disease that has spread beyond the prostatic capsule. When the disease metastasizes, it can do so via both the blood and lymph-nodes, the latter particularly along the pelvic and abdominal great vessels. Early metastatic nodal tumors from prostate cancer are usually tiny, measuring less than 1 cm, and so they are frequently missed by high-resolution, anatomically based imaging procedures such as the CT scan and the MRI. Nevertheless, it is important to distinguish patients with locally confined prostate cancer from those with lymph-node disease, cancer that has spread to other areas of the body, or both. This is essential so that the appropriate treatment is chosen. In addition, it is important for the physician to distinguish local residual or recurrent disease in the prostatic fossa from lymph-node or distant metastases in treated prostate cancer patients who have a rising PSA.

To date, staging recently diagnosed patients with prostate cancer or restaging those patients with suspected recurrent or residual disease has been difficult. The ability to accurately diagnose patients with extracapsular lesions in newly discovered prostate cancer by means of the PSA level is very limited. In addition, ultrasound imaging by itself is also limited because half of the patients with presumed localized prostate cancer are found to have extracapsular disease based on pathologic review. The DRE, which is somewhat specific, fails to be sensitive. Currently, imaging methods such as the CT scan have poor sensitivity for detecting capsular penetration as well as lymph-node and seminal-vesicle involvement. Sensitivity of the CT scan has been estimated to range from 6 to 30 percent. MRI using an endorectal coil has been shown to improve the ability to determine local staging. As a result, most patients with lymph-node involvement can be accurately assessed only with bilateral pelvic lymphadenectomy (pelvic lymph-node dissection). Many of the same staging limitations noted in patients with newly detected disease also exist for patients with recurrent prostate cancer.

Describing the ProstaScint Scan

Developed in the 1990s, the ProstaScint scan detects prostate cancer anywhere in the body. An antibody, derived from mice and chemically modified so that it can carry a radioactive tracer called Indium-111, is injected into the vein. After the injection, a gamma camera is used to locate the tumor tissue in the body by recording the radioactivity of the tracer. At least two times after the injection, the gamma camera is used to depict images. Usually, the first imaging session begins 30 minutes after the injection. Delayed imaging is performed from 3 to 5 days later.

Advantages

Following are the advantages of ProstaScint:

- It is one of the few noninvasive diagnostic modalities that can detect prostate cancer outside the capsule, especially in the lymph nodes.
- It may be cost-effective. When one of the coauthors was suspected of having prostate cancer outside the capsule, he had a skeletal X-ray, two CT scans, two bone scans, a bone biopsy, and an MRI. If the ProstaScint had been available, it might have been the only detection technique needed (See Figure 9-1)

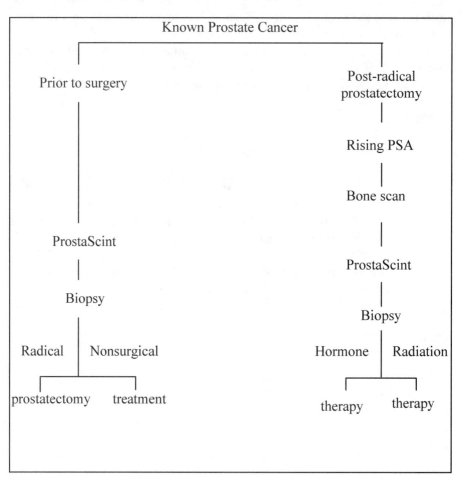

Figure 9-1.

- A study involving a large series of patients suggests that ProstaScint was six to ten times more sensitive than either the CT scan or MRI.
- The absence of any detection of prostate cancer appears to correlate well with the absence of the disease.
- The ProstaScint scan appears to detect more prostate cancer patients who had their disease outside the capsule than previously thought.
- It can detect both locally recurrent and distant prostate cancer.
- To ensure appropriate administration and interpretation, ProstaScint is available only at hospitals that have undergone specific training in the protocol.
- It appears to work for patients undergoing hormonal therapy.

- Before ProstaScint, there was no way to find out whether a tumor had metastasized unless it had spread to the bone, which would show up on a bone scan.
- The ProstaScint is the first scan that is specific for prostate cancer. It looks for prostate cancer cells and goes right to them.
- It helps eliminate doubt when other tests are inconclusive.
- The ProstaScint scan can distinguish prostate cancer from benign tumors.
- The ProstaScint images can show where the cancer has spread outside the prostate gland.
- The ProstaScint scan can help determine the most appropriate treatment.
- The ProstaScint scan has a 70 percent accuracy rate; although not great, it's one of the best available.

Disadvantages

The drawback to ProstaScint is that a bone scan tends to be – but is not always — more accurate for detecting bone metastases.

How Is ProstaScint Used?

The ProstaScint scan is used for staging purposes and to detect a recurrence of prostate cancer, as described below.

Staging Presurgical Patients

When prostate cancer is detected in a patient, a complete clinical staging should follow. Staging procedures may include a bone scan, digital rectal exam (DRE), transrectal ultrasound (TRUS), and CT scan or MRI or MRSI of the pelvis and abdomen.

The attempt to accurately stage the extent of a tumor has frustrated physicians for decades. Despite the dramatic increase in the number of men with clinically organ-confined disease during the past decade, recent large series have demonstrated the risk of stage T3 disease to be between 40 and 50 percent. Paulson, M.D. and colleagues demonstrated the poor prognosis of such patients.

The evaluation of pelvic lymph nodes is critical in the management of patients with presumed localized disease. The presence or absence of metastases to the pelvic lymph nodes is one of the most important prognostic factors for patients with prostate cancer. Gervasi and colleagues reported the risk of metastatic disease at 10 years as 31 percent ($\pm$7 percent) for those patients with no lymph-node involvement and 83 percent (±7 percent) for those with at least one malignant node. Because the status of the pelvic lymph nodes is so important to the prognosis, urologists routinely perform pelvic lymph-node dissections prior to prostatectomy. CT and MRI of the pelvis are generally not used to evaluate lymph nodes – these tests on an increase in nodal size as the indicator of possible neoplastic involvement. Normal-size nodes with microscopic metastases and enlarged nodes with benign processes are inaccurately diagnosed by these tests.   However, MRSI may be an exception to this statement.

Determining the Location and Extent of Recurrence

Unfortunately, many patients who have undergone treatment will develop a recurrence of prostate cancer. Relapse can occur locally, in the prostatic fossa; regionally, in the lymph nodes; or distantly, in the bones. Measuring PSA is the most effective way to follow patients who have been treated for prostate cancer. Treatment failure is most often heralded by detection of serum PSA, which had been previously undetectable, or by a rising serum PSA, which had previously been stable. A detectable PSA after radical prostatectomyand a rising PSA after radiation therapy are both associated with high rates of clinical recurrence. A critical concern in these men is whether the disease recurrence is confined to the prostatic bed or is present in lymph nodes or bones. The distinction is important because the patient with local relapse is a potential candidate for radiotherapy or salvage prostatectomy (in patients who had radiotherapy as a primary treatment). Patients with regional or distant metastases are best treated with hormonal therapy. A ProstaScint scan can clarify the extent and location of recurrent disease to aid in choosing the most rational therapeutic approach for patients with a rising PSA who have undergone prior treatment.

The initial results with ProstaScint in patients with a rising PSA have been favorable. A total of 181 postprostatectomy patients with elevated PSA levels underwent ProstaScint imaging. These patients had CT and bone scans and were considered candidates for local salvage radiation therapy. Prostate cancer was localized to prostatic fossa only in 32 (18%) patients, to fossa and other sites in 30 (17%) patients, and to other sites alone in 46 (25%) patients. Thus, ProstaScint scan showed that 76 of 181 (42%) patients had evidence of regional or distant metastases or both.

ProstaScint performed favorably during clinical trials in the evaluation of pelvic lymph-node disease. One hundred and fifty-two patients with clinically localized prostate cancer, who were at high risk for presence of lymph-node metastases and who were scheduled for pelvic lymph-node dissection prior to definitive primary therapy, underwent ProstaScint imaging. Sixty-four patients had lymph node metastases that were confirmed at surgery. At least one surgically confirmed lymph-node metastasis was detected by the ProstaScint scan in 40 patients for a sensitivity of 62 percent. CT detected lesions in only 4 percent of the patients. The improved sensitivity of this noninvasive test to detect pelvic lymph-node involvement may lead some physicians to use this scan as part of the presurgical staging regimen of prostate cancer patients.

Presurgical Evaluation

John K. Burgers, M. D., Urologic surgeon at Riverside Hospital, Ohio, performed a study of 65 prostate cancer patients who were imaged with ProstaScint and CT prior to surgery. Of the 21 patients with surgically confirmed lymph-node metastases, ProstaScint detected disease in eleven patients (sensitivity: 52%), while CT detected disease in two patients (sensitivity: 10%). Five of the nine lymph-node metastases detected by ProstaScint and missed on CT were smaller than 1 cm. According to Dr. Burgers, "The information provided by ProstaScint regarding the presence and location of prostate cancer, which currently goes undetected by other modalities, is potentially significant in determining the optimal treatment for these patients. ProstaScint may provide opportunities to enhance patient management in a cost-effective manner."

Prostatectomy Follow-Up

Richard D. Williams, M.D., chairman of the Department of Urology of the University of Iowa Hospitals and Clinics, followed 23 men who had undergone a radical prostatectomy, had a rising PSA, and were scheduled to have a biopsy. Prior to the biopsy, they were evaluated with the ProstaScint scan, which detected a recurrence in the original tumor bed in 11 of the 23 patients. Five of six patients with positive biopsies of this area had a positive scan, whereas nine of eleven patients with negative biopsies had negative scans. Dr. Williams stated, "The scan is highly accurate and potentially clinically useful in detecting recurrent prostate cancer in the tumor bed after a radical prostatectomy."

The Procedure

A ProstaScint test requires a minimum of two visits to the nuclear medicine office. On the first visit, the technologist obtains a detailed medical history and then injects ProstaScint into the bloodstream. There are no special instructions for the first visit. A scan to visualize the pattern of blood distribution may be performed approximately 30 minutes after the injection.

The second imaging session, from 2 to 5 days after the injection, can take up to three hours. There are no dietary restrictions, but other preparations are necessary. The patient will need to have an enema on the evening before because it decreases the chance of ProstaScint uptake in the colon obscuring or mimicking disease spread. On the second day of imaging, the patient may be asked to perform another enema or undergo bladder catherization if there is excessive activity in the rectum or urinary tract. The patient will then be placed on a table where a camera will rotate around him, obtaining the images. When the imaging is complete, a nuclear medicine physician will review the scan and establish whether the patient will need to return for more imaging. If additional images are not required, the scan will be processed and displayed in three planes on the computer for interpretation.

Sensitivity and Specificity of the ProstaScint

Several factors are responsible for improving the sensitivity and specificity of the ProstaScint scan, which were the main limitations of the original scan. These are described below.

Physician Experience

Evidence exists that performance improves as experience with the ProstaScint scan is gained. In clinical trials, the sensitivity and specificity for detecting pelvic lymph-node metastases were significantly higher at clinical sites performing 10 or more scans (65 and 78 percent, respectively) versus sites performing fewer than 10 (58 and 62 percent).

Dual Isotope Procedure

In the original ProstaScint procedure, some physicians found that the accurate alignment of corresponding sections from days 1 and 5 was a problem. Jerry J. Sychra and colleagues described the results of images of the ProstaScint scan of 20 patients who on day 5 underwent the original procedure plus an additional data acquisition of the pelvis with a second isotope (the technetium-99m-labeled red blood cells, or RBCs. All patients were required to take a cathartic on the afternoon and evening of day 4 after the infusion. If significant colonic activity was seen on the initial abdominal image of the patient on day 5, the examination was discontinued, and the patient was advised to take an additional cathartic and return for imaging on day 6 or 7. On the day of delayed imaging, a 5-cc sample of blood was taken from the patient for RBC labeling with the ultra-tag kit. During the RBC labeling, a whole-body image of the patient's chest, abdomen, and pelvis were completed. This alteration in the sequence of imaging tasks decreased the imaging time needed for the examination and greatly improved any alignment problems between the blood-pool and antibody images. Therefore, when these two imaging sets of data are acquired simultaneously, computer subtraction of the blood-pool activity from the antibody is made possible, thus making image interpretation easier.

Quantitative Spect Imaging

In an effort to obtain improved sensitivity and specificity with the ProstaScint scan, D. Bruce Sodee, M.D. and colleagues developed a quantitative spect imaging technique, designed to separate benign tumor tissues from cancerous tumor tissues. It uses a region-of-interest (ROI) analysis on reconstructed transaxial images. Researchers maintained that if the ROI could be localized and defined, then semiquantitative uptake-intensity information could be used to develop a prostate-to-background ratio or a prostate-to-back-muscle ratio. They also thought that this ratio, a result of biopsy-positive versus biopsy-negative ROI in patients with prostate cancer, can also be used to assess areas of uptake in the prostate bed of patients after surgery. By using the dual-isotope technique, these researchers established a standard 30-pixel ROI on delayed transaxial images of the prostate bed. To view the ROI, all of the slices were magnified by a factor of 3 prior to ROIs being placed on a computer screen. Anywhere between four to six ROIs were situated on either side of the prostate gland. ROIs were also set posteriorly to the bone marrow of the symphysis pubis and anterior to rectal activity. Background counts were also obtained by placing the ROIs in the external obturator muscle. The total counts in each ROI were used to get the P/M ratio. As a result, a ratio is obtained to indicate the presence of specific tumor uptake versus nontumor. These collective reports should reveal a substantial increase in the specificity of the ProstaScint scan for the presence of prostate cancer whenever a P/M ratio is greater than 3.

Another factor that led to an increase in the sensitivity and selectivity of the ProstaScint scan was the infusion of other images with the ProstaScint spect images. Research revealed that even with the dual-isotope imaging and the substraction software, the interpretation of the pelvic SPECT data is still difficult.

The CT scan and MRI images of the pelvis provide an excellent presentation of the anatomic structures. The bone and tissue structures in the images provide a framework within which the tumor, prostatic bed, pelvic lymph nodes, seminal vesicles, and the bladder, which are indicated by the In MoAb examination, and can be interpreted. In addition, the bone marrow in the In MoAb images can be compared with the bony structures cited on the CT scan.

Bruce Sodee, M.D., of University Hospitals of Cleveland/Case Western Reserve University has pioneered a major advance in the ProstaScint technique. First, he dramatically improved the resolution (sharpness) of the images. Second, he fused the ProstaScint scan with the CAT scan. As a result, positive findings can now be clearly attributed to specific body structures visible on the CAT scan. It is now easy to identify antibody uptake into lymph nodes, seminal vesicles, or parts of the prostate gland, rather than into urine in the bladder or stool in the colon. This advanced form of the ProstaScint scan has been being widely implemented at cancer centers throughout the United States.

How to Use This Information

If it is important in deciding upon treatment to know if you have extraprostatic disease, consider the following:

1. Ask your physician to use the Partin tables to determine the probability of your disease being outside the capsule. If the probability is high, ask for a PAP test to help determine the likelihood of extraprostatic disease.
2. If there is a high probability of extraprostatic disease and/or if your treatment regimen will be changed by its presence, then a ProstaScint scan may add meaningful data to help you and your physician make appropriate decisions.
3. ProstaScint scans are generally reimbursed by most public and private insurance companies. The Cytogen Corporation, which manufactures the ProstaScint imaging agent, has established a reimbursement hotline for patients and physician. After the ProstaScint scan has been prescribed, the hotline can provide information on insurer coverage, coding, reimbursement, or help with preauthorization letters. To contact the Cytogen reimbursement hotline, call 1-800-833-3533 between 9 A.M. and 5 P.M. EST, Monday through Friday. In the metropolitan Washington, D.C. area, call 202-508-6572.

Chapter 10

USING MRI AND MRSI TO STAGE PROSTATE CANCER

Before the use of the PSA test became widespread, most organ-confined prostate cancer was discovered by a digital rectal exam (DRE) or a transurethral resection (TURP). While use of the PSA test increased the detection rate of prostate cancer, revealing cancer that would not have been detected by a DRE, there was no effective way to pinpoint its exact location.

Although imaging studies to determine tumor size and location would be invaluable in the clinical staging of the disease, most methods (except the MRSI) were not particularly useful. The ability to correctly determine whether cancer had spread outside the prostate was 63 percent with the TRUS, 71 percent with the body-coil MRI, and 83 percent with the endorectal MRI. The CT scan was effective in staging cancer only when there was extensive lymph-node disease — and only when the PSA was over 10 ng/ml and the Gleason score was more than 7.

Doctors typically reviewed the patient's PSA, Gleason score, and other conditions of the patient and then made an educated guess about his stage. As a result, doctors were incorrect 50 to 60 percent of the time, causing the patient a great deal of anxiety - and money. To improve their batting average, physicians began referring to the Partin tables, to determine the location or extent of the disease. These tables increased the chance of correct staging to 85 percent.

Importance of Staging

A patient's prostate cancer must be staged before any decision can be made about treatment. Staging is based on the extent of the primary tumor, the pathologic examination of the tissue, whether cancer is found in the lymph nodes, and whether the patient has metastatic disease.

Clinical staging is done preoperatively using laboratory tests, including biopsy, and a physical examination of the patient. *Pathologic staging,* which is done by assessing surgically removed tissues and organs, finds that the extent of the disease is greater than had been estimated.

61

Treating Localized Prostate Cancer

The goal of treating localized prostate cancer is to cure it: that is, as stated at a prostate cancer meeting held in Antwerp, Belgium, to give the patient the best chance of dying of something else. Several factors should be considered when deciding whether a patient is suitable for such therapy. Chief among them is pinpointing the location of the cancer. While it may be impossible to determine the location with 100 percent accuracy, physicians should certainly attempt to do so.

Combined MRI/MRSI

Tumor volume refers to the size of the tumor; it is often indicated in centimeters. *Organ-confined* refers to cancer that is located within the prostate gland or its capsule. This cancer has the best cure rate. *Capsular penetration* is the spread of the tumor beyond the prostatic capsule. The extent of penetration is defined in terms of the maximum length of the tumor that has penetrated the capsule. If the cancer has affected the seminal vesicles, there is often cancer at other sites in the body.

The combination of (1) the high specificity of MRSI to metabolically identify prostate cancer with (2) the high sensitivity of an endorectal MRI has improved the ability to determine the location and extent of cancer within the prostate, as well as its spread outside the gland.

The Spectroscopic MRI

Modified MRI

Magnetic resonance imaging (MRI) uses a magnetic field and radio waves to obtain three-dimensional images of internal organs. The images can be contrasted so that the cancer appears as a reunion of low-signal intensity when compared to surrounding regions of healthy tissue. The degree of signal intensity is due to changes in the structure of the normal tissue. In the case of prostate cancer, prostatic ducts (sacs containing fluid) are replaced with densely packed, cancerous epithelial cells. However, in some cases, the diagnosis of cancer based on an MRI is erroneous because other factors can cause a decrease in signal intensity (e.g., postbiopsy hemorrhage, chronic prostatitis, benign prostatic hyperplasia, intraglandular dysplasia, trauma, and therapy). These factors limit definitive diagnosis by MRI alone, and in some cases, they lead to overestimation of tumor presence and capsular penetration.

The endorectal coil combined with the four external coils is used to acquire anatomic images with much higher resolution than what was previously possible. The endorectal coil provides the necessary sensitivity to focus on the prostate and surrounding structures. The pelvic phased-array (for external coil 5) allows for a larger field of view in order to assess the pelvic lymph nodes and bones for metastatic disease. Improving the magnetic resonance technology has allowed for a reduction in the time required for this component.

Previous studies have reported that the endorectal MRI immobilized is quite accurate in detecting seminal-vesicle invasion and intracapsular extension of prostate cancer (81% and 96%, respectively). However, the accuracy of finding cancer within the prostate gland with the MRI alone is reduced because other factors can cease and decrease in signal intensity similar to cancer.

An exciting study was published in the <u>New England Journal of Medicine</u> (2003) by Mukesh Harisinghani, M.D., and colleagues. Researchers from Massachusetts Hospital and the University Medical Center in the Netherlands found that an intravenous contrast agent called Combidex was highly effective in imaging by MRI clinically occult lymph-node metastases in patients with prostate cancer. The intravenous contrast agent was highly lymphotrophic (lymphnode-seeking) superparamagnetic nanoparticles. These particles gain access to lymph nodes by means of the lymphatic fluid, and when Combidex is used in conjunction with high-resolution MRI small nodal metastases were detected that were otherwise undetectable with the contrast material.

Eighty patients with presurgical clinical stage T1, T2, or T3 prostate cancer who underwent surgical lymph-node research or biopsy were enrolled in the study. All patients were examined by MRI before and 24 hours after the IV administration of Combidex. The imaging results were then correlated with findings at surgery or by biopsy.

A total of 334 lymph nodes from 33 patients (41%) that underwent resection on biopsy showed metastatic disease. Sixty-three of the 334 (71.4%) lymph nodes did not fulfill the usual imaging criteria for malignancy. MRI with the Combidex infusion correctly identified all patients with nodal metastatic disease, and a node-by-node analysis had a significantly higher sensitivity than did conventional MRI (90.5% vs. 35.4%, P<0.001) or nomograms. Overall, MRI with Combidex had 100 percent sensitivity in identifying lymph-node metastases and 95.7 percent specificity, giving an overall accuracy of 97.5 percent. This finding is probably the greatest single advance in imaging studies for the staging of prostate cancer described thus far.

If these numbers hold up in other studies, it will be a great step forward in our ability to decide who the candidates for aggressive primary therapy of prostate cancer are, and who already has nodal metastatic spread, indicating systemic disease. We will thus be much more accurate in our ability to predict who will benefit from an aggressive attempt to control cancer that is localized to the prostate.

MRSI

The development of magnetic resonance spectroscope imaging (MRSI) has expanded the diagnostic assessment beyond the anatomic information provided by the MRI. The MRSI uses a magnetic field and radio waves to obtain pictures (spectra) based on the concentrations of cellular chemicals (metabolites). The MRSI provides metabolic information specific to the prostate by detecting the cellular metabolites citrate, creatine, and choline.

Using the same endorectal technology for imaging, three-dimensional spectroscopic studies have become possible. The entire prostate can be evaluated in one study, and excellent images can be obtained from glands as small as 0.24 ml. As a result, by superimposing the spectroscopic, three-dimensional data set on corresponding images, the exact location of the tumor may be determined and the volume estimated.

The endorectal MRI alone is quite accurate in detecting seminal-vesicle invasion (96%) and the spread of prostate cancer outside the capsule (81%). However, detecting localized cancer within the prostate with MRI alone is limited because factors such as chronic prostatitis, benign prostatic hyperplasia, intraglandular dysplasia, trauma, and therapy can cause a decrease in signal intensity

Multiple Uses of the MRSI

Since the 1990s, the University of California at San Francisco has used the MRSI for multiple purposes:

- To identify the location and extent of the disease within the prostate gland.
- To determine if cancer has spread outside the capsule.
- To find any involvement of nearby tissues, such as nerves, blood vessels, and seminal vesicles.
- To indicate any lymph-node or bone involvement within the pelvis. In 1999, a total of 69 percent of patients received the MRSI prior to therapy for a variety of reasons:

64

- To determine the location, extent, and potential for spread and thus to determine the best treatment.
- To improve therapeutic planning and evaluation.
- For diagnostic purposes – in some men with negative biopsies elevated and rising PSAs, the technology was used to identify areas for guiding the ultrasound for performing a biopsy.

A growing number of patients who suspect a recurrence of prostate cancer are also opting to have a MRSI for restaging purposes. In fact, in 1999, a total of 34 percent of MRSIs were performed after treatment for the following purposes:

- A total of 103 patients had the image study after combination hormonal therapy.
- A total of 76 patients had the MRSI after brachytherapy.
- A total of 27 patients had the MRSI after external beam radiation.
- A total of 11 patients had the MRSI after surgery.
- A total of 40 patients had the MRSI before and after nutritional and lifestyle changes.

Advantages of Combined MRI/MRSI

The addition of the MRSI to MRI has already demonstrated several advantages:

- MRSI will probably have the greatest impact on determining prostate cancer treatment and on the selection of additional therapy. Treatment often causes structural changes that limit assessment of other modalities such as MRI and ultrasound, which rely on structural changes to identify cancer.
- The MRSI can distinguish residual or recurrent prostate cancer from normal and necrotic tissue after cryosurgery. Evidence indicates that the same is true for hormone ablation, radiation, and chemotherapy, and that the MRSI can detect residual cancer in the prostatic bed after prostatectomy.
- Postbiopsy hemorrhage, a major impediment to MRI interpretation, occurred in 28 percent of all patients studied and was extensive, involving more that 50 percent of the sites sampled in 63 percent of these patients.

- The addition of an MRSI sequence to an MRI staging exam significantly increased specificity and accuracy of tumor detection when the patient had a postbiopsy hemorrhage.

- A review of MRI data suggests that the addition of MRSI can improve staging of prostate cancer prior to treatment. Studies on MRI/MRSI staging after therapy are ongoing.

- In a study of 85 men who had a combined MRI/MRSI prior to radical prostatectomy, significantly higher choline levels and significantly lower citrate levels were observed in regions of cancer as compared to areas of BPH and normal prostatic tissue. The ratio of these metabolites in regions of cancer had minimal overlap with normal and BPH values.

- In 25 patients studied before and after cryosurgery, MRSI was able to distinguish residual cancer from necroses and other residual tissues.

- The metabolic information obtained from MRSI may also allow tumor aggressiveness and the risk of disease progression to be determined.

- The endorectal coil provides the necessary sensitivity to focus on the prostate and surrounding structures.

- The pelvic phased-array (four external coils) allows a large enough field of view to assess pelvic lymph nodes and bone for metastatic disease. However, one problem with multiple-surface coils is variability in image quality and subsequent interpretation, mostly because image intensity dramatically decreases with distance from the surface coil.

In a study of 62 patients undergoing MRI/MRSI evaluation prior to radical prostatectomy, prostate cancer was localized to a sextant of the prostate gland with a specificity of up to 91 percent. When both the MRI and MRSI were positive for cancer, and a sensitivity of 95 percent when either the MRI or MRSI were positive for cancer.

A Caveat

A patient called one of the coauthors for guidance, saying he wanted to undergo a radical prostatectomy for stage T2 prostate cancer. He was told that *New Guidelines for Surviving Prostate Cancer* says, "Don't rush to surgery." In addition, he was strongly advised to have an MRSI to pinpoint the location of his tumor before opting for surgery. So the patient took the advice and asked his physician to prescribe an MRSI. However, his physician refused because he did not want to display his ignorance about the test. The patient went ahead and had a prostatectomy. Two weeks later, he learned his disease was actually T3 and that he had seminal-vesicle invasion. A spectroscopic MRI would have imaged the seminal vesicles, and he would have been spared unnecessary surgery.

Accuracy of the MRSI

The most important parameters used when assessing any imaging modality are sensitivity, specificity, and positive predicted value. *Sensitivity* is the proportion of men with prostate cancer who have an abnormal imaging test. *Specificity* refers to the proportion of men who do not have prostate cancer and have a normal imaging test. *Positive predicted value* is the probability that an abnormal imaging test is due to prostate cancer.

The addition of three-dimensional MRSI to MRI provides better detection and localization of prostate cancer alone. ROC analysis showed significantly improved tumor localization for both readers when MRSI was added to MRI. High specificity (up to 91%) was obtained with both MRI and 3D-MRSI indicated cancer, whereas a positive result of either test provided high sensitivity (up to 95%). Additionally, combining MRSI with MRI improves diagnostic accuracy and decreases the interobserver variability of MRI in the diagnosis of extracapsular prostate cancer. Adding MRSI to MRI for the most experienced reader improved accuracy over the use of MRI or MRSI alone. Adding MRSI to MRI for the less experienced reader improved accuracy to a level comparable to the more experienced MRI reader.

Why Choose an MRSI?

An MRSI is the best technique for staging localized prostate cancer because:

1. It has the highest degree of accuracy for pinpointing the staging of localized prostate cancer.
2. The number of patients who are understaged or overstaged will be minimized.
3. The MRSI can distinguish prostate cancer from normal tissue and BPH better than any other technique.
4. The entire prostate can be evaluated in one study with excellent clarity.
5. The potential is unlimited.

How to Use This Information

1. If your pathologic grade, clinical stage, and biochemical parameters (PSA, PAP) pinpoint your disease as definitely localized or definitely metastatic, you may not need an MRI/MRSI. However, for cancers that fall in between, or for those patients who need a baseline for a less aggressive approach, additional local staging is important. Don't undergo a radical prostatectomy before getting an MRI/MRSI to determine the exact location of your prostate cancer. If the results indicate your cancer has spread outside the gland, do not have surgery.
2. Don't have a CT scan or a bone scan if your PSA level is less than 10 ng/ml. Instead, get an MRSI as a reference point or baseline.
3. After treatment, monitor your disease with the MRSI.
4. Have an MRSI if you are undergoing any treatment for prostate cancer.
5. Don't be alarmed if your physician is not aware of the MRSI. This imaging test is relatively new, and doctors are still learning about it.

PART III TREATING PROSTATE CANCER

Chapter 11

BALANCING THE BODY'S pH

When was the last time your physician took your pH level? Western doctors are not taught in medical school that the pH exerts broad control over every aspect of body chemistry. In fact, total healing of chronic disease takes place only when and if the blood is restored to a normal, slightly alkaline pH.

The body's pH affects everything. When the pH is imbalanced, microorganisms in the blood can shape, mutate, become pathogenic, and thrive. Enzymes that are constructive can become destructive. Oxygen to the cells suffers, and organs such as the brain and heart can become compromised. When the pH is imbalanced, mineral assimilation can get thrown off, and prostate cancer is allowed to grow and thrive in an acidic internal environment. The internal environment becomes a playground for bacteria, viruses, fungi, and so on to destroy the body. Calcium in the bones becomes brittle, and the bones eventually break. And when the pH continues to be imbalanced, the body slowly deteriorates and eventually succumbs.

What Is the pH?

The pH is a measurement of hydrogen potential — that is, how much the negative ions (alkaline-forming) and positive ions (acid-forming) push against each other.

The human body is composed of 70 percent water, a medium that transports nutrients, oxygen, and other biochemicals from place to place. This water contains either acidic or alkaline properties. These are measured by a graduated scale called pH (potential hydrogen), which runs from zero to 14. Levels below 7 represent increasing acidity, and levels above 7 represent increasing alkalinity. Most biological fluids are between pH one and 14; however, there are a few exceptions — for example, stomach acid. The internal pH of most living cells is close to 7. Whenever there is a slight change in the pH, it can be extremely dangerous because the chemical processes of the cells are sensitive to the concentration of hydrogen and hydroxide ions. Biological fluids can resist a change to their own pH when acids and bases are introduced because of the presence of buffers. Buffers in human blood, for example, maintain the blood pH at 7.40. A person cannot survive if the pH of the blood drops to 7 or rises to 7.8. Under normal circumstances, the buffering capacity of the blood prevents such swings in the pH level.

Maintaining alkalinity is so essential for surviving that the body mobilizes its special buffering system to neutralize excess acidity whenever the scale tips. A vital link in this complex buffering system is the body's alkaline reserve. The body draws on alkaline mineral elements to help restore alkalinity in the system. However, the minerals in the alkaline reserve must be replenished regularly through alkaline-forming foods.

How Glands and Organs Depend on Alkalinity

The pH level is the most basic and broad control of every aspect of body chemistry, says Arthur C. Guyton, M.D., author of <u>Medical Physiology</u>. The mechanisms of action by which pH controls work are chemical, hormonal, and electric. These biochemical controls are mediated through enzymes, which are catalysts for all biochemical activity. Enzymes are very pH sensitive. Hormones also are very sensitive as well as electricity by very pH sensitive. Together, enzymes, hormones, and electricity affect many body functions. Nine organs and two glands function properly in precise proportion to the alkaline and acid levels in the body.

Heart

The heart depends more on alkalinity than does any other organ. It is partly supplied with blood by the vagus nerve, which functions best in an alkaline environment. The function of the heart is to pump about 13,000 quarts of blood a day. When this pumping is performed in a toxin-free environment, there is little or no strain on the heart. If, on the other hand, the body is beset with toxins, a tremendous strain is imposed on the heart. As a result, the proper heartbeat is altered by acid wastes because the waste dispels the necessary oxygen from the heart, causing it to falter. In any case, an internal body environment that is alkaline creates an ideal milieu for the heart to function in.

Lungs

The purpose of the lungs is to keep the body in an alkaline environment, breathe in oxygen, and release carbon dioxide. They also aid in the elimination of fluids settling in the blood system. A contaminated or slightly acid blood system can cause a host of problems.

Stomach

The purpose of the stomach is to use the hydrochloric acid stored within it to digest and assimilate ingested foods. When this food is too acidic, a multitude of problems result.

Liver

The liver has about three hundred functions. Its primary functions are to process acid toxins from the blood, produce a number of enzymes for the body, and defend the body against any poisons. In addition, any nourishment obtained from the gastrointestinal tract enters the blood via the liver.

The workload of the liver is difficult when acidic waste products are floating in the blood. It is essential to clean up this "river of life" and to prevent it from becoming too congested with protein acidic wastes. If an alkaline internal environment is not maintained, death is imminent.

Pancreas

The pancreas, which produces alkaline enzymes and sodium bicarbonate, is highly dependent on an alkaline environment. All aspects of pancreatic function are devoted to reducing excessive acidity. The pancreas also regulates blood-sugar balance, which creates energy in the body. In order to achieve proper blood-sugar balance, an alkaline-forming internal environment must be maintained.

Small Intestine

The small intestine is responsible for many bodily functions and is necessary for maintaining good health. Peyer's patches, located in the upper portion of the small intestine, are essential to life. The small intestine is important for the proper assimilation of food throughout the body, and it is an important link between the autonomic and cerebrospinal nervous system for producing lymphocytes for the lymph-node network.

The small intestine also produces large amounts of <u>chyle</u>, the major alkalizing substance in the body. The uninterrupted flow of chyle into the body is important. Too much acid waste produced by acid-forming foods affects the Peyer's patches and diminishes the production of chyle. How well the Peyer's patches function can determine the length of a person's life.

Kidneys

The primary function of the kidneys is to form and excrete urine and excess acid in the body. In an adult, about one liter of blood passes through the kidneys per minute. By performing this function, the kidneys keep the blood alkaline and rid the body of acid albumin. It should be obvious that the kidneys should not be overburdened with too much acidity.

Kidney stones are composed of waste acid cells as well as mineral salts. Reducing acid-forming products from entering the body will prevent this acid-induced condition.

Spleen

The spleen processes old blood cells. In order for the spleen to perform at its best, it must have an alkaline environment. Otherwise, it becomes enlarged or fails to completely detoxify the body.

Colon

The colon must be kept clean of any accumulated acid wastes. Poisons are likely to collect on the walls of the colon because of constipation. They then become hardened and are reabsorbed into the bloodstream. Regular bowel movements are important to good health.

Colon cancer is the second leading cause of cancer death in the United States. Why? Well, many ailments and diseases begin as the result of inadequate ingestion, poor assimilation, and lack of excretion.

Thyroid Gland

The thyroid gland must function in an overall alkaline environment because it (and other organs) guard and activate the brain. The thyroid is dependent on iodine, which helps in eliminating acid wastes that could be transported to — and affect — the brain.

Adrenal Glands

The adrenal glands are like a multitude of tiny workhorses that produce hormones for the human body. Together they create an alkaline reaction by increasing energy, thereby helping the liver and pancreas to regulate blood sugar, which is an alkaline-forming activity.

E. Roy Berger, M.D., F.A.C.P. and James Lewis, Jr., Ph.D

Why Maintain an Alkaline Body?

Many people do not understand the reason for maintaining an alkaline body. Nor do they understand that the pH of their bodies needs to be in balance — if the pH is too alkaline, they will feel unwell, and if the pH is too acidic, they will feel tired and fatigued. As a result, their eyes will begin to burn, and they will be more prone to getting cancer and other diseases.

Most prostate cancer patients have a pH level of about 7.4. Maintaining an acidic body is not good for their health, and an imbalanced pH can lead to cardiovascular diseases such as diabetes, cancer, high blood pressure, high cholesterol, kidney stones, urinary incontinence, arthritis, and osteoporosis.

The standard American breakfast is acidic, leaving an ash within the body - when the body metabolizes food, it leaves chemical and metallic residues, which cause either an acid or alkaline internal environment. When the diet is imbalanced with an excessive amount of acidic residue, the body's pH is directly affected, causing it to remain continuously within the acidic range.

Rebalancing the pH

A _buffer_ is a supplement that helps the body naturally and safely balance an overly acidic or overly alkaline system. The alkalizing complexes and phytomedicinals within the buffer help it to remove overly acidic and alkaline residues from the body, as well as to dissolve toxin-laden plaque, thus helping the body's ability to cleanse and repair tissues more quickly.

By using pH test strips, you can determine your urinary pH, which is a good indicator of total body pH. When your urinary pH ranges continuously from 6.5 in the morning to 7.5 by evening, you are functioning in a healthy range. When your pH is continuously above this range, you are too alkaline, and when it is continuously below it, you are too acidic.

A Balanced pH

A balanced pH provides many health benefits:

- proper calcium absorption, lessening the probability of osteoporosis and osteoarthritis
- proper fat metabolism, weight control, and healthy insulin production

- reduced urinary problems
- healthy oxygen flow to tissues to flush out toxins and protect against premature aging
- smooth blood flow throughout arteries, veins, and heart tissue
- proper blood-pressure regulation
- critical lipid, fatty acid, and hormonal metabolism
- cellular regeneration and DNA-RNA synthesis
- proper electrolyte activity
- access to energy reserve
- appropriate cholesterol levels so plaque does not form

The Most Important pH Levels

A number of pH levels are crucial for maintaining good health. Ignore them, and you will be beset with many ailments.

- The normal saliva pH value prior to eating — or two hours after eating — should be 6.4.
- Immediately after eating, the pH should be 7.2.
- When urine pH is constantly higher than 6.4 and saliva pH is constantly lower than 6.0, many health problems occur.
- The best time to take your urine pH and saliva pH is in the morning.
- The first reading of urine pH should be from 5.5 to 6.0, and saliva pH should be from 6.2 to 6.4.
- The most dangerous pH readings are when saliva pH is acid (below 6.0) or urine pH is very alkaline (over 6.8).

Imbalanced pH

An imbalance in pH or *acidosis* can cause serious problems, especially as a person grows older. Although it may go undetected for years, an imbalanced pH can lead to the progression of most, if not all, degenerative diseases. These include cardiovascular disease, cancer, and diabetes, as well as the never-ending frustration of excessive weight gain.

Acidosis disrupts general lipid and fatty acid metabolism within the body, which could lead to neurological problems, including multiple sclerosis. It can also cause hormonal imbalances within the endocrine system, leading to urinary incontinence and urinary-tract infections.

From 25 to 30 percent of all people in nursing homes are there because of a hip fracture. The rate of hip fractures has doubled in the last 50 years, and worldwide, there are now millions of such fractures a year. The risk of fracturing a hip is greater than that of developing cancer. One out of every six women will fracture a hip during her lifetime. And among men, fractures from osteoporosis result in more deaths than those caused by cancer.

This new epidemic of osteoporosis is not due to a drug deficiency. In addition to other factors, our acid-forming diets are to blame. Researchers have found that men eating a high acid-producing diet had more rapid bone loss and a greater risk of hip fracture than did men eating fewer acid-producing foods.

An imbalanced pH has considerable influence over the majority of metabolic problems, including weight gain, diabetes, and obesity. A habitually acid pH can cause weight gain by triggering a condition known as insulin sensitivity, which causes erratic insulin production by the body. When the body is flooded with insulin, it diligently converts every calorie it can into fat. Thus, an acid pH will likely direct more insulin to be produced and subsequently demand that the body store more fat than usual.

Men with osteoporosis have a loss of calcium due to the body's ability to "rob Peter to pay Paul" when the pH level is imbalanced. Because calcium is the most abundant mineral in the body and plays an important role in maintaining an acid alkaline balance, adequate calcium in the blood is required to ensure that the serum pH level is maintained at the critical level of 7.4. When a chronic overacid condition in the body produces a drop in blood calcium, hormones produced by the parathyroid gland stimulate a mechanism that takes calcium from the bones. As a result, unless blood levels of this mineral are raised through calcium assimilated from foods and minerals, the calcium is not replaced, and the bones become soft and brittle. The person then has osteoporosis.

An alkaline-forming diet that includes plenty of calcium-rich, green leafy vegetables ensures the mineral's optimal use and is both the best source as well as the best preserver of calcium in the body.

Colon Health

A natural-health pioneer over 50 years ago used colon therapy to avoid surgery in all but 20 of 40,000 patients afflicted with gastrointestinal disease. In fact, in the early 1900s, colon therapy was an accepted practice by mainstream medical professionals.

Colon problems are at the root of most health problems. Most of the nutrients the body needs are absorbed through the walls of the small intestine. One of the colon's jobs is to squeeze waste in order to push it out of the body. However, if the bowel isn't working properly, not everything gets pushed out, and gradually the residue coats the walls of the colon. It also creates a toxic liquid, which goes into the bloodstream. This condition, *autointoxication*, is the root cause of many diseases and illnesses.

It is quite interesting to see what is expelled during a normal colonic treatment. Mucus, parasites, and fecal material may have been in the patient's colon for years. The feces looks like vulcanized rubber and have that kind of consistency.

There is probably no more effective way to stay healthy than to take good care of the bowels, and yet the colon is one of the areas most neglected by the medical establishment. Digestive-system and colon health have reached an all-time low in the United States. Diseases of the digestive tract are on the rise, including colorectal cancer among men and women.

The intestinal wall is lined with villi, tiny fingerlike projections that absorb nutrients from digested food. However, mucus on the villi blocks this absorption. Sometimes the mucus gets so thick and tough that it is almost like plastic film. As a result, almost no nutrition can get through to the body. One could take a thousand dollars' worth of supplements a month and follow a good diet yet still get almost no nutritional value. If there were only one kind of pill that would help everybody, it would be a mucus dissolver.

Symptoms of Parasites

Organs can be blocked by the presence of worms. Normal elimination may no longer occur when worms block the common bile duct and intestinal tract.

Some of the symptoms of colon buildup and toxins in the body are:

- constipation or diarrhea
- chronic yeast infections
- chronic fungus on nails, or nails become brittle or lose their luster
- frequent sickness, including colds (depressed immune system)
- weight problems or rapid weight gain
- acne, skin disorders, or dry or pale skin
- mood swings or depression
- low sex drive
- lack of concentration, short-term memory problems
- sleeping problems
- frequent headaches
- chronic urinary-tract irritation or infection
- arthritic bone pains or rheumatism
- allergies

- gas, bloating, flatulence
- general weakness, frequent or chronic fatigue, lack of energy, or apathy

From James Lewis: We Disagree

My coauthor disagrees with me about the importance of this chapter. I don't fault him. It's how he was trained. The pH is just not emphasized in the curriculum in our medical schools. This is unfortunate, because an unbalanced pH is dangerous. Our bodies are exposed to an overly acidic pH medium, such as the diet we ingest, the lack of emphasis in our medical schools and the lack of concern by patients. Just as acid rain can destroy forests and alkaline wastes can pollute lakes, an imbalanced pH debilitates the body, slowly bringing destruction to it's more than fifty-thousand miles of veins and arteries. If left unchecked, an imbalanced pH will cause havoc to all of the body's cellular activities and functions, threatening life itself. How can our wonderful medical system ignore this process?

Louis Pasteur, who was given credit for the germ theory, said on his deathbed in 1895, "It is not the germ that is the problem, it is the internal environment, the internal milieu that allowed the germ to develop in the first place that is the problem." He was referring to the importance of balancing the pH, which helps regulates the internal environment.

I included this chapter in Updated Guidelines for three reasons:

1. Balancing the pH level in the human body is recognized by all medical physiology texts as one of the most important biochemical balances in the body's chemistry.

2. Otto Warburg won the Nobel prize for showing that all degenerative diseases - such as cancer and osteoporosis - are scientifically linked to acid in the body. According to Warburg and many other scientists, many diseases thrive in an acidic environment but cannot survive in an alkaline environment. In fact, Warburg won the Nobel prize in medicine for his discovery that cancer is anaerobic – that is, it occurs in the absence of free oxygen. In chemistry, alkali solutions (pH over 7.0) tend to absorb oxygen, while acids (pH under 7.0) tend to expel oxygen. Therefore, when the body becomes acidic by dropping below pH 7.0, oxygen is driven out of the body, thereby inducing cancer.

3. I believe modern medical schools do not stress balancing the pH, in part because of a scientific and philosophical debate that occurred in the nineteenth century between Antoine Bechamp and Louis Pasteur. Pasteur promoted the theory of disease that described it as

being caused solely by bacteria that invade the body from the outside.

On the other hand, Bechamp theorized that microorganisms go through different stages of development and evolve into various growth forms. He discovered bacteria in the blood and maintained that these bacteria would change shape as the patient became diseased. As a result, he believed that the cause of disease came from inside the body.

Another scientist, Claude Bernard, entered the debate and took sides with Bechamp. He theorized that bacteria change according to the environment in which they are exposed, thereby supporting the theory that disease is due to the internal biological terrain of the body. The core of the terrain is the pH factor.

Pasteur went to great lengths to prove his theory and disapprove Bechamp and Bernard's theory. Finally, in 1895 when Pasteur was on his deathbed, he acknowledged Bechamp's work and said, "Bechamp was correct. The microbe or bacteria is nothing; the internal terrain is everything." But modern medicine has failed to heed this.

Alkaline-Forming Food

These foods have a pH of 6.0 or slightly higher:

apricot	grapefruit
avocado	guava
banana	kiwi
berries	kumquat
breadfruit	lemon
cactus	lime
citron	mango
currant	melon
date	nectarine
fig	papaya
gooseberry	passion fruit
grape	

Acid-Forming Food

These foods have a pH ranging from 2.5 to 1.0:

barley	pork
basmati rice	rabbit
beef	refined pasta
bleached wheat	refined sugar
brown rice	rye
buckwheat	spelt (a kind of wheat)
corn	tapioca
cream of wheat	turkey
oats	white rice
popcorn (with salt)	whole wheat

Acid-Forming Health Conditions

acne	metallic taste in mouth
agitation	mild headaches
bloating	multiple sclerosis
cancer (all forms)	muscular pain
cold hands and feet	myasthenia gravis
colitis	numbness and tingling
constipation	obesity
Crohn's disease	overall fatigue
diarrhea	pain in upper chest
dizziness	panic attacks
excessive hair loss	rapid heartbeat
food allergies	rapid panting breath
heartburn	rapid rise in blood pressure
hives	rheumatoid arthritis
Hodgkin's disease	sarcoidosis
hot urine	scleroderma
hyperactivity	sinusitis
impotence	stress
joint pain that travels	strong-smelling urine
lack of sex drive	stuttering
learning disability	tuberculosis
leukemia	urinary difficulties
low energy	urinary infection
lung pain	white-coated tongue

Factors Influencing the pH Level

The following factors can influence the pH level:

- Acid-Forming Food: Fast food, meats, certain grains, greens, most fruits, refined salt, sugar, condiments, and soda have a pH range of 2.8 to 5.5, which is extremely acidic.
- Alkaline-Forming Food: Almonds, melons, nonpasteurized honey, bee pollen, maple syrup, figs, dates, natural yogurt, cheese, dairy, most vegetables grown in the earth, apricots, avocados, coconuts, grapes, molasses, raisins, and lemons have a range of 5.6 to 7.0.
- Emotions: Not only is the body's pH level influenced by the food you ingest, but by emotions such as happiness, love, and joy, which create an alkaline-forming chemical reaction in the body. Emotions such as hate, fear, anger, and jealousy create an acidic-forming chemical reaction in the body.

How to Use This Information

1. Check your pH level before eating, immediately after eating, and two hours after eating. If it deviates from normal, take a pH buffer to normalize them. For the blood pH buffer, take one or more of the following: water, dark green vegetables, barley, wheat grass juice, or a low sodium vegetable juice spiked with Tabasco sauce. For the saliva pH buffer, take a tablespoon of blackstrap molasses three times a day, dark green vegetables, lemon juice, olive oil, carrot tops, or beet tops. For a urine pH buffer, take a tablespoon of one or more of the following: flax oil, olive oil, butter, cod liver oil, evening primrose oil, most nuts and seeds, or pectin.
2. Pretend that your saliva pH is below 6.0 and your urine is 5.5. What foods should you eat to produce a normal saliva and urine pH?

Chapter 12

DETOXIFYING THE BODY

All around the world, industries have changed the external - and to some extent, the internal — environments we live in. For example, millions of pounds of chemicals are released in our dear earth everyday, poisoning the soil and contaminating our food, the air we breathe, and the underground water tables that supply our drinking water. It has been estimated that over 188 million pounds of chemicals have been dumped into our lakes, rivers, and oceans. In addition, chemical emissions from both our factories and automobiles are pumped into the air. In just one year, more than 5 million pounds of pollutants are released into the environment. Moreover, much of the nutritional value of our food supply has been refined away and replaced with artificial coverings, preservatives, flavorings, and conditioners, causing numerous diseases and ailments. These chemicals can weaken our immune system with side effects that are subtle, chronic, or long-term. Once in the body, these chemicals act as toxins to block receptor-ligand binding stress; bind to proteins, lipids, and nucleic acids, thereby altering the expression of critical gene products; cause changes in calcium homeostasis; and selectively kill cells. Just a tiny bit of these toxins can affect organs, altering their structure and function.

What Is Detoxification?

Detoxification is the process of eliminating toxins from the body, neutralizing or transforming them by clearing excess mucus, congestion, and bodily waste. On an internal level, these toxins are oxidized fats, cholesterol, free radicals, and other irritating molecules due to poor digestion, colonic sluggishness, and dysfunction, poor or reduced liver function, poor elimination, and poor functioning of the kidney, respiratory tract, and skin.

Detoxification also involves dietary and lifestyle changes that reduce the intake of toxins and improve elimination. Minimizing the toxin load involves the avoidance of chemicals from refined food, sugar, caffeine, alcohol, tobacco, drugs, and other sources. In addition, consuming purified water and increasing fiber by eating more fruits and vegetables are important steps in the detoxification program.

Purposes of Detoxification

There are several purposes of detoxification:

- It enables you to take control of your body, thereby improving your health.
- It provides the body with all the energy it needs to operate.
- It rids the body of the toxins accumulated over years of neglect.
- It cleanses the internal and external systems.
- It improves the circulation and the immune system.
- It makes you feel more vital, creative, and open to emotional and spiritual energies.
- It helps you to rest or heal your overloaded digestive organs.

Why Detoxify?

Some reasons for cleansing and detoxifying the body are:

- prevent disease
- treat disease
- rest and relax organs
- reduce symptoms
- lose weight
- purify the body
- rejuvenate the body
- increase energy
- become more motivated
- clean the skin
- slow the aging process
- improve flexibility
- enhance the senses
- become spiritual
- become more creative
- relax
- attune to the environment

Why Does the Body Become Toxic?

When the body is healthy, it is able to clean itself by detoxifying and disposing of all toxins. However, we often confuse this normal detoxification process with symptoms of disease. In our efforts to treat the disease, we may actually suppress vital eliminative functions. As a result, the body may become retoxified. For example, many autoimmune conditions may result from retoxification. Toxins that should have been eliminated are suppressed and are reincorporated into the new tissues of the body. These tissues may become tainted and so may be recognized as foreign by the immune system; an autoimmune condition may result. This retoxification process is hypothetical; however, it may explain the dramatic increase in autoimmune-related diseases.

Common Toxicities

The two most common toxicities are caused by chemicals and metals. Viral toxicity is a close third. Some viruses may actually result from the normal internal cleansing of the body.

Using Vitamins and Minerals to Detoxify

The following vitamins and minerals can protect you against a toxic world:

- Lecithin (1 to 2 tbsp a day) helps neutralize body poisons.
- Vitamin A (25,000 USP units a day) improves the body's oxygen economy and protects against smog.
- Vitamin D (25,000 USP units a day) improves the body's use of calcium, one of the most important antitoxin materials.
- Yogurt and other soured milk (1 pint to 1 quart a day) neutralizes such poisons as DDT and strontium 90, thus minimizing damage to the body.
- Brewer's yeast (1 to 3 tbsp a day) helps the liver to detoxify.
- Vitamin B-1 (25 mg a day) protects against the damaging effects of lead.
- Vitamin B-15 (100 mg a day) protects against the damaging effects of carbon monoxide.
- Vitamin C (3,000 mg a day) helps the body withstand toxic assault better and prevents damage to organs and glands.
- Vitamin E (600 IU a day) protects the body against polluted air, food, and water, and helps the liver to detoxify.
- Calcium (1,000 mg a day) and magnesium (500 mg a day) helps the body to neutralize and eliminate toxic substances such as lead, mercury, strontium 90, radioactive iodine, and cadmium.
- Kelp (5 to 10 tablets, or 1 to 2 tsp of granules a day) protects against radioactive fallout.

Protecting against Toxins

The following measures will help you survive in a polluted environment:

1. Avoid eating animal products.
2. Wash inorganic foods with soap and water.

3. Do not use cleaning sprays. Use only soap.
4. Avoid automobiles, factories, and smoggy cities.
5. Eat only organic foods.
6. Fortify your diet with the necessary vitamins and minerals.
7. Follow an alkaline diet.
8. Do not use toxic chemicals in your household.
9. Stay away from preservatives and artificial sweeteners.
10. Balance your pH factor daily.

Toxins and How to Get Rid of Them

Healing cannot take place unless we detoxify and cleanse our bodies of any dead cells, poisonous substances, and waste materials. The following pages describe toxins, the organs they harm, and how to protect them from harm.

- **Carbon Monoxide** is one of the most damaging agents found in the air we breathe. It damages all of our cells by preventing oxygen from being absorbed by the lungs and cells. In addition, it can cause headaches, loss of memory, respiratory disorders, irritability, shortness of breath, angina, emphysema, anemia, heart disease, and cancer.

Affected organs: lungs and bloodstream.

Eradication:

1. Take 400 to 600 IU a day of vitamin E to increase the oxygenation of tissues and to decrease the body's other oxygen needs by preventing the undesirable oxidation of lipids in the bloodstream.
2. Take 30 mg of vitamin B-15 three times a day, or 50 mg morning and evening, to increase the body's tolerance to oxygen deficiency caused by the toxin.
3. Take 25,000 to 50,000 USP units a day of vitamin A, which increases the permeability of blood capillaries and facilitates improved delivery of oxygen to the cells.

- **Ozone and nitrogen dioxide** are the result of smog and have a damaging effect on your health.

Affected organ: lungs

Eradication:

1. Take 50,000 units a day of vitamin A to protect the mucous membranes.
2. Take up to 1200 IU a day of vitamin E to keep the ozone from destroying vitamin A in the body.

- **Lead,** one of the most toxic metal contaminants, can be fatal in small amounts. It also has a cumulative effect on the body, causing damage to the kidneys, liver, heart, and nervous system.

Affected organs: kidneys, liver, heart, nervous system, eyes, and brain

Eradication: This toxin can be eliminated by at least 10 vitamins or minerals.

1. Take 5 to 10 tablets of bone meal or calcium lactate daily to rid lead from your body.
2. Take 25,000 units of vitamin A to activate enzymes that help detoxify lead poisons.
3. Take 25 to 100 mg of vitamin B, as well as one high-potency B-complex tablet a day to protect against the damaging effect of lead.
4. Take 1 to 2 tbsp of lecithin a day in granular form to neutralize any poisons and protect the myelin sheaths.
5. Eat generous doses portions of legumes to reduce lead in the body.
6. Take potassium iodide and combine it with lead in the body to rid it from the system.
7. Take 1,000 to 3,000 mg a day of vitamin C to neutralize lead and protect muscle tissue.

- **Mercury** is very deadly and has a cumulative effect on the body.

Affected organs: kidneys, liver, brain, eyes, and nervous system

Eradication:

1. Take 3 to 5 tbsp of brewer's yeast a day to destroy mercury in the body.
2. Take up to 1,000 mg of calcium a day to neutralize mercury and rid it from the body.
3. Take 1 to 2 tbsp of lecithin granules a day.
4. Take large doses daily of vitamins A, C, E, and B complex to protect the body from mercury.

- **DDT** is a cumulative poison stored in the fat tissues of the body.

Affected organs: all body tissues and intestines

Eradication:

1. Take vitamin C to neutralize DDT in the body.
2. Consume yogurt and other soured milk to neutralize DDT in the body.
3. Take 2 to 3 tbsp of lecithin in granular form to rid DDT in the body.

- **Cadmium** is extremely toxic and can cause harm to our waters and to shellfish. It is found in automobiles.

Affected organs: heart, lungs, and kidneys

Eradication:

1. Take 3,000 mg a day of vitamin C.
2. Avoid white flour.
3. Avoid using enameled utensils.
4. Avoid drinking tap water.
5. Include in your diet raw seeds, nuts, whole grains, and zinc.

- **Strontium 90** is produced by nuclear tests and explosions:

Affected organs: bones and intestines

Eradication:

1. Eat lots of raw sunflower seeds each day.
2. Take 5 to 10 tablets of kelp a day.
3. Consume 1 quart of yogurt or soured milk a day.
4. Take brewer's yeast and vitamins E, C, and B complex.
5. Take calcium and magnesium.

- **Radioactive iodine** is found mostly in milk and is more toxic than strontium 90.

Affected organs: thyroid gland

Eradication:

1. Take 1 to 2 tsp of granules or 5 to 10 tablets of kelp.
2. Consume 1 quart of yogurt or soured milk a day.
3. Take brewer's yeast and vitamins E, C, and B complex.
4. Take calcium and magnesium.

- **X-rays** are cumulative, as they add to the total amount of radiation received from all sources.

Affected organs: whole body

Eradication:

1. Take 100 to 200 mg a day of rutin to strengthen the capillary walls and reduce hemorrhaging.
2. Take large doses of vitamin C with rutin.
3. Take 25 to 50 mg of pantothenic acid to prevent radiation injuries.
4. Take 2 to 3 tbsp a day of lecithin to counteract the radiation.
5. Take insoltol to prevent damage.

- **Drugs** All drugs are toxic and can cause harmful side effects.

Affected organs: liver, kidneys, and sex organs

  Eradication:

  1. Take vitamins C and E to protect against aspirin.
  2. Take 2 to 3 tbsp a day of lecithin.
  3. Take up to 10,000 mg a day of vitamin C.
  4. Take high-potency vitamin B complex.

- **Nitrates and nitrites** Many foods have been preserved with these toxic chemicals to enhance their appeal to customers.

Affected organs: liver, stomach, brain, esophagus, bladder, kidneys, heart, and other organs

  Eradication:

  1. Take 5,000 mg a day of vitamin C to neutralize and destroy nitrites and to prevent their conversion into nitrosamines.
  2. Take vitamins B complex, A, and E and lecithin to neutralize the damaging effects of both toxins.

- **Parasites** Numerous parasites can lurk in the body.

Affected organs: colon, small intestine, heart, eyes, brain, lungs, muscles, joints, esophagus, and skin

  Eradication:

  1. Cook all foods.
  2. Take some chlorophyll and noni fruit concentrate.
  3. Consume colloidal silver.
  4. Take rhodium and iridium.
  5. Combine and take n-acetyl cysteine, L-taurine, and organic sulfur.

- **Overstress** is a harmful physical and emotional response that occurs when the requirements of life do not match the capabilities, resources, or needs of the person. It can lead to poor health and even injury.

Affected organs: heart, kidneys, lungs, colon, liver, brain, breasts, stomach, circulatory system, skin, lymphatic system, pancreas

Eradication:

1. Balance your pH factor.
2. Get plenty of rest.
3. Practice yoga.
4. Engage in deep abdominal breathing.
5. Meditate and practice tai chi.
6. Try hypnotherapy or biofeedback.
7. Believe in a higher power.
8. Take 250 mg of vitamin C a day.

From James Lewis: We Disagree

This is another area in which the two authors have some problems agreeing. Deselecting toxins, dead cells, and other waste materials from the body are extremely important if dead prostate cancer cells are to be kept from infecting the body.

How to Use This Information

1. Ask your doctor which toxin may be affecting you most and be guided by the contents of this chapter.
2. Inspect your home for various types of toxins and dispose of them.
3. Purge your body of parasites at least twice yearly.
4. Clean your colon at least once a year.

Chapter 13

ADOPTING A WATCHFUL WAITING STRATEGY

Researchers in Europe and the United States advocate a watchful waiting strategy for some older men. For example, in a study reported in 1994, University of Chicago researchers determined that men in their late sixties, seventies, and eighties who were diagnosed with prostate cancer but not treated for it but who were regularly monitored with the DRE and the PSA test, usually did not die of prostate cancer. These men were offered hormone therapy only if their tumor progressed.

Ten years later, researchers found that only 13 percent of men with stage A and B tumors had died as a result of prostate cancer, while many more had died from other causes. These statistics were similar to those for men who had undergone surgery or radiation. In addition, those men who opted for watchful waiting did not endure the severe side effects of these two treatments. These researchers concluded that, if their life expectancy is 10 years or less, men with stage A or B clinically localized prostate cancer could follow a watchful waiting strategy.

Defining Watchful Waiting

Watchful waiting, or observation-deferred treatment, is a strategy in which a patient with prostate cancer is monitored periodically but receives no treatment. Generally this strategy is advised for older men with limited life expectancy, those with localized prostate cancer who do not want to experience the side effects of conventional treatment, and those who have cancers that are not likely to kill them.

Using a Watchful Waiting Strategy

The question of whether to watchful wait or treat prostate cancer will continue to be asked by early-diagnosed prostate cancer patients until there are definitive answers from randomized clinical trials, such as the Prostate Cancer Intervention Versus Observation Trial (PIVOT study). This multi-institutional cooperative study involves comparing randomized early or clinically localized prostate cancer patients who undergo radical prostatectomy or watchful waiting alone. This study will monitor and report patients in terms of progression-free survival, freedom from metastatic disease, disease-specific survival, and overall survival, as well as quality of life.

Willet F. Whitmore, Jr., M.D., asked an all-important question, "When treatment is possible, is it necessary, but when treatment is necessary, is it possible?" The PIVOT and other trials comparing watchful waiting to such modalities as external beam radiotherapy, seed implantation, and cryosurgery must be completed and reported in order to answer with any degree of certainty Dr. Whitmore's oft-quoted question.

Formulate a Treatment Plan

Patients who are newly diagnosed with prostate cancer need to proceed with a treatment plan, so it is important they understand watchful waiting and its implications. This is especially cogent because men are being diagnosed earlier due to the advent of the PSA test.

Watchful Wait or Treat?

Metastatic prostate cancer may either be symptomatic or not. A patient who is suffering from symptoms due to prostate cancer metastases deserves palliation or relief, so watchful waiting in this circumstance is not an option. The best treatment at present is CHT (combination hormonal therapy). It has been clearly shown that CHT improves progression-free survival. Therefore, it would be hard to believe that CHT would not be vastly better than observation alone in patients with metastatic disease.

However, we must confess that a study of "maximum androgen blockade in advanced prostate cancer," an overview of 22 randomized trials with 3,282 deaths in 5,710 patients, disagrees with our claim. This study was conducted by the Prostate Cancer Trialists Collaborative Group, the Biomedical Department of The Netherlands Cancer Institute, and was cited in Lancet. It concluded that CHT does not result in longer survival than that provided by conventional castration or monotherapy with an LHRH agonist alone. This, however, does not address the multiple problems with the paper, especially that the conclusion is based on a large number of small trials without statistical power, which diluted the results of the large randomized controlled trials. We maintain that survival for men treated with CHT is based on the number of lesions: the lower the number, the higher the survival rate; the higher the number, the lower the survival rate. This was confirmed by Fernand Labrie, M.D., et al. and E. David Crawford et al., respectively.

In a study by Dr. Labrie et al. entitled "Major Advantages of Early Administration of Endocrine Combination Therapy in Advanced Prostate

Cancer," 286 men with advanced prostate cancer were evaluated according to the number of lesions each had. Bone lesions were present for 261 men, while the other 25 had prostate cancer in their soft tissue. The 261 patients were organized into three groups: (1) those with 1 to 5 lesions, (2) those with 6 to 20 lesions, and (3) those with 11 to 40 lesions. All patients received CHT, with the exception of 11 who were orchiectomized and received flutamide. In April 1992, a total of 261 patients were eligible for assessment. Of these patients, 80 had a complete response to the CHT, while 75 and 87 patients showed partial and stable responses, respectively. Only 17 patients showed no response. A total of 123 men died from other causes, thus leaving 111 patients alive. When survival time is analyzed in terms of the severity of the disease at the beginning of treatment, it is apparent that patients with minimal disease according to clinical symptoms, as well as those who had a small number of bone lesions, had a much better chance for long-term survival. The median survival time for the group who had minimal symptoms was 5.47 years, compared to 2.71 for those with moderate symptoms and 2.1 years for those who had severe symptoms.

The median survival time was 8 years in the group of patients who had one to five bone lesions, while it was reduced to 3.56 years for men who had six to ten. This represents a difference in overall survival time of more than 4.4 years. For patients with 10 to 40 bone lesions, the calculated median survival time was 2.36 years. This study clearly demonstrates a dramatic difference in life expectancy when CHT is administered early in prostate cancer patients with bone lesions. It should be clear from this study that the addition of a small number of bone lesions has a major impact on survival time. When the number of bone lesions exceeds five, CHT has less impact on the duration of survival, thus demonstrating that delaying the treatment of advanced prostate cancer is not prudent.

Dr. Crawford et al. have reported that patients who had minimal disease displayed a much better response to CHT. In fact, an analysis by the Intergroup Trial, which was sponsored by the National Cancer Institute, revealed an advantage of 19.5 months in survival time for patients with minimal disease who received CHT versus leuprolide and a placebo. The median survival time of the CHT group of patients was improved. It has also been reported that patients with one or two lesions survive much longer than do those with three or more lesions.

Immediate or Delayed CHT?

Patients with metastatic disease who are asymptomatic must consider whether to begin CHT immediately or delay it. There has not been a good randomized control trial using these two treatments. A good way to understand these two options is by looking at the data from the NCI Intergroup Trial, which randomized patients with minimal metastatic disease to monotherapy versus CHT. The survival time appears to be much greater with CHT. Furthermore, the survival rate was much greater for the men with widespread metastatic disease using CHT. These two observations, in the absence of more direct evidence, lead us to conclude that early treatment with CHT in patients with minimal metastatic disease will improve their survival time, compared to waiting until symptomatic metastasis occurs. In fact, there is now a trend in the oncologic and urologic communities to treat patients earlier, before symptoms develop.

Dr. Labrie observed that when patients with stage D disease are treated with CHT, local control takes place in about 98 percent of them. It is extremely rare for a patient to progress at the level of the prostate when on CHT. This is another reason for early administration of CHT, as it also controls local symptoms and prevents urinary obstruction as well as other local complications from the growth of the prostate.

Should Stage C Patients Watchful Wait?

Stage C patients often have micrometastatic disease; however, long-term control is possible. A number of trials have demonstrated a definitive advantage of the use of hormonal therapy in conjunction with external beam radiation. Bolla et al. published in the New England Journal of Medicine their study of 415 patients with locally advanced prostate cancer who were randomly assigned to receive either radiation therapy alone or radiation plus immediate treatment with an LHRH agonist lasting 3 years. The hormonal therapy group had an antiandrogen for the first month and the LHRH-agonist was continued for a total of three years. Overall survival at 5 years was 79 percent in the combined treatment group versus 62 percent in the radiation therapy group. The proportion of patients surviving who were free of disease at 5 years was 85 percent in the combined treatment group and only 48 percent in the radiation group. The authors concluded that adjuvant treatment with an LHRH agonist (in this case, goserelin, acetate, or Zoladex) when started simultaneously with external beam radiation therapy improved local control and survival in patients with locally advanced prostate cancer. Most of the patients in this trial were in fact stage T3 or stage C.

In another trial, conducted by Pilepich and the RTOG (Radiation Therapy Oncology Group), 468 patients received external beam radiation therapy alone and 477 patients received adjuvant Zoladex plus flutamide. There was significantly improved progression-free survival in the hormonally treated group compared to those receiving radiation therapy alone. At 5 years, 84 percent of the patients with adjuvant hormonal therapy showed no evidence of progression, compared to 71 percent undergoing radiation only. Figures for freedom of distant metastases and disease-free survival in the two therapies were 83 versus 70 percent and 60 versus 44 percent, both favoring adjuvant hormonal treatment. Biochemical freedom from disease was also significantly increased, with 53 percent free of disease (PSA level less than 1.5) versus only 20 percent on the observation arm. Survival data are still pending; however, patients with a high Gleason score had a lower rate of survival.

An additional study by Laverdiere showed that advanced local prostate cancer when radiation therapy was combined with 3 months of neoadjuvant hormonal therapy showed that the positive biopsy at rate 2 years decreased to 28 percent from 65 percent (without 3 months of hormonal therapy). More impressively, he noted that only 5 percent of biopsies were positive if 3 months of combined hormonal therapy preceded radiation and was continued for a total of 10.5 months of combined androgen blockade.

The preceding data support the use of hormonal therapy either before, during, or after radiation therapy. Further studies are being conducted to determine the best time and best dose of hormonal adjuvant and neoadjuvant treatment. Should Stage D1 Patients Watchful Wait?

There are now data indicating that early combination hormonal therapy improves patients' quality of life as well as their overall survival.

The Medical Research Council Prostate Cancer Work Party Investigators Group published their findings in the British Journal of Urology. They studied men who had advanced or locally advanced prostate cancer who were asymptomatic and who were treated with either (1) immediate orchiectomy or an LHRH agonist or (2) delayed treatment with the same modality. They found that fractures, spinal cord compressions, urethral obstruction, and extraskeletal metastases was significantly decreased in patients who had immediate hormonal treatment. There was also an improvement in survival rates in these patients. This group had a disease-specific death rate of 81/256 (31.6%) versus 119/244 (48.8%) at the 5-year interval. This group of patients probably had a large number who had nodal involvement but nodal biopsies were not performed.

A study by Messing published in the New England Journal of Medicine, involved 98 men who were radical prostatectomy candidates and who were found to have pelvic lymph-node involvement. They were randomly assigned to (1) immediate LHRH q.28 days or bilateral orchiectomy or (2) observation until disease progression. The end points in this study were overall survival, prostate cancer–specific survival, and progression-free survival. There was a median follow-up of 17 years. The death rate from prostate cancer in the immediate hormonal therapy group was 4.3 percent; it was 30.8 percent in the observed group. In the immediate group, cancer progressed in 18.8 percent, while in the observed group, it progressed in 75 percent. "No evidence of disease" was much higher in the immediate hormonal therapy group, as one would expect.

These two studies give added evidence that immediate hormonal therapy in stage D1 patients should be the treatment of choice rather than delaying treatment until the progression of disease, symptoms, or both.

Should Stage B Patients Watchful Wait?

Stage A and B tumors are the stages in which most physicians who believe cure is possible by primary modality therapy advocate its use.

The rationale for the aggressive treatment of localized prostate cancer is based upon the observations of several researchers. They found that survival for patients who, for example, undergo radical prostatectomy and have organ- or capsule-confined disease is similar to that of a normal age-matched population. However, when the disease is outside the prostate, there is a marked decline in progression-free and overall survival.

Currently, the major reason why radical prostatectomy and other primary modalities for treating prostate cancer fail is due to our inability to stage the disease accurately. Approximately 50 to 60 percent of cancers thought to be localized at diagnosis, have, in fact, already spread beyond the confines of the prostate, and, therefore, they are unlikely to be cured by radical prostatectomy.

Data from Drs. Fernand Labrie, William R. Fair, and Mark S. Soloway have shown a 25 to 30 percent decrease in positive margins at radical prostatectomy when the patient is treated with CHT for three months prior to surgery. In the Soloway group, after 5 years there were no differences in survival rates. A number of surgeons believe, therefore, that adjuvant hormonal therapy adds nothing to survival time when coupled with radical prostatectomy. There are, however, other results that make one believe that this is not true. The early adjuvant breast cancer studies showed no difference between 3 days of early chemotherapy at the time of mastectomy versus observation for the first 5 years. However, between years 5 and 10, and especially after years 10 to 15, the survival curve diverges, showing a significant survival difference in favor of the chemotherapy group. This chemotherapy was not the most effective one available; however, this was not known at the time. So, too, the analogy in prostate cancer can be made: patients did not receive enough hormonal therapy and the follow-up has not been long enough to show that there is no benefit to using it prior to radical prostatectomy.

Although we do not have good studies comparing external beam radiation therapy with watchful waiting, we do have at least two radiation trials adding an LHRH agonist to external beam radiation therapy. Both of these were positive in terms of disease-free and overall survival in a subset of patients favoring the addition of hormonal therapy to radiation. Final conclusions cannot yet be made about the appropriate timing of treatment. However, combination hormonal therapy plus external beam therapy does seem to be of value. The major question is, When should it be applied? The answer depends upon the age and overall medical condition of the individual patient.

Many studies have assessed groups of patients with clinically localized prostate cancer who have been followed by watchful waitingand deferred treatment. These observations were, of course, made on a heterogeneous group of patients with differing volumes, stages, and grades of cancer. There have been two attempts at a randomized controlled trial comparing radical prostatectomy with watchful waiting. One study did not show a benefit in favor of radical prostatectomy; however, critics point to a number of limitations in the study largely invalidating its conclusions. The latest study addressing this question is whether a stage B patient should watchful wait or treat.

Lars Holmberg at University Hospital in Uppsala, Sweden, randomized patients who had palpable prostate cancers to (1) radical prostatectomy and (2) observation, foregoing treatment unless and until the cancer spread. After an average of 6.2 years of follow-up, 16 of the 347 men who had surgery had died of prostate cancer, or 4.6 percent. But 31 of the 348 men assigned to watchful waiting had died of prostate cancer. This was 8.9 percent, a statistically significant difference.

The researchers calculated that 17 men would have to have the operation to prevent one death from prostate cancer over an 8-year period. This study, of course, did not include any other treatments for prostate cancer, only radical prostatectomy. While the prostate cancer death rate was reduced in the Swedish study, the overall death rate from all causes including prostate cancer was not. Fifty-three men who had surgery died, compared to 62 men in the watchful waiting group, a statistically insignificant difference. There were two possible reasons for this: (1). To make an impact on the overall death rate, there would have to be a much greater decline in prostate cancer deaths than occurred in this study. (2). Men who had the surgery might die at a higher rate from causes other than prostate cancer – for example, from a blood clot a month after surgery or a stroke related to the surgery.

Of interest is that 80 percent of the men who had a radical prostatectomy were impotent, compared with 45 percent of those who had watchful waiting. Men were also more likely to be incontinent if they had the surgery than if they followed watchful waiting. They were, however, less likely to complain of difficulty urinating if they had the surgery. Men in both groups had similar assessments of the overall quality of their lives.

It should be stressed that, because of PSA screening, prostate cancer in men in the United States is usually discovered at a much earlier stage than it is in other men. We cannot extrapolate the data of the Swedish study to men whose cancer is picked up by a PSA test. For this, we await the results of the PIVOT study in which a total of 735 men with localized prostate cancer were randomized to watchful waiting versus radical prostatectomy. The results will not be evident until approximately 2008. Five years into the study, however, no survival advantage had been noted.

Other nonrandomized studies have reported the results of conservative management of men with clinically localized prostate cancer. Jon Johansson, M.D., observed the clinical course of 223 patients of all ages for a mean time of 12.5 years. Patients whose disease progressed were hormonally treated if they had symptoms. At 12.5 years, 23 of 223 patients (10%) had died of prostate cancer, while 125 of 148 (84%) had died of other causes. The 10-year, disease-specific survival rate was 85 percent, and it was equally high in a subgroup of 58 patients who met current indications for radical prostatectomy. The progression-free 10-year survival rate was 55 percent, but in 49 of 77 patients, local growth provided the only evidence of progression, and endocrine treatment (monotherapy) was generally successful in these cases. Johansson concluded that the low disease-specific death rate, especially in men with well- and moderately differentiated tumors, means that any local or systemic therapy intended for patients with early prostate cancer must be evaluated in clinical trials with untreated controls for comparison.

One such trial in progress in Sweden and Finland is evaluating deferred treatment versus radical prostatectomy. Since the early 1990s, over 330 patients have been evaluated. Again, there were flaws in certain areas of the study, such as patient selection and the use of localized radiation therapy in about half of the men under 75. However, the overall results indicate that most patients with early prostate cancer and a life expectancy of 10 years or less are unlikely to live longer by undergoing aggressive local therapy.

Jon Adolfsson, M.D., et al. came to a similar conclusion. They followed 172 patients with stage T1 to T3 prostate cancer on watchful waiting, with deferred treatment until symptomatic progression. Of these, 58 percent had local and 19 percent had distant metastases; 52 percent had received treatment at follow-up. The disease-specific survival rate at 10 years was 80 percent for the total series, 84 percent for the subgroup of stage

T1 or T2 tumors, and 92 percent for those with T1 or T2 who were less than 70 years old at diagnosis. For the subgroup with stage T3 tumors, the disease-specific survival rate at 9 years was 70 percent. In all subgroups deaths from other causes were higher than those from prostate cancer. Therefore, deferred treatment appears to be acceptable for patients with tumors confined to the prostate and who have a life expectancy of 10 years or less.

Another study of conservative management compared with radical surgery or radiation in men with localized prostate cancer was reported by the Prostate Patient Outcomes Research Team (PPORT). A decision-analysis model was used to assess the relative benefits of therapy for early-stage disease based on the probability of cancer progression, death, and therapy-related side effects. These parameters were determined from a review of published results of surgery, radiation, and watchful waiting studies. While the authors concluded that aggressive therapy may benefit younger men with higher-grade tumors, the overall improvement in "quality-adjusted life expectancy" was limited in most cases. Specifically, patients with moderately or poorly differentiated cancer may receive up to 3.51 additional years of quality-adjusted life, but men over 70 and those with well-differentiated prostate cancer were unlikely to benefit from radical surgery or radiation therapy in comparison with watchful waiting.

Flaws in this study include false assumptions of sexual activity, use of studies more than 20 years old, use of hormones in the conservatively treated group, and use of a series involving men with only stage A prostate cancer. Therefore, the conclusions may not reflect the long-term results seen in contemporary studies of men who are candidates for aggressive local therapy.

In an attempt to minimize the effects of selection bias on the reported results of conservative management of early prostate cancer, a pooled analysis of the disease progression and survival rates of 828 patients from six institutions has been published. The disease-specific survival rate after 10 years of follow-up was 87 percent for men with both well-differentiated and moderately differentiated (grade 2) tumors, and 34 percent for those with high-grade malignancy (grade 3). However, the rate of development of distant metastases was significantly different based on tumor grade, with evidence of disease spread after 10 years noted in 19, 42, and 74 percent of the men with well-, moderately-, and poorly differentiated tumors, respectively. While this pooled analysis is also retrospective and nonrandomized and reflects the patient-selection biases at each participating institution, the reported results add significantly to the conclusion that the overall survival of most men with a life expectancy of 10 years or less is unlikely to be improved by aggressive treatment of early prostate cancer.

However, since distant metastases have more poorly differentiated tumors, younger and healthier men with grade 2 malignancies have a significant risk of developing incurable disease and eventually dying of prostate cancer with conservative management.

Jonas Hugosson, M.D., et al. studied 490 men from a population of 3,081 diagnosed with prostate cancer between 1960 and 1979. A total of 62 percent of the men surviving longer than 10 years ultimately died of prostate cancer. According to Hugosson et al.'s calculations, the cancer-specific survival rate at 15 years was only 15 percent. Thus, they concluded that watchful waiting is difficult to justify for men with localized prostate cancer who have a long expected survival time.

Should Stage A Patients Watchful Wait?

Currently, stage A1 disease (well-differentiated cancer and less than 5 percent of the chips involved at transurethral resection of the prostate, or TURP) is associated with a normal life span. Most physicians believe that watchful waiting can be used in this group. However, recent studies show that 20 percent of patients with A1 disease develop metastases within 10 years.

Stage A2 disease (poorly differentiated cancer or more than 5 percent of chips involved at TURP) is associated with a much more aggressive clinical course and frequently disease outside the prostate. Decisions about observation versus therapy involve considerations similar to those for stage B prostate cancer.

According to Dr. Labrie, an inescapable conclusion derived from all studies, including those based on watchful waiting, is that prostate cancer progresses slowly; however, it inevitably leads to distant metastases and death if left untreated and sufficient time elapses. Such a progressive increase in volume is associated with increased de-differentiation and malignancy with an increased number of genetic alterations. When prostate cancer reaches a certain size, it migrates outside the prostate and becomes de-differentiated, and a cure is no longer possible. There is no means of determining the exact stage or grade of the cancer or of predicting which cancers will become incurable if left untreated for some more time. In fact, N.J. George, M.D., reported an 84 percent local progression rate within approximately 4 years, whereas Dr. Adolfsson et al. reported that 55 percent of patients progressed to stage T3 within 10 years. The bias toward tumors of low grade in Dr. Adolfsson's study can explain the apparent difference, although the progression rate in his study is still very high.

J.I. Epstein, M.D., et al. and M.L. Blute, M.D., et al. showed that young patients who are not treated, even those with low-grade tumors who are in the best prognostic category, would eventually show progression if they survive and are followed for a sufficient time. Similarly, John E. McNeal, M.D., indicates, "There are not two types of prostate cancers with different biological potential but a simple species having a slow growth rate and a logarithmic growth curve. There is a gradual increase in biologic malignant potential that is closely linked to tumor size." In fact, in men younger than 50 years diagnosed with stage A2 or stage B prostate cancer, the probability of living 10 years is 70 percent and 15 years is 60 percent, thus indicating that patients remain at risk for death from prostate cancer more than 15 years after diagnosis.

The ultimate decision regarding therapy versus watchful waiting and delayed therapy is up to the patient and his family. One must carefully consider a patient's general health, his overall expected survival from other medical problems, and the degree of side effects and adverse events that may accompany particular treatment. For many men with clinically localized prostate cancer, there is an important risk in making assumptions based upon low-grade histology on biopsy. In fact, the very useful data on watchful waiting collected by E. David Chodak, M.D., et al. shows that 13 percent of men with stage 1 or 2 prostate cancer will die within 10 years from prostate cancer, and distant metastases will develop in 19 percent. In stage 3 tumors, on the other hand, 63 percent died from the disease within 10 years, and distant metastases developed in 74 percent. Similarly, at 10 years a follow-up of stage B patients treated with signs of progression in the study of Dr. Whitmore et al. showed that 20 percent died from prostate cancer, whereas 50 percent had distant metastases and 70 percent had local progression.

The risk of dying from prostate cancer at 10 years if not immediately treated after the diagnosis of localized prostate cancer is estimated as being at least 15 to 20 percent. A value such as this is unlikely to be overestimated when one considers the 13 percent cancer-specific death rate estimated by Dr. Chodak for a series of patients who were biased toward low-grade disease. Although the estimates for local progression, distant metastases, and death from prostate cancer can have a significant error, the objective is to say that there is a 15 to 20 percent risk of death from prostate cancer within 10 years. A 70-year-old man with a life expectancy of less than 10 years will probably not die from prostate cancer if initially observed and then treated upon progression. However, a 55- to 65-year-old man in good health with a life expectancy of 10 years or more needs to be treated more aggressively, because the risk of dying from prostate cancer is very high in a population of healthy men who are relatively unlikely to die from other causes. There is in fact about a 40 percent risk of distant metastases at 10 years of follow-up and a 60 percent risk of local progression as well.

Perhaps a more viable option than watchful waiting is immediate combined hormonal therapy). For men aged 70 years or more or those having a life expectancy of less than 10 years, Dr. Labrie's data showed that CHT alone can control the disease and should prevent death from prostate cancer. In addition to overall survival benefits, combination therapy alone in older men prevents complications of local recurrence, including urinary tract obstruction and other signs and symptoms related to enlargement of the prostate, thus adding important benefits to the quality of life. It is unlikely that a patient with localized prostate cancer treated by combination therapy will have progression of his disease during a 10-year period. It seems reasonable, therefore, to administer CHT alone to these patients, thus avoiding the side effects and risks of radical prostatectomy and radiation. Studies are in progress to determine the efficacy of intermittent administration of CHT to these patients using serum PSA as an indicator of prostate cancer control. This will decrease the side effects and toxicity of the therapy and improve quality of life. Again, randomized controlled trials are necessary to compare local control as well as disease-free survival and survival figures using (1) CHT alone versus (2) observation versus (3) any primary therapy, including use of CHT as neoadjuvant therapy (therapy given before the primary treatment in order to shrink the tumor).

If you have a life expectancy of greater than 10 years, watchful waiting may be a viable strategy. Watchful waiting involves having a digital rectal examination and a PSA blood test every 3 to 4 months. If the PSA continues to progressively rise or the DRE reveals the growth of a previous tumor or one or more new masses, the doctor and patient should take appropriate action.

Advantages of Watchful Waiting

There are four advantages of watchful waiting:

1.   It allows men to maintain their current quality of life, and to avoid the complications that can occur following conventional therapies.
2.   It enables men to make an informed decision by reviewing the research and speaking with informed physicians and patients.

Guidelines for Watchful Waiting

A patient who follows a watchful waiting approach should be mindful of the following:

1. Lower-grade tumors usually grow more slowly than do higher-grade tumors.
2. Younger men have more years than do older ones for their cancer to grow and become aggressive.
3. If their disease is not systemic, men in their late seventies and eighties will probably die <u>with</u> prostate cancer, not <u>of</u> it.

Who Is Eligible for Watchful Waiting?

A good candidate for watchful waiting is a man:

1. in his late seventies or eighties, with a limited life span.
2. in his sixties or seventies, with a potentially life-threatening health problem.
3. who has less than 5 years to live.
4. who has a cancerous tumor that is low-grade (i.e., well-differentiated).
5. who has a low PSA level (and a Gleason score under 7).
6. who has a diploid tumor.
7. who has a stable PSA level with a low PSA velocity.

When Is Watchful Waiting Not Recommended?

Watchful waiting has the following disadvantages:

1. The patient takes the risk that his cancerous condition may worsen or that other problems may occur.
2. It can be dangerous and shortsighted.
3. Disease progression causes morbidity.
4. The window of "curability" is not indefinite, and a patient cannot be assured that the initiation of therapy upon progression will provide an opportunity for cure.
5. Catastrophic events, such as spinal cord compression, pathological fractures, and urethral obstruction may occur.
6. Treatment tends to be more effective while tumor bulk is smaller.
7. Prostate cancer may become less hormone-sensitive as it progresses.

8.   Waiting too long after symptoms have worsened can cause irreversible kidney damage.
9.   Prostate enlargement may block urine flow through the urethra.
10. There is no foolproof way to determine in advance if the growth is imperceptible and remains confined to the prostate gland.
11. The patient may miss the opportunity to be cured of the disease.
12. It does nothing to stop the growth of prostate cancer.
13. It may not be feasible for men who want to live more than 10 years.

When Is Watchful Waiting Recommended?

There are many advantages to watchful waiting:

1.   The patient does not have to undergo any invasive treatment.
2.   Treatment is relatively inexpensive.
3.   The patient avoids the side effects of conventional therapy, such as impotence, incontinence, and loss of libido.
4.   It gives the patient time to consider conventional as well as complementary therapies.
5.   It requires only quarterly examinations and PSA tests.
6.   It is best for older men whose tumor is low-grade and of small volume.
7.   It does not require drugs, hospitals, or loss of work.

What to Do While Watchful Waiting

While following a watchful waiting strategy, a patient can:

1.   Study the conventional and complementary options available.
2.   Consider adopting an alkalarian or other diet (see Chapter 37) to halt the growth of cancer.
3.   Follow an exercise program.
4.   Avoid sugar, alcohol, and all dairy products.
5.   Monitor his cancer by getting a PSA blood test periodically.
6.   Join a support group to learn what treated patients have to say about various facets of prostate cancer.
7.   Search the Internet to enhance his knowledge about cancer.

Making the Decision to Watchful Wait

In considering whether or not to treat his prostate cancer, a man should consider the following questions:

1. How long do I have to live?
2. How aggressive is my prostate cancer?

If the patient has a short period to live, he should spare himself the probability of experiencing the serious side effects that can accompany conventional therapies.

The second question will be more difficult to answer, and the patient will have to depend on the skill of his doctor. However, it is impossible for the doctor to know precisely how aggressive the cancer is or if it will metastasize. Fortunately, he will have the following guidelines:

- Because there is a relationship between tumor volume and the degree of cell differentiation, the tumor volume may be a useful indicator of whether tumors have metastasized.
- A tumor of less than 1 cubic centimeter (cc) has a low metastatic potential; tumors smaller than 3.5 cc seldom penetrate the prostate capsule and invade the seminal vesicles.
- Prostate tumors exceeding 5 cc usually contain more poorly differentiated cells and therefore may be more metastatically aggressive.

Learning from Studies

Several studies seem to suggest that watchful waiting is effective; however, it is not a superior approach when compared with more aggressive treatment for localized prostate cancer. Unfortunately, many of these studies have some flaws, thereby providing some unreliable or inaccurate conclusions.

In the United States, doctors usually recommend watchful waiting to older patients with low-grade, early stage prostate cancer. This is because it frequently takes a well-differentiated, small-volume tumor many years to become harmful. Scandinavian studies show that even when patients have low-grade tumors, more than 50 percent show progression of their tumor within 10 years if watchful waiting is selected. Unfortunately, 60 percent of patients diagnosed with prostate cancer at the age of 70 died of the disease if watchful waiting was employed. If prostate cancer was diagnosed at the age of 55 or younger, 100 percent of the patients in the study died of the disease when watchful waiting was selected.

How to Use This Information

If you adopt watchful waiting, you should:

1. Be monitored regularly by your physician.
2. Know its benefits and disadvantages.
3. Understand what the watchful waiting studies suggest.
4. Be ready to give up watchful waiting if there are signs your disease has progressed.

According to the research on watchful waiting versus treating prostate cancer, the following is recommended:

1. Stage A and B prostate cancer patients who have well-differentiated tumors and no other serious medical conditions, and who are older than 70, should consider watchful waiting.
2. Stage C and D prostate cancer patients should opt for treatment, which usually includes CHT.
3. Advanced prostate cancer patients with few lesions should opt for CHT to help control the disease.
4. Men who are 70 or older should consider CHT as a primary therapy in order to prevent or delay death from prostate cancer.
5. Intermittent CHT may be a viable treatment choice in the future, not only for improving a patient's quality of life, but also for increasing his survival time.

Chapter 14

UNDERGOING A RADICAL PROSTATECTOMY

A radical prostatectomy, the surgical removal of the prostate, is performed to treat localized prostate cancer. After prostatectomy, the patient's PSA should drop to an undetectable - or virtually undetectable - level. If it does not do so within a month or so after surgery, it is usually assumed that there is residual cancer in the prostatic fossa or elsewhere in the body. Frequently, this cancer is within the area where the prostate gland used to be, and external beam radiation therapy may be helpful. This will often decrease the PSA to an undetectable level. Approximately 25 to 30 percent of patients whose PSA level is undetectable following radical prostatectomy will have a gradual rise in PSA within 4 or 5 years. This usually means that prostate cancer has recurred. Because no test will indicate with certainty where the recurrence is located, the recommended treatment is often external beam radiation to the area where the prostate used to be. If the physician believes that the recurrent cancer is elsewhere in the body, he or she may recommend external beam radiation, hormonal therapy, or both. The goal with any treatment is to get the PSA level as close to undetectable as possible and to keep it at that level for as long as possible.

The goals of this chapter are to review the indications for radical prostatectomy, to describe the procedure, and to discuss how to avoid a recurrence, and what actions to take if one occurs.

Radical Retropubic Prostatectomy

Three different approaches can be used to perform a radical prostatectomy. The first approach, radical retropubic prostatectomy, accounts for 85 percent of prostatectomies.

The operation begins with an incision through the skin and muscle in the abdomen that extends from the pubic area to the navel. At the beginning of the surgery, the pelvic lymph nodes are excised. They are then rushed to a pathologist for a frozen section analysis. The tissue are frozen and then sliced into very thin sections, which are viewed under a microscope and examined for cancer cells. If the lymph nodes are cancerous, the operation is usually discontinued, and other treatment options are explored.

Radical Perineal Prostatectomy

The radical perineal prostatectomy is used for those patients who do not need a pelvic lymph-node dissection. This operation begins with a semicircular incision made between the scrotum and the anus. Usually, less bleeding occurs with this type of prostatectomy, and there is no visible scar associated with it. However, with this type of incision, it is difficult to save the nerves in the neurovascular bundles, which usually affect the ability to have an erection. Frequently, the lymph nodes are sampled laparoscopically. (If however, the lymph nodes cannot be operated upon by laparoscope, a separate incision is made in the lower portion of the abdomen.)

Laparoscopic Prostatectomy

The laparoscopic prostatectomy does not represent the standard of care in this country. This type of operation requires five small (5 to 10 mm) incisions. One is made just below the navel, and two each are made on either side of the lower abdomen. Carbon dioxide is then passed into the abdominal cavity, where a small tube is placed into the incision below the navel. This gas lifts the wall of the abdomen to give the surgeon an improved view of the abdominal cavity when the laparoscope is in place. The surgeon uses a laparoscope, which transmits a picture of the prostate into a video monitor.

The urologists who perform this procedure believe that patients experience less blood loss, less need for pain medication, less time in the hospital, quicker return to regular diet and activities, and a quicker recovery.

Regardless of the type of radical prostatectomy, the outcome and side effects depend on the expertise and experience of the surgeon. That's why a patient should select a doctor based on the quantity and quality of his or her experience. This treatment option depends also on the PSA level, Gleason score, and stage of the cancer. Although the MRSI cannot detect microscopic extracapsular disease, it is the best diagnostic test we have for indicating whether cancer is contained within the prostatic capsule (see Chapter 10). In fact, some urologists prescribe this test before performing a radical prostatectomy. Candidates for this surgery should ask their doctor to consider having them undergo an MRSI.

Next, the major vein system that overlies the prostate and urethra is excised. Blood loss is kept to a minimum so that the operation can be performed in a bloodless terrain and enable the doctor to see what's happening. The next step is a delicate procedure that involves cutting through the urethra, which runs through the prostate gland. If the doctor cuts too close to the prostate, sometimes some cancer is left behind. On the other hand, if the surgeon cuts the urethra too far from the prostate, it may damage the urethral sphincter, causing urinary problems. Depending on the amount of cancer, the surgeon will need to make a decision that will most likely affect the patient's potency. This decision involves whether or not to remove one or both of the neurovascular bundles in order to excise all the cancer. If the surgeon decides to preserve the neurovascular bundle, it is based upon a clinical decision that the cancer can be fully extracted without removing them. If, however, one or both of the neurovascular bundles must be removed, the surgeon will excise them near the urethra, next to the rectum.

Next, the surgeon will begin to focus on the prostate by making an incision to separate it at the base of the bladder, which connects the bladder to the prostate. The doctor will then remove the seminal vesicles, vas deferens, and any surrounding tissues as well as the prostate gland. The final step will involve rebuilding the urinary tract connecting the bladder to the penile urethra and the urethral sphincter. Often the doctor will use sutures to reduce the size of the neck of the bladder so that it is equal to the size of the urethra. As a result, a Foley catheter will be inserted into the urethra leading to the bladder.

Open Versus Laparoscopic Surgery

OPEN SURGERY	LAPAROSCOPIC SURGERY
Hospital stay: 2 to 4 days.	Hospital stay: 1 to 2 days.
1-2 units of blood may be lost, which can be replaced through a transfusion of the patient's own blood or donor blood.	Significantly less bleeding.
Recovery can take as long as 6 to 7 weeks.	Most patients can return to work within 2 to 3 weeks.
Some postoperative pulmonary and gastrointestinal complications.	Postoperative pulmonary and gastrointestinal complications, possibly greater than with open surgery.
More pain and scarring after surgery.	Less pain and scarring after surgery.
Urethral catheter for 10 to 14 days.	Removal of urethral catheter in 3 to 6 days.

OPEN SURGERY	LAPAROSCOPIC SURGERY
Operation leaves a long incision.	Operation leaves five small (5-10 mm) incisions.
Rectal injury in less than 1 percent of patients.	Higher risk of rectal injury.
Avoid lifting of anything over 10 pounds for 9 months or more.	Lifting heavy items is permitted.
Many qualified surgeons available.	Only a few qualified surgeons available.
Normal urinary function returns within 3 months.	Normal urinary function returns within a shorter period of time; however, there are no data to prove this.
Began in 1904.	Began in early 1970s.
May take 6 to 9 months to regain urinary control.	May take 6 to 9 months to regain urinary control.

Who Qualifies for Open Surgery?

To qualify for open surgery, the following criteria should be met:

- The patient must have a life expectancy of 10 years or more, and he should usually be under 70 years of age.
- The cancer must be localized.
- The patient should not have cancer in the seminal vesicles, lymph nodes, or bones.
- The patient's PSA level should not exceed 10 ng/ml.
- The patient should not have a serious medical condition such as congestive heart failure.
- The patient should not have undergone an abdominal surgery within the past 6 months. If he has, the operation should be postponed several months.

Advantages of Surgery

The advantages of radical prostatectomy follow:

- There is a probability of a cure.
- The postoperative PSA test can be used to determine whether there is a recurrence.

- The patient has the emotional benefit of knowing that prostate cancer and the prostate have been removed from his body.

Who Qualifies for Laparoscopy?

Laparoscopic surgery is appropriate for:

- Young and middle-aged men with pressing career or family responsibilities, or both.
- Active men who are unable to endure a long recovery period.

Before Surgery

Only patients who are in excellent health should select a radical prostatectomy to treat their prostate cancer. For example, surgery is not recommended for men older than 70 who have less than 10 years to live or who have serious heart or other disease.

Before surgery, patients should stop taking aspirin and other blood-thinning medications. Sometimes patients will be asked to donate several units of their blood. All patients will be required to have an enema or take a laxative right before the surgery. They will also have to stop eating for a number of hours as well. The anesthesiologist will meet with the patient before the operation to ask about his health. The patient will be asked if he is on any medications and if he has ever had any unusual problems with bleeding.

How to Use This Information

If you are thinking of undergoing a radical prostatectomy:

- Consider getting an MRSI to determine if your prostate cancer is localized.
- Ask your urologist to give you a list of patients on whom he or she has performed a radical prostatectomy. The list should include both patients who did well and those who did poorly.

Chapter 15

IMRT: AN IMPROVED VERSION
OF EXTERNAL BEAM RADIATION

External beam radiation started in the 1970s with the use of box-like fields, which often missed the prostate but gave a significant dose to nearby structures. This caused acute and long-term side effects. However, with the advent of 3D conformal radiation in the early 1990s, radiation oncologists were able to shape the radiation field much more precisely to the region of the prostate, allowing more radiation to be delivered to the prostate and less to the normal tissues nearby, improving not only the cure rate, but also reducing the side effects of the treatment. In the late 1990s, the advent of intensity-modulated radiation therapy (IMRT) increased this advantage, allowing clinicians to increase the radiation dose to the prostate to a level where cure rates approached or equaled those of surgery while reducing side effects to levels equal to or less than those of surgery. However, there are no moderate- to long-term data, which demonstrates the superiority of IMRT or compares it to surgery. Previous applications of external beam radiation involved a single large radiation dose passing through the body to reach cancerous tumors. On the other hand, intensity-modulated radiotherapy IMRT allows the delivery of very precise external beam radiation treatments. It involves the modulation of the radiation beam within a given radiation portal. As a result, this application delivers a high dosage of radiation to the tumor cells and a lower dosage to the healthy cells. IMRT allows radiation oncologists to treat prostate cancer with a high dose of radiation and to safely treat prostate cancer located near dangerous areas of the body. It allows for better control, lower side effects, increased flexibility of radiation delivery, and improved results.

What Are the Purposes of IMRT?

The goals of IMRT are:

1. To improve the efficiency and efficacy of external beam radiation.
2. To optimally treat individual patients without damaging the tissues and organs around the tumor.
3. To adjust the dose according to the needs of each patient.
4. To eradicate the tumor, thereby improving the probability of curing the patient.

5. To precisely model the patient's internal anatomy and disease using CT and/or MR, so that external beam radiation can be aimed with greater accuracy and radiation treatment defined with greater certainty of effect.

What Is IMRT?

IMRT is a three-dimensional conformal radiation treatment that combines the power of today's computers with advanced delivery devices to produce a highly focused radiation dose that conforms to the area of disease identified by the radiation oncologist and reduces the radiation received by nearby normal tissues. IMRT radiation beamlets are combined by the computer into a precise treatment delivery that results in a high dosage to the cancerous tumors and a lowered dose to the surrounding healthy tissues.

In addition, IMRT also treats tumors that are located very close to sensitive body organs such as the spinal cord. IMRT is, without a doubt, the most updated technologically advanced external beam radiation method available.

Understanding the Need for the IMRT

The medical linear accelerator was first used in the 1950s, which revolutionized the way external beam radiation was delivered to treat prostate cancer. Linear accelerators accelerated electrons to produce radiation that could be aimed with greater precision. By using electromagnetic waves, the device accelerated electrons through a specially designed tube to generate X-rays. However, until the advent of digital diagnostic imaging capability, powerful computers, and specialized software, it was almost impossible for radiation oncologists to conform the external beam radiation to the shape of the tumor. Prior to the advent of CT-based treatment planning, it was possible to miss the target. Heavy lead blocks and cerrobend were used and constantly repositioned for each patient. In addition, the therapist had to leave the radiation room to change the direction of the machine and the field size and to insert a new block and any other field changes. The introduction of the multi-leaf collimator (MLC) and other devices has changed the dynamic role of external beam radiation in treating prostate cancer.

Early radiation treatment techniques were unable to aim radiation in such a way as to allow conformation of the radiation to a target volume. In addition, early diagnostic imaging techniques were unable to precisely determine the exact region of cancer that needed to be irradiated. As a result, radiation therapy used larger beams and treated more healthy tissue in order to be sure that the cancerous tumors were adequately treated. IMRT, which had been proposed as early as the 1960s, only became a treatment reality with (1) the advent of MLCs, which allowed faster, more precise shaping of the radiation beam, (2) advances in computer technology, allowing medical physicists to produce radiation beams with more complex shapes to use the MLCs, and (3) better diagnostic imaging, using CT and MR to more clearly identify the regions of disease to be treated as well as the regions of normal tissue most prone to radiation damage.

Advantages of the IMRT

The advantages of IMRT include:

- Greater reduction of dose to surrounding healthy tissues, thus reducing side effects.
- Increased flexibility in treating difficult lesions surrounding critical organs.
- Improved conformal dose distributions around the cancerous area.
- Advanced approach to 3-dimensional radiation therapy.
- It is a more expensive treatment requiring much greater physic support.
- Improved potential for curing patients.
- Higher tumor controls and lower normal tissue toxicity.

Planning the Treatment

IMRT treatment planning is very complex. As a result, the standard trial-and-error planning method used by most physicians has been replaced by more complicated computer algorithms to optimize dose distribution. Current IMRT methods can be divided into three distinct groups:

- The use of general-purpose MLCs, either by a static or segmental technique, or by dynamic motion of the MLC, to shape the radiation beam within a given portal while the radiation gantry and table remain stable.
- The use of rotational techniques, generally called tomotherapy, where not only is the radiation field shaped dynamically, but the radiation source rotates around the patient as well.
- The use of static compensators, which are inserted for each treatment field and which vary the intensity of radiation reaching the patient by varying levels of shielding material placed on the

compensator. Image fusion techniques, using CT, MRI, and/or PET scans, are employed to better delineate the target volume.

The planning process is basically the same: imaging, structure and target segmentation, prescription, and computer-controlled plan optimization. Planning for IMRT begins identically to planning for conformal radiation therapy. A treatment-planning CT scan or an MRI is obtained.

The margin to take into account the motion and uncertainty in the setup of the patient is a key part of the IMRT process. Each additional "rind" of healthy tissue that must be treated due to the uncertainty of the setup and delivery of the radiation decreases the ability of the radiation oncologist and the computer to improve the gap between "killing" radiation doses to the cancer and nonlethal doses of radiation to the healthy tissues nearby. Thus, reducing the rind is highly important but not at the expense of missing the tumor.

Once all the data are entered into the computer, the software simulates the delivered dose using mathematical models to search for treatments that best satisfy the radiation oncologist's multifaceted prescription. After the computer renders an initial plan, a physician evaluates it by reviewing isodose contours. If the tumor is not adequately covered or if the dose close to the normal tissue areas is unacceptably high, the dose is changed and the initial treatment plan re-optimized until a final treatment plan is reached.

Delivering the Treatment

With the more complex delivery of IMRT, there are now too many treatment parameters to be transferred by nonelectronics means; information must be sent from the treatment-planning computer to the delivery device using media such as a floppy disk or by direct network connection. Once delivered to the treatment machine, key parameters are verified by the clinic's medical physics staff to insure a correct delivery.

Positioning the Patient

Careful attention must be given to the movement of both the patient and the internal organs. In addition, the position of the prostate gland relative to fixed bony landmarks will vary due to the fullness of the bladder and rectum, which is constantly changing. External marks on the skin or anatomic landmarks of the pelvis cannot accurately determine what is going on inside the pelvis. Therefore, it is essential that the daily positioning of the patient account for the exact location of the prostate itself in order to optimize therapeutic effects as well as to minimize toxicity resulting from the radiation of healthy tissues. The prostate position is also sensitive to the position of the patient. In particular, the angle of the ankles and the bend of the knees should be reproducible during treatment. This requires either excellent immobilization or another technique to determine the position of the prostate. In the early 2000s, a number of ways were being considered for identifying the prostate gland on a daily basis such as:

- imaging of marker seeds within the prostate
- CT scanning prior to, during, or after treatment
- ultrasound imaging of the prostate at the time of treatment

The B-mode acquisition and targeting (BAT system) is used by a number of centers around the United States to help identify the location of the prostate on a daily basis prior to radiation treatment with the patient in the treatment position. This is important because the patient may move during transfer from the CT-simulation suite to the treatment machine, creating a potential source of error.

BAT, an ultrasound-based targeting system, localizes the prostate in relationship to its planned position. The position of the prostate can change from one treatment day to another. With conventional radiation, important margins are added to the volume of the tumors to account for the day-to-day variation. Although this may increase the likelihood of covering the tumors, it also creates greater exposure to increased percentages to the surrounding structure of high doses of radiation, which will increase the risk of complications. BAT uses an ultrasound to image the prostate and associated organs at the time of treatment. The ultrasound probe is calibrated both to the treatment plan approved by the physician and to the treatment machine. As a result, the position of the target can be compared to the position that existed at the time of planning. The center of the treatment plan (ISO center) can be adjusted to compensate for any prostate motion. In this way, margins added to the target volumes can be reduced, and this can theoretically reduce normal tissue irradiation.

BAT is appropriate for any organ that can be visualized by the ultrasound, especially the prostate, liver, bladder, kidney, and pancreas and for metastatic disease.

Positioning the patient in the proper position is extremely important. Once done, the patient (and therefore the target) must remain stationary for the duration it takes to deliver the radiation. Therefore, as for all external beam radiation treatments, proper patient positioning and immobilization, including proper treatment-couch repositioning, are critical for successful treatment. However, since the BAT immobilization technique needs only to retain positioning information for the length of a single treatment, which takes about 15 minutes, devices can be used that are much more comfortable for the patient. As a result, treatment is more precise than previous techniques.

Computer Optimization

The treatment planning for the target volumes that are removed from the surrounding normal structures can be accomplished with conventional treatment-planning techniques that use a trial-and-error approach. In this typical planning process, the radiation physicists and physicians design a treatment plan and make use of a computer to display the dose that would be received if the plan were delivered. This plan, which consists of a number of beams from several directions, as well as their relative weights, is changed until which time an adequate dose is achieved.

IMRT takes a different approach. Certain dose prescriptions and dose constraints are given to the computer, and the computer generates a plan that meets these dose goals. There are a number of optimization of types. Each one allows the computer to determine the "best" solution among millions of possible combinations of beam directions and weights. This particular process is called "inverse planning." The physician and physicist determines what doses to deliver to the tumor and what limits on dose should be applied to nearby organs, and the computer determines how to deliver that dose. The process is similar to the one used in image reconstruction in computed tomography (CT). The specific task of the CT scan image reconstruction is to calculate the underlying density distribution in the transverse slices based on the measured X-ray projections of a number of angles through the patient.

Inverse planning systems must translate the physician's requirements into a set of beam, angles, and the modulation necessary to achieve these goals. The Corvus treatment planning system of NOMOS Corporation is the first inverse planning system to be used in radiation therapy. Currently, it is used by more than a hundred hospitals and clinics around the world to create complex treatment plans used with IMRT. However, other inverse planning systems are now in clinical use, and it is anticipated that soon all treatment planning for IMRT will be of the "inverse mode."

Essentially, the only (but real) difference between earlier planning models and the inverse model is who implements the planning step - the computer or the user? In the latter planning model, the doctor implements the planning steps. As a result, the success of the plan is based on the experience and knowledge of the doctor. With the inverse planning model, the computer implements the planning steps based on techniques that are uniform from doctor to doctor.

Complications

Complications from radiotherapy to the prostate gland are mainly related to radiation damage to the prostatic urethra, bulbo-membranous urethra, anterior rectal wall, lower portions of the bladder, or neurovascular bundles. Following are other side effects:

- Increased urination throughout the treatment.
- Temporary decrease in urine flow.
- Bleeding from the bladder (usually uncommon).
- Most urinary symptoms are resolved within 2 to 3 months, but some patients may have symptoms that last for 9 to 12 months.
- Rectal bleeding or proctitis (rare).
- Pain during ejaculation (in a minority).
- Impotency can occur, but it is influenced by such factors as age, diabetes, or preexisting erectile dysfunction.
- Late complication may include diarrhea (in fewer than 5%).
- Mild fatigue.
- Temporary increase in nocturia, the need to urinate frequently during the night.

Using IMRT for Advanced Prostate Cancer

Treating prostate cancer with IMRT is an ideal application of this technology. It can be viewed as a very advanced form of 3D conformal radiation therapy. The capacity of IMRT to reduce the radiation dose to organs such as the rectum and bladder allows for a further decrease in complications and the potential for dose escalation. The ability to safely deliver higher doses of radiation to the prostate gland is very important for patients with certain tumor characteristics, a Gleason score of 7 or higher, a PSA level over 10 ng/ml, and extracapsular extension.

The information in the Resource section identifies the IMRT centers and clinics showing their locations, telephone number, physicians, and number of patients treated.

Retaining Erectile Function

One of the side effects of being treated for prostate cancer is erectile dysfunction. Dr. John Robinson et al. from the University of Calgary found that brachytherapy (seed implantation) was the treatment that afforded prostate cancer patients the highest probability of maintaining potency. This was followed by brachytherapy plus external beam radiation, external beam radiation alone, nerve-sparing radical prostatectomy, standard radical prostatectomy, and cryotherapy. The probability of erectile dysfunction after each of the treatments varied significantly, with one possible exception: brachytherapy plus external beam radiation had the same results as external beam radiation alone.

When the results were adjusted for age, the probability of erectile function after all radiation therapies increased; however, for standard and nerve-sparing prostatectomy patients, age adjustment decreased the probability of maintaining erectile function. Cryotherapy probabilities were not affected by age adjustments.

Robinson et al. concluded that men concerned with retaining erectile function have "reason to choose one treatment over another." Patients need to be advised that any advantages brachytherapy has over external beam radiation in preserving potency appears to be lost when it is combined with that therapy.

Brachytherapy alone is recommended only for men with low-risk prostate cancer. Thus the choice for many men is often between external beam radiation, radical prostatectomy, and cryotherapy. Of these, external beam radiation therapy appears to offer the best chance of retaining erectile function, according to Dr. Robinson and his team.

How to Use This Information

1. If you are to undergo external beam radiation, consider going to a center with IMRT technology. Members of the Education Center for Prostate Cancer Patients may ask to speak with Dr. Lewis at the Education Center for Prostate Cancer Patients.
2. Go to a center with experience with the IMRT.
3. If you are going to undergo brachytherapy and external beam radiation, see item 1.

Chapter 16

CRYOSURGERY

A study of 590 patients treated with cryosurgery of prostate cancer for localized advanced prostate cancer from March 1993 to September 2001 was reported in Urology. The patients were stratified into three risk groups according to clinical characteristics. Biochemical disease-free survival after cryosurgery, biopsy results, and morbidity after cryosurgery were calculated and presented. The mean follow-up for all patients was 5.43 years. The percentage of patients in the low-, medium-, and high-risk groups was 15.9, 30.3, and 53.7 percent, respectively. The biochemical disease-free survival for a PSA cutoff of 1.0 ng/ml for low-, survival for low-, medium-, and high-risk patients using the American Society for Therapeutic Radiology and Oncology (ASTRO) definition were 92, 89, and 89 percent, respectively. The percent of positive biopsies was 13 percent.

After a positive biopsy, 32 patients underwent repeat cryosurgery. For these patients, 68, 72, and 91 percent remained biochemically disease-free using a definition of 0.5 ng/ml, 1.0 ng/ml, and the ASTRO definition, respectively, after a mean follow-up time since repeat cryosurgery of 63 months. The rate of complications was modest, and no serious ones were observed. Primary therapy with curative intent was shown to be equal to or greater than the outcome figures for external beam radiation, 3-dimensional conformal radiation, and brachytherapy in other reported series. A randomized controlled trial, however, would need to be done to confirm these results.

Cryosurgery for Prostate Cancer

In the 1990s, with the advent of new technologies and procedures, doctors began to return to two treatments that had not been successful in the past: seed implantation and cryosurgery. Although many physicians advised patients that these treatments were experimental and should be avoided, many patients chose to ignore them. Today, as a result of the ease of the operation, the minimal side effects, and lowered cost, these two approaches are getting a great deal of attention. In many cases, urologists are being trained to perform either cryosurgery or seed implantation. These physicians are at the forefront of what are potentially more acceptable and, hopefully, more effective therapies for prostate cancer. It is possible that radical prostatectomy and external beam radiation will become obsolete in the future because of the success of investigational treatments such as cryosurgery. Why? Because these treatments are getting results similar to or better than those for radical prostatectomy and external beam radiation. They have less morbidity, they can be used as salvage treatments, and they can be repeated. Patients can receive these treatments in less time, and they are less costly.

What is Cryosurgery?

Cryosurgery, also called *cryoablation surgery*, is a technique in which six to eight *cryoprobes*, small tubes utilizing argon gas, are inserted between the scrotum and anus. They enter the prostate gland to freeze and thus kill prostate cancer cells.

Freezing of the prostate was first done about 30 years ago; however, it was abandoned because of severe side effects. With the advent of transrectal ultrasound, it reemerged as a viable technique and an alternative to radical prostatectomy and radiation. During cryosurgery, a 2-hour procedure performed under anesthesia, the prostate is frozen with argon gas circulated in cryoprobes. The physician monitors the procedure using transrectal ultrasound and thermosensors to assure a killing temperature (-20 °C to -40 °C) at the site of the cancer.

Pioneers in Cryosurgery

Cryosurgery has been used for more than 29 years in such fields as dermatology, gynecology, and liver cancer. Richard J. Ablin, Ph.D., and Maurice Gonder, M.D., were pioneers in the application of cryosurgery in the 1960s. Although it had the same survival rates as radical prostatectomy and external beam radiation, it was soon abandoned because of damage to the adjacent normal structures. Fred Lee, M.D., internationally known for using transrectal ultrasound to detect prostate cancer and for using transrectal biopsy techniques, provided the precise applications needed for the success of the freezing process.

When Cryomedical Science, Inc., of Rockville, Maryland, developed the liquid-circulating probe (under the name of CMS Acu-Probe), several hospitals throughout the United States began to experiment with cryosurgery. The first medical center to do so was Allegheny General Hospital in Pittsburgh, spearheaded by Gary Onik, M.D., and Jeffrey Cohen, M.D.

In March 1992, Dr. Onik reported in <u>Cancer</u> that 15 patients with prostate cancer were treated with cryosurgery, and 14 (93.3%) showed no residual prostate cancer on a short-term basis.

For any definitive treatment, patients should first use combination hormonal therapy for 3 to 6 months to debulk and downstage the disease and to decrease the overall gland size.

- Efficiency and safety is due to transrectal ultrasound imaging and use of thermosensors to assure adequate killing temperatures.
- It is applicable for stages T1 to T3, and there has been unexpected good success with late-stage (stage C+T3) prostate cancer.
- It is ideally suited for patients who have other medical problems.
- Severe fistula and total incontinence occur in less than 1 percent of patients, but impotence has been reported to be as high as 100 percent. Sloughing of tissue may be greatly reduced (less than 10 percent) by use of a Foley catheter for 3 weeks.

Advantages and Disadvantages of Cryosurgery

The advantages of cryosurgery are:

1. No incisions are required. The probes are inserted directly through the skin between the scrotum and anus.
2. The procedure requires a hospital stay of only 1 to 2 days. Frequently, patients are discharged the same day.
3. The procedure can be repeated once or twice.
4. It is less expensive than either radical prostatectomy or external beam radiation (Medicare's total payment in 2003 was $7,000).
5. There is no blood loss.

The disadvantages are:

1. Its effectiveness has not been supported by either a 10- or 15-year statistical survival study.
2. Follow-up biopsy of the prostate is needed to assure total removal of the cancer.
3. The PSA level should be near zero if some the gland has been removed. Most studies to date report PSA levels of less than 0.5 to 1.0 ng/ml.
4. Seventy percent of patients will be impotent one year after the treatment.

Medicare and Cryosurgery

When the first edition of this book was written, Medicare did not cover the cost of cryosurgery. Since then, patients at Patient Advocates for Advanced Cancer Treatments (PAACT) worked diligently to have it paid for by insurers. The following is a press release about Medicare covering the cost of cryosurgery for localized prostate cancer.

Eligibility

All patients who have no documented evidence of distant spread are eligible for cryosurgery. Patients going to get treatment out of state will probably be asked to bring the results of their CT scan, bone scan, PSA levels over time, and pathology slides.

Preliminary Treatment

Depending on the physician performing the treatment, the prostate will be measured by a transrectal ultrasound. If the gland is more than 40 grams, the patient will most likely undergo a preliminary treatment of CHT for 3 to 6 months to debulk and shrink the prostate. (The authors believe this should be done regardless of the size of the gland. Also, staging biopsies to determine the extent of the disease allow one to tailor the procedure for each patient.)

Before Treatment

Before you are admitted to the hospital, your blood pressure, heart rate, pulse, and weight will be checked. The purpose of these tests is to uncover any serious medical problems that need to be treated. Then your surgeon or another physician will examine you.

On the day before the operation, a mechanical bowel preparation and antibiotics will be administered.

Some time before the surgery, an anesthesiologist will ask if you are allergic to any drugs and if you have had any experience with anesthesia. The procedure for anesthetizing will be explained.

Shortly before surgery, a nurse will insert a needle for intravenous antibiotics and fluids into your arm, take your vital signs, and give you a shot to control any nausea after the anesthesia wears off.

The drugs will be introduced into the intravenous drip and begin to take effect. A tube will be inserted into your windpipe to control your breathing and to deliver the proper mixture of oxygen and anesthesia. A mask will be placed over your face and the anesthesiologist will closely monitor you. Once you are fully anesthetized, some physicians will insert a suprapubic (below the navel) tube, guided by a cystoscope and a guidewire, into the bladder in order to allow the urine to bypass the prostatic urethra; others use only a Foley catheter. A urethral warming catheter will be inserted through your penis into the bladder to protect the bladder neck, prostatic, urethra, and external sphincter from freezing.

Prior to the operation, your prostate gland is measured, and the tumor location confirmed using transrectal ultrasound. These data are then used to directly place cryoprobes guided by the ultrasound into predetermined areas of cancer. Six to eight cryoprobes are used at temperatures between -175 °C and -196 °C. A confluent iceball is formed within the prostate gland and is monitored with ultrasound. To more precisely monitor the freezing process, Dr. Lee strongly advises that thermometers surround the gland to assure the tumor kill (less than 20 °C). The probes are thawed and retracted, in some cases to freeze the apex of the prostate, and a repeat freezing cycle is performed, thus covering the entire prostate. The ultrasound is used to bringing the iceball up to, but not including, the rectal wall.

After Surgery

The usual stay in the hospital is overnight, and your doctor will discharge you as an outpatient with either a suprapubic or Foley catheter in place. The Foley may be left in for 2 or 3 weeks, though this is variable to institutions. Dr. Fred Lee and D. Bahn note less than 10 percent clinical sloughing when no voiding occurs through the prostate, and the Foley drains the urinary bladder for 2 to 3 weeks. Possible complications and symptoms are also monitored in detail every 6 months for up to 2 years. Follow-up visits are as needed.

"Cryosurgery may be a viable treatment option for patients with localized prostate cancer and failure of radiation therapy," reported the first state of Michigan consensus conference of prostate cancer for 1996. According to Lee, Bahn, et al., as more scientific papers are published, the results for local prostate cancer obliteration appear to be approximately 100 percent for stage T1, 90 percent for T2, and 74 percent for stage T3. Mean PSA for those with negative biopsies is 0.5 ng/ml.

Major complications of rectal injury or total incontinence are rare (less than 1%). But potency after cryosurgery rarely returns, and erectile aids are usually needed.

In summary, cryosurgery for prostate cancer continues to show promising results after 7 years of follow-up. It appears equal to outcomes of other current treatments, and has a low incidence of complications. Most will consider it user-friendly.

Citing the Statistics

Is cryosurgery as effective as radical prostatectomy? We cannot answer this. We can only cite some statistics and let you decide for yourself. PAACT (Patient Advocates for Advanced Cancer Treatments) maintains that it is and has been coaching scores of prostate cancer patients to consider it as a viable treatment. In fact, this international organization believes that cryosurgery is an acceptable alternative for the many reasons already cited.

What are the statistics? Some would say that it is too early to know. To date, the longest long-term study (7 years) confirms cryosurgery as a viable first-line treatment, especially because it can be repeated. Dr. Jeffrey Cohen maintains that initial follow-up biopsy and PSA data are encouraging, and this treatment approach deserves further investigation.

Though it is too early to tell, initial results seem to indicate that cryosurgery may be as effective as radical prostatectomy or external beam radiation for treating stage A and B patients and possibly better than both procedures for treating stage C patients. In terms of side effects, cryosurgery seems to be better than radical prostatectomy, but it may not be better than external beam radiation as far as impotence is concerned. Whether 5- and 10-year follow-up studies will get similar results is unknown.

Should you opt for cryosurgery over the traditional treatments of radical prostatectomy or external beam radiation? Yes, if you are willing to take the risk to possibly enjoy a better quality of life. A problem most patients do not consider when choosing radical prostatectomy or external beam radiotherapy is that once you opt for either of these treatments, you markedly diminish your other choices. Making cryosurgery your first choice leaves open several other treatment options if you have a recurrence. For example:

- If cryosurgery fails, you can repeat it one or two times.
- If prostate cancer has invaded your neurovascular bundles, cryoprobes can be placed near them to destroy the cancer cells.
- If the disease has invaded your seminal vesicles, probes can be used to destroy it.
- You may also be a suitable candidate for seed implantation.
- If your disease remains localized, you may be a candidate for radical prostatectomy, or external beam radiation therapy.

Seven-Year Study Results

In an article in <u>Urology</u>, "Cryoablation of the Prostate" by Daniel B. Rukstalis, M.D., and Aaron E. Katz, M.D., it was reported that the 7-year results showed that cryosurgery is an effective treatment for locally confined and locally advanced prostate cancer.

A scientific rationale for future modifications of cryosurgery by Daniel B. Rukstalis, M.D., et al. investigated potential directions for the future of cryosurgery. This paper indicated that:

- The most common areas for potential alterations in the cryosurgery technique include modifications that would further simplify the procedure, continue to reduce real and perceived toxicity, and augment efficacy.
- Modifications designed to reduce treatment-related side effects could conflict with efforts intended to improve the eradication of prostate cancer.
- Pathologic analysis revealed multifocal cancer in 80 percent of the samples, with 66 percent of cases exhibiting cancer within 5 mm of the urethra.

Cryosurgery As a Salvage Treatment

As mentioned previously, cryosurgery can be used as a salvage treatment. In fact, one hospital in the United States performs cryosurgery only on patients who have failed external beam radiation. However, since this updated treatment approach is relatively difficult, selection of a doctor is extremely important. The most complex part of the treatment is the analysis and interpretation of the images on the transrectal ultrasound in order to place the probes in the proper location.

In a study by Gregory T. Bales, M.D., et al. "Initial Outcome with Cryosurgery in Prostate Cancer Patients Having Failed Radiation Therapy", cryosurgery emerged as a potential treatment option for prostate cancer patients who failed external beam radiation. Eighteen patients were involved in this investigation. All of them had a rising PSA level and a positive prostate biopsy but no evidence of metastatic disease on a CT and bone scan. The median PSA level prior to cryosurgery in these patients was 7.6 ng/ml (range: 0.1 to 43.9). All patients underwent cryosurgery with five to eight cryoprobes, with careful attention directed to treating the seminal vesicles. A PSA level and biopsy were performed on each patient 3 months after treatment. The 12-month PSA results available for 11 patients revealed a median PSA of 0.5 ng/ml (range: 0.1 to 28.3). Of these, only three PSA levels were below 0.1 ng/ml, and 3 of the 11 patients had a higher PSA level after the 3 months. No prostate cancer was detected in 8 of 11 patients (67%), as demonstrated by the postcryosurgery biopsies. Complications were high, partially due to the doctors' attempts to treat the seminal vesicles and the apex of the prostate gland. Complications included impotence (49%), incontinence (44%), constipation (17%), retention (17%), epididymitis (11%), tissue sloughing (5%), and death (5%). The study proved that cryosurgery appears to eradicate tumors in a high percentage of patients who failed external beam radiation; however, significant complications occur when the seminal vesicles are treated.

How to Use This Information

Before choosing cryosurgery as a treatment for prostate cancer, consider the following information:

1. Don't be a guinea pig. Use only doctors who have performed many cryosurgery procedures, preferably a radiologist/urologist team with access to thermometers to monitor the freezing process. Remember, this procedure is extremely "operator-dependent."
2. Before undergoing cryosurgery, insist on being placed on CHT for 3 to 6 months to both downsize the gland and downstage your disease.
3. Before undergoing CHT, get a transrectal ultrasound to determine the precise location of your tumor, and undergo biopsies if needed to determine seminal-vesicle or lymph-node involvement.
4. Get the names and telephone numbers of several of your physician's patients who have undergone cryosurgery. Call them, ask if they have had a recurrence, and ask about side effects.
5. Ask for the results of your physician's cryosurgical experience.

Chapter 17

UNDERGOING HIGH-DOSE RADIATION

High-dose radiation (HDR) became more widely known in 1996 when Andy Grove, CEO of Intel, was diagnosed with prostate cancer. Rather than taking his urologist's advice to have a prostatectomy, he decided to explore all of the available treatments. After reviewing published medical papers and research results, Grove plotted graphs showing the performance results of each treatment to determine its success, benefits, and complication rates. Finally, he chose HDR brachytherapy. Grove's HDR physician coined the term "smart bomb" for this kind of treatment, as against the "carpet bombing" approach and unknown certainty of dose with permanent seed (see Chapter 20).

What Is High-Dose Radiation?

High dose radiation is a temporary form of internal radiation. A single, tiny (4 mm) iridium-192 source is introduced into thin, plastic treatment catheters, called *flexiguides*, which the brachytherapy physician has positioned around and through the prostate. A computer guides the source in and out of each of these catheters, and it moves along each catheter in 5-mm steps, called *dwell positions*. By controlling how much time the source spends in each dwell position, the radiation dose can be shaped to conform to the prostate while minimizing the dose to the nearby structures, such as the bladder, urethra, and rectum. This ability to shape the radiation means that there are no "hot and cold spots," areas that receive too much or not enough radiation. The ability to regulate or modify the dose after the catheters are placed, but before any radiation is given, is one of the great advantages of HDR over permanent seed implantation. HDR is considered a temporary form of brachytherapy because after a treatment is completed, the source retracts back into the afterloader, or source of radiation. There is no radiation left behind in the patient. Unlike with permanent seeds, radiation exposure to others is eliminated.

Criteria for the Use of HDR

This chapter will identify which patients qualify for HDR treatment, indicate what HDR involves, compare permanent and temporary seed implantation of HDR, discuss what takes place during the treatment, and relate the results of some research.

HDR can be used for prostate cancer stages T1 through T3. Early-stage cancers, where the disease is confined to the prostate, can be treated with HDR monotherapy – that is, HDR alone. Later stages (T2b through T3) are usually treated with a combination of HDR and external beam radiation. With these stages, there is an increased chance that the disease has broken through the prostate capsule (i.e., extracapsular extension). If extracapsular extension is expected, the physician will place the catheters outside the gland. With permanent seeds, the radiation "reach" is about 3 mm, and if the seeds are not positioned accurately just inside the capsule, the extension will not be adequately treated. Permanent seeds shift around after implantation due to prostate swelling and bleeding, so their actual position isn't known until a CT scan or X-ray is taken sometime after implantation. Permanent seeds are also known to migrate to the lungs in about 20 percent of cases, if they get into the venous system. Some seed-implant physicians have inserted seeds outside the gland to try to treat extracapsular extension. In these cases, a Mayo Clinic study reported a migration or pulmonary embolization rate of up to 55 percent. If seeds can shift around inside the firmer prostate tissue, then seeds that are placed in the looser periprostatic connective tissue are much more likely to shift and migrate, delivering unknown doses to the tissues.

If the cancer has penetrated the capsule, the HDR will be followed by a short course of external beam radiation. If the disease is known to be in the pelvic lymph nodes, antiandrogen hormones might also be given. This is called *triple modality therapy*.

HDR is also used as a salvage treatment for men whose cancer has locally recurred after either prostatectomy, external beam radiation (X-ray or proton), cryosurgery, or permanent seeding. As long as the cancer has not invaded areas such as the bones or lymph nodes, and any prior radiation damage to the surrounding tissues is not too severe, HDR salvage can be used.

Who Qualifies for HDR?

In general, HDR brachytherapy can be used for prostate cancer patients with the following conditions:

- Any size prostate gland; however, an extremely large gland will need hormone therapy to shrink it prior to implantation.
- Any cancer that has not spread to the lymph nodes and bones.
- Unlimited PSA value.

- All Gleason grades.
- Prior TURP (transurethral resectioning) does not exclude the use of HDR. However, any radiation treatment can increase the incidence of urinary incontinence.
- Either extracapsular penetration or seminal-vesicle involvement.
- Perineural invasion.
- Localized recurrent prostate cancer.

Who Does Not Qualify for HDR?

Prostate cancer patients do not qualify for HDR if they have the following problems:

- Spread of cancer to specific organs (metastases).
- Significant radiation damage to nearby organs (usually the rectum) caused by prior radiation treatments.

Side Effects of HDR

Physicians who have used both permanent seeds and HDR are unanimous in their opinion that HDR produces side effects of shorter duration than those associated with standard brachytherapy. According to published long-term studies, major complications are uncommon:

- Serious cases (grade 3 to grade 4) of long-term rectal injury are unusual.
- Grade 3 and 4 urinary morbidity is rare in previously untreated patients and is less than 5 percent in men who had prior TURPs.

Typical acute side effects of HDR, which last for a few weeks, may include:

- urinary frequency
- blood in the urine
- some urinary retention
- rectal irritation
- perineal discomfort

Pretreatment

The prospective patient is required to complete a preconsultation checklist before to scheduling an appointment so that the medical staff can determine if he is an appropriate candidate. Medical history, physical exam, urologic exam (DRE, ultrasound), PSA history, any CT/MRI and bone scan reports, and pathology reports are all necessary in order to assess the patient's disease. Sometimes the patient is required to get other tests such as the endorectal MRI. Before Andy Grove underwent HDR, he had an endorectal MRI to determine if the cancer had broken through the prostate. This diagnostic procedure is a step above any other diagnostic technique in determining extracapsular penetration.

Consultation

Upon reviewing the patient's medical history and most recent test results, the patient and the doctor mutually agree to proceed with HDR. The procedure is explained, and possible side effects are mentioned. The physician may also do a digital rectal examination and a pre-implant ultrasound. HDR is administered in multiple treatments or fractions. Some HDR centers do one implant and deliver three or four treatments per implant, so they require a two-night hospital stay. Other centers perform two implants, separated by a week, where only two to three treatments per implant are delivered, and only a one-night hospital stay is needed. The reasons for the variations in treatment delivery are discussed with the patient during the consultation.

HDR Procedure

In the operating room, the patient is given a spinal anesthetic, numbing him from the waist down. Using fluoroscopy, cystoscopy, and ultrasound to guide him or her, the physician inserts thin, flexible plastic catheters around and through the prostate. The catheters are held in position by a rubber template that is sutured to the perineum, the space between the scrotum and the anus. The template will remain in place until all the treatments are complete. After a brief time in the recovery room, the patient undergoes radiographic imaging, usually a CT scan. The images of the implant and the internal structures are then entered into the "treatment-planning" computer and the patient waits while the radiation dose plan is devised. The physicist or dosimetrist adjusts the time the source spends in each of the dwell positions in each catheter in order to shape the radiation so that the prostate is totally encompassed by the prescription dose; the doses to the bladder, urethra, and rectum are minimized. Once the physician approves the treatment plan, the instructions are programmed into the afterloader. The afterloader guides the single, tiny radioactive iridium-192 source in and out of each of the catheters. The patient can hear the motor as it guides the source in each of the catheters. The patient is also in audio and visual contact with the physician during the treatment.

Before the patient goes to his hospital room, stabilizer rods are inserted into the flexiguides. The patient is told he can roll from side to side, and elevate the head of the bed a little, but not to sit upright or put pressure on the template.

Before each treatment, the implant is checked using fluoroscopy to make sure that the catheters have remained in the same position since the previous treatment.

After the treatments are completed, the template and catheters are removed. The patient may have some soreness in the perineal area for a few days, so activities like bicycle riding should be avoided.

Advantages of HDR over Permanent Seeds

• Because of the ability to control the time the source spends in each dwell position, cold and hot spots are eliminated with HDR. With permanent seeds, once they are implanted, they cannot be adjusted or moved; thus the doses cannot be adjusted.

• With HDR, the doses to the surrounding tissues are known before any radiation is given. Due to the shifting of permanent seeds, the actual doses to the surrounding tissues are not known until they "settle," which takes about a month. A post-seed implant CT scan is done to identify the seeds and do the dose calculations to see what the surrounding tissues and the prostate actually received. If there is a cold or hot spot, nothing can be done to rectify the situation.

• HDR does a better job of treating any extracapsular disease with doses that are accurate and adequate.

• With HDR, radiation exposure to others is eliminated, and there are no seeds to migrate into the lungs. The side effects of HDR are of shorter duration than are those of permanent seeds.

How to Use This Information

Although HDR is not supported by a 10-year study, consider this treatment if you are a high-risk prostate cancer patient.

Chapter 18

LIVING WITH HORMONE-REFRACTORY PROSTATE CANCER

When metastatic prostate cancer is refractory to hormonal therapy (stage D3), it is not always amenable to successful treatment. Although initial response rate of 75 to 80 percent for either surgical or chemical castration are common, when patients are hormonally sensitive, most patients with metastatic hormonally refractory prostate cancer will progress within one year. Usually, the goal of doctor is to try to give the patient more time, as well as to diminish his symptoms and relieve him of any pain. Studies that are ongoing will hopefully show both efficacy and improve both quality of life and survival.

If initial hormonal therapy fails, the doctor will attempt what is frequently referred to as *second-line hormonal manipulation therapy* by doing two things:

1.   The doctor will take the patient off any antiandrogen he may be taking and observe his PSA level. In about 30 percent of patients, treatment is usually not needed until the PSA increases.
2.   When the PSA level begins to rise, the patient may be placed on Nizoral with or without hydrocortisone. If this procedure fails, the doctor may suggest clinical trials.

Defining the Hormonally Refractive Condition

Hormonal refraction describes a condition in which the once-dominant hormonally sensitive, or dependent, cells become subordinate to hormonally insensitive, or independent, cells. These cancer cells will begin to increase and grow in areas where they are already located and may spread to other areas, such as bones and other organs.

Most, if not all, of the information on combination hormone therapy (CHT) states that it will not cure prostate cancer but will only palliate it. The survival ratefor stage D2 patients on CHT is said to be between 2 and 3 years. However, for some reason about 5 to 10 percent of the patients receiving CHT actually live for 10 years or more. In fact, in some patients who have undergone CHT for years, a physical examination, including biopsy of the prostate, demonstrated that cancer cells could no longer be found. Some of these patients elected to discontinue therapy and be

133

monitored carefully. The biggest problem, which physicians have not solved, is how these patients can be identified.

Hormonally Refractory Prostate Cancer: Two Theories

There seem to be two schools of thought about the origin of androgen or hormonally insensitive or independent prostate cancer cells, as illustrated in Figures 18-1 and 18-2.

Figure 18-1. Homogeneous Model for Hormonally Refractory Disease

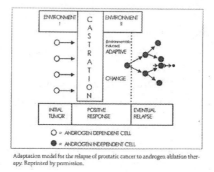

Adaptation model for the relapse of prostatic cancer to androgen ablation ther-apy. Reprinted by permission.

Adaptation Model for the Relapse of Prostate Cancer to Androgen Ablation Therapy. Reprinted with permission.

The homogeneous theory suggests that initially, prostate cancer cells are homogenous in terms of their requirements for androgen. Following either surgical or medical castration, most of these cells stop reproducing and die, thus producing an initial response to hormonal deprivation. However, some of these hormonally dependent cells randomly adapt as a result of environmental conditions to become hormonally independent. Thus, these hormonally independent cells begin to grow and repopulate the tumor, producing a rise in the PSA. This homogenous theory postulates that changes in the host's environmental milieu following hormonal therapy are critical in introducing a change in an initially hormonally dependent cell to a hormonally independent tumor cell.

Dr. Fernand Labrie, the "father" of CHT, believes that all prostate cancer cells are initially hormonally responsive. He maintains that some cells are much more sensitive than others and that, unless all forms of androgen can be eliminated from the body, the ultrasensitive cells will continue to multiply and divide. Theoretically, then, the more complete the androgen blockade treatment, the more effective the therapy will be against these clones of cells. Eventually, however, these cells mutate to become hormonally insensitive, or refractory. The second theory espoused by many doctors is that prostate cancer cells are heterogeneous in their need for androgens to grow.

Figure 18-2 Heterogeneous Model for Hormonally Refractory Disease

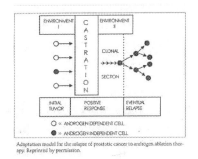

Adaptation model for the relapse of prostatic cancer to androgen ablation therapy. Reprinted by permission.

Adaptation Model for the Relapse of Prostate Cancer to Androgen Ablation Therapy. Reprinted with permission.

The heterogeneous model maintains that prostate cancer cells are composed of preexisting clones of both hormonally dependent and independent prostate cancer cells. As a result, hormonal deprivation would cause the death of hormonally dependent cells without affecting the growth of hormonally independent tumor cells. Even if the hormonally independent cells represented only a small portion of the original tumor, they would, however, eventually replace any tumor loss due to the death of hormonally dependent cells and would contribute to the expansion of the prostate cancer cell population.

This theory seems to be echoed by Dr. Stephen B. Strum. In "How Do You Beat Disease Progression When Primary Hormonal Therapy Is No Longer Effective?" (1995), he writes: "Prostate cancer will involve clones of androgen sensitive, androgen insensitive, and possible androgen-altered cells. This heterogeneity may be related to tumor size in what is called tumor bundles. With increased tumor bundles, the frequency of gene mutation increases, which in turn may lead to hormone resistance." He continues, "Mutations involving activation of oncogenes are probable." He identifies a sequence for his theory: "Increased tumor burden produces gene mutation that stimulates oncogenes, which results in hormonally independent or insensitive cells."

Drs. Patrick C. Walsh and Leonard G. Gomella believe this theory, too. They seem to agree that prostate cancer consists of a mixture of cells, dependent or independent. According to Dr. Walsh's book The Prostate (1997), prostate cancer cells are a bunch of different cells mixed up together, so a drug treatment that targets one band of cells, for instance, will not have any effect against another group. The cancer is made up of many different landscape cells, and some of them have learned to be resistant, to grow in the absence of androgens (male hormones).

Yousuf Sharief, M.D., et al. maintain that if androgen receptor gene mutations play a role in androgen-independent prostate cancer growth, the cells with androgen receptor mutations should be found more often in hormone-refractory prostate cancer than in radical prostatectomy specimens. However, this was not the case. Researchers in the Netherlands obtained fresh tissue from the primary tumors of 20 prostate cancer patients with hormonally refractory disease. In 11 of the patients, DNA was isolated and amplified by polymerase chain reaction (PCR). No mutation was found. In 15 patients in whom RNA was extracted, splicing errors were not detected by RT-PCR. Studies therefore suggest that mutations of the androgen receptors are not associated with hormonally refractory prostate cancer. In the final analysis, the hormonal therapy will not affect those cancer cells thought to include as many as 10 to 20 percent that are not hormone dependent.

According to Dr. Walsh, "Scientists believe that these adaptive-independent cells probably inhabit the prostate for years." They do not just suddenly appear one day after the cancer is diagnosed. The big questions are: (1) Does hormonal treatment produce mutation of hormonally dependent cells to hormonally independent cells? (2) If it does, at what point does this occur? There is recent evidence that prolonged hormonal therapy can produce an androgen receptor mutation, which may be one of the mechanisms leading to hormonally refractory disease. Therefore, another important question is: Does intermittent hormonal therapy help prevent this from occurring?

Dealing with Hormonally Refractory Disease

The six phases for dealing with hormonally refractory prostate cancer presented here could well be called a systematic approach. The omission of one phase or a poorly developed phase could shorten the life of the prostate cancer patient. Each phase should be attended to in sequence.

Phase 1: Monitor Disease Stage

To understand the stage pertinent to hormonally refractory disease, you should understand its subdivision. Essentially, hormonal refraction deals with stage D3; however, all of stage D is described below:

- D0: In stage "D-zero," prostatic acid phosphatase is elevated, suggesting that the cancer has spread to the pelvic lymph nodes despite negative X-ray tests such as CT scan.
- D1: In this stage, tumor cells have spread to lymph nodes in the lower pelvic area adjacent to the prostate but have not spread any further. This is usually documented by open or laparoscopic biopsy, but sometimes by obviously positive CT scan, MRI scan of the pelvis, or ProstaScint scan.
- D2: In this stage, cancer has spread to the skeleton (bones), organs, or other tissues.
- D3: In this stage, at least some of the cancer cells are no longer responsive to hormonal manipulation.

Once you are aware of the stage of your disease, your next step is to identify one or more methods with which to monitor yourself. As stated throughout this book, markers that are useful for monitoring your disease are the AP (alkaline phosphatase) for bone metastases, as well as the PAP and PSA for metastatic disease. Stage D patients should monitor their disease at least on a quarterly basis; however, a monthly monitoring schedule may be required.

Other monitoring methods include:

- CT scan
- MRI
- X-ray
- bone biopsy
- ProstaScint scan or spectroscopic MRI
- PET scan may soon be approved, but at present it is still experimental

These tests are usually used less often than the PSA test.

Phase 2: Monitor Disease Progression

As mentioned previously, PSA is the best marker for diagnosing and following the results of the treatment of prostate cancer patients. A continuous rise in the PSA on two or three consecutive occasions indicates a treatment change may be mandated. However, a stabilizing of, or decline in, the PSA would suggest that the treatment has been effective or should remain unchanged.

If you are on CHT and your PSA increases on two or more occasions, your doctor should strongly consider withdrawing the antiandrogen (Casodex, Eulexin, or Nilandron). Approximately 30 percent of patients who stop the antiandrogen will show a decline in their PSA level. This phenomenon, referred to as a *rebound regression,* lasts an average of 3 to 4 months but can last much longer in some patients.

Phase 3: Try Hormonal Manipulation Again

If after 4 to 8 weeks of antiandrogen withdrawal there is no decline in the PSA level, other hormonal manipulations may be tried, including treatment with antiandrogens that have not yet been used, use of progestational agents such as Megace, and treatment with Nizoral in conjunction with hydrocortisone.

Phase 4: Treat Hormonally Refractory Disease

Doctors use a variety of approaches to treat hormonally refractory patients. However, it is usually wise to seek the expertise of a medical oncologist, especially one who subspecializes in treating prostate cancer patients. Although no hormonal or chemotherapeutic regimen has yet shown a clear-cut survival difference in randomized controlled trials (once the disease had become hormonally refractory), it does not necessarily mean that individual patients cannot benefit from a secondary treatment. Indeed, several studies in the literature and anecdotal case reports indicate that there are still effective treatments for individual patients.

Phase 5: Consider a Clinical Trial

When all else fails, your doctor should determine if you are eligible to participate in a clinical trial. Some patients involved in clinical trials have had a few years added to their lives.

Phase 6: Consider a Complementary Treatment Plan

A complementary treatment plan is one that involves a supplement to your medical treatment such as herbs, vitamins, or other substances that do not interfere with your medical therapy. Usually, complementary treatment will cause you no harm, and it may help your condition. (See Chapters 26 and 41.)

Dr. Mario A. Eisenberger of the University of Maryland states that "current data suggest that prostate specific antigen (PSA) is a marker that may be helpful in defining active disease and is likely to represent a major and valuable therapeutic benefit." He continues, "Data from large prospective studies indicate that major PSA decreases are seen with hormone ablative treatments and that the degree of PSA drop may be of major predictive value with regard to survival of stage D2 patients. This same observation is less well-defined in hormonally refractory patients, especially since the activities of hormonal treatments have been much superior to combination cytotoxic chemotherapy."

Monitoring the Prognosis of Your Stage D Status

Some patients with advanced prostate cancer are eager to know how long they have to live. That is, they want to know as accurately as possible the prognosis of their disease. In the near future, doctors will be able to input pertinent medical data into a computer and retrieve a printout of the probable prognosis. In the meantime, these patients should have a basic understanding of the prognostic indicators that will give the best prediction of their longevity.

A variety of potential prognostic factors have been studied in prostate cancer, including the following:

- age
- weight loss
- pain from metastases
- performance status
- hemoglobin level
- stage D0, D1, D2, or D3
- Gleason grade and sum
- extent of metastatic disease
- number of hot spots on bone scan
- presence of soft-tissue deposits
- estimate of "minimal disease" versus "severe disease"
- serum testosterone
- acid and alkaline phosphatase levels
- creatinine (kidney test)
- PSA level
- changes in PSA level following treatment

139

However, of all of these prognostic indicators, hemoglobin level, alkaline phosphatase level, and pain score appear to be the most important.

Using these indicators, a study is currently being conducted that has developed a formula that separates three prognostic groups - namely, good, intermediate, and poor prognoses - with a median survival time of 5.4, 2.9, and 1.7 years, respectively. However, more work has to be done before the formula is ready for use by physicians.

In the meantime, your doctor should carefully study the following points in order to give you a gross estimate of your prognosis:

1. *PSA*: The PSA level is a useful prognostic indicator for patients with advanced prostate cancer in two different contexts:

   - Researchers have found that patients with a PSA level less than 10 ng/ml rarely have skeletal metastases, regardless of clinical stage or grade. A bone scan, however, would certainly be useful if you are one of the few patients who do have bone metastases and are about to undergo radical surgery or any other invasive treatment. Remember, it is better to be safe than sorry - it is better to have too much information about your condition than too little.

   - As an indicator of response to treatment, PSA level usually declines after treatment in most patients. Research has shown that the lowest PSA level 3 to 6 months after treatment is an effective prognostic indicator. One study observed that 48 percent (20 of 41 patients) with a PSA level less than 10 ng/ml progressed for an average of 2 years compared to 91 percent (20 of 22 patients) whose PSA level did not fall below 10 ng/ml. Another study found that stage D patients whose PSA level was normal or undetectable after 6 months of treatment had the best chance of long-term survival.

1. *Extent of disease*: A few studies have demonstrated that patients with five or fewer bone metastases gain the most from CHT when this therapy is compared to orchiectomy or a LHRH agonist alone. However, further study of a larger number of patients is necessary to confirm this finding.

2. *Bone scan:* Some researchers have reported that the number of hot spots observed on bone scans in over 100 patients revealed that survival correlated with the number of metastases. Those patients with fewer than six deposits had a significantly longer survival time than did those with more. It appears that the earlier CHT is initiated

in these cases, the more effective treatment is. Delaying the onset of hormonal therapy is rightfully becoming a thing of the past.

When treatment is indicated, many doctors prescribe CHT for their patients. The best time to start hormonal therapy is still being debated. However, if the number of hot spots on a bone scan is the basis for making a decision, it would probably be wise to begin hormonal therapy before six or more hot spots appear. Theoretically, the less cancer there is, the more effective therapy should be. Therefore, most physicians who treat prostate cancer no longer wait for the disease to become symptomatic but instead treat it as soon as metastatic disease (or sometimes recurrent disease) is evident. This follows a general oncologic principle: the earlier you use an effective treatment in the course of the disease (i.e., the fewer cancer cells present), the more effective the therapy will be. This concept has led to advances in the treatment of other cancers such as breast and testicular cancer and so should be applicable to prostate cancer as well.

Recently, doctors have given more consideration to providing patients with intermittent hormonal therapy, not only to possibly prolong their lives, but also to improve the quality of their lives. However, more studies have to be done to prove the efficacy of this theory.

As discussed throughout this section, several prognostic indicators seem to be indicative for long-term survival of a patient with advanced prostate cancer:

- Five or fewer bone metastases on the bone scan.
- The lowest PSA level is achieved after 3 to 6 months of treatment and continues to stay at that level.
- Hormonal therapy is started prior to the development of five bone metastases or ten metastases of any kind.

These indicators are only guidelines and should not be considered as definitive for maximizing longevity. There are patients with a large number of metastases who have survived for many years. In other words, there are always exceptions to the rule, so patients should not give up hope.

Treating Hormone Refractory Disease

This section presents a variety of techniques and drugs that two doctors use to treat hormone refractory patients. Discuss these treatments with your physician to arrive at one that may help your condition.

Options for Therapy in Hormone-Refractory Prostate Cancer by E. Roy Berger, M.D., F.A.C.P.

The way I approach the disease is based upon a combination of my experience as well as that of other medical oncologists and urologists who treat this perplexing disorder and, of course, the medical literature.

First, I would like to make it clear that my overall approach in treating hormone-refractory prostate cancer is based upon the overall clinical picture of the patient. For example, the therapy prescribed for a patient whose PSA is rising after receiving hormonal therapy, without any evidence of gross metastatic disease and who is asymptomatic, will be very different than the treatment given the patient who has symptomatic disease that is hormone-refractory. Generally, I try to walk the fine line between (1) the anxiety of patients and their families when the PSA rises in an asymptomatic patient and the "need" to treat that patient versus (2) the side effects and toxicity and potential decrease in quality of life that the treatment might cause. This is especially important when one considers the literature that shows that no treatment to date has yet shown a survival benefit once a patient becomes hormone refractory. My personal belief is that the latter statement is not correct; however, it must be taken into consideration when an individual physician is prescribing treatment for an individual patient.

I will now review some of the major treatment options available to hormone-refractory patients without going into great detail about the multiple and exciting research that is being done in several areas, including gene therapy, vaccine therapy, and new drug treatments.

First, it is important to define hormone-refractory prostate cancer, a definition that to most of us is a rising serial PSA with two to three values at least two to three weeks apart in the presence of castrate levels of testosterone. In patients who have metastatic disease and meet this criterion, the median survival is generally less than one year.

There are many different presentations of hormone-refractory prostate cancer, and the preceding statement only applies to men who have gross metastatic disease. Therefore, extent of disease becomes quite important – that is, does the patient have measurable or gross metastases versus biochemical PSA progression? is the patient asymptomatic versus symptomatic? Is the patient totally hormone-refractory versus hormone insensitive?

Metastatic disease is usually made up of three different cell lines composed of hormone-dependent cells, partially hormone-dependent cells, and hormone-independent cells. As a patient's tumors proceed from hormone sensitive to partially hormone responsive to hormone-refractory, the number of hormone-dependent cells decrease and the number of hormone independent cells increase. During this continuum, there remain some partially hormone-dependent cells, which can be manipulated through a variety of mechanisms.

The first question that must be addressed is, Should primary hormonal therapy be continued? To date, there have been no prospective trials to answer this question. Retrospective data are somewhat conflicting and address survival instead of quality of life. We do know that patients who are given exogenous testosterone have symptomatic worsening in 95 percent of cases. Because, as stated previously, there are hormone-dependent cells usually still present in most tumors, most of us who treat prostate cancer continue an LHRH agonist or some form of primary hormonal therapy if the patient has not undergone bilateral orchiectomy in order to treat those hormone-dependent cells.

In general, the options for treating this disease once it has become hormone-refractory include:

1.   second-line hormonal manipulation
2.   chemotherapy
3.   radiation
4.   investigational approaches on clinical trials

When considering what to do with a patient who has become hormone refractory, one must consider his performance status, symptoms, and comorbidity, as well as the location of the metastatic disease, cost, and, finally, logistics.

With all this in mind, one must be able to determine whether or not the patient is responding. We generally evaluate responses in hormone-refractory disease by evaluating (1) measurable disease, (2) PSA decline (greater than 50% or greater than 75%), (3) time to progression, (4) quality-of-life issues, and (5) survival.

PSA level has been shown to be a prognostic factor in hormone-refractory disease. No absolute number correlates with survival, but a greater than 50 percent decrease in PSA is considered a partial response and appears correlate with increased survival.

Second-line hormonal manipulations that are frequently used include:

- antiandrogen withdrawal
- antiandrogen addition
- estrogens

143

- ketoconazole (Nizoral)
- aminoglutethimide
- corticosteroids

The antiandrogen withdrawal syndrome was first observed with flutamide; however, it has also been reported with bicalutamide, nilutamide, ketoconazole, DES, and Megace. It is used when PSA rises on total androgen blockade. At that time, the antiandrogen is stopped, and within weeks the PSA begins decreasing depending upon the antiandrogen. The PSA response rate varies between 13 and 30 percent for a median of 3.5 months, with a range of 1, to 12 months or longer. Four to 8 weeks is necessary to see if this withdrawal is in fact working by virtue of a PSA decrease.

Secondary hormonal manipulation can come in a few forms; high-dose bicalutamide (Casodex 150 – 200 mg) has been shown to give responses in the range of 15 to 40 percent. The median duration of response is 3.5 to 4 months.

DES and other estrogens, which have been used for years, work by hormonal suppression as well as direct cytotoxicity, often with a decrease in pain and a lowering of PSA. Since DES has been associated with a number of hypercoagulable complications including myocardial infarction, deep vein thrombophlebitis, and pulmonary emboli, it has generally fallen out of favor and in fact is not commercially available. There is, however, a trend toward using low-dose DES (diethylbestrol) in some patients among some physicians who have it compounded by specialty pharmacies.

Until 2001, PC SPES, a Chinese herbal compound sold as a dietary supplement, was available and was believed to be useful in the treatment of hormone-refractory disease. I have used this compound quite often and quite successfully. Its mechanism of action is debated, but it probably has estrogenic, immune-stimulating, and cytotoxic and cytostatic properties. We know that it induces programmed cell death by down-regulating the protein that is associated with continued life of the malignant cell (BCL-2). PSA declined over 50 percent in 100 percent of 31 patients who were hormone-naïve and in 54 percent of 35 patients who were androgen-insensitive. The major side effects were thromboembolic events, gynecomastia, some nausea, and loss of libido. Most of us who have used this drug placed patients on low-dose Coumadin to help prevent the hypercoagulable side effects. Currently, various manufacturers are trying to duplicate this product, as it is no longer available due to governmental restrictions. The original company, BotanicLab, is no longer operating.

Ketoconazole (Nizoral) is an antifungal agent that inhibits cytochrome P-450 enzymes and therefore blocks testicular and adrenal androgenesis. It also probably has direct cytotoxic (cell-killing) effects on the cancer cell, and it has been used by a number of us in association with low-dose hydrocortisone. Ketoconazole is taken on an empty stomach in an acid environment, which is required for absorption (1 gram of vitamin C is especially useful if the patient is on acid-lowering drugs). It is available generically. A total of 60 to 70 percent of men on ketoconazole had a reduction in PSA level of over 50 percent. The main side effects are nausea, liver function test abnormalities, and "sticky skin."

Cortocosteroids have been quite useful to hormone refractory prostate cancer patients over the years. There is an approximately 20 percent PSA response after antiandrogen withdrawal therapy. The optimal dose and the optimal drug are still not known. We do know that prednisone (5 mg twice a day) or low-dose dexamethasone as well as hydrocortisone have all been used, and they all improve appetite and decrease symptoms, especially pain, as well as causing a decrease in PSA as noted previously. The side effects include high blood sugar, edema, and skin and mental-status change. Longer-term effects include cataracts and osteoporosis.

One must ask, "At what point should chemotherapy be considered?" Currently no definite guidelines exist: however, most of us who are students of this disease use it when patients are symptomatic, except in clinical trials. Systemic symptoms include loss of appetite, weight loss, and severe fatigue as well as pain. When the disease goes to organs other than bone, especially liver and lung, chemotherapy should also be considered.

The goals of therapy for hormone-refractory patients include treating their pain and improving their quality of life, or at least maintaining it; increasing symptom-free survival; and if at all possible, increasing survival time.

Chemotherapeutic options include:

- mitoxantrone and steroids
- estramustine combinations
- taxanes: Taxol and Taxotere
- other single-agent chemotherapy agents or combinations
- investigational approaches

Mitoxantrone and prednisone have been shown to improve palliative response approximately twofold greater than steroids alone with a threefold improvement in pain. It was approved by the FDA for use in hormone-refractory disease on the basis of this palliative effect. Although it has no survival benefit, it has been shown to be well-tolerated and useful in decreasing symptoms and improving quality of life. It should not, however, be used in patients who have decreased cardiac ejection fraction, but it is otherwise tolerated very well, even in patients who have poor performance status.

Estramustine phosphate (Emcyt) and either VP-16 or Velban have been shown to decrease PSA in approximately 50 to 60 percent of patients, and adding Emcyt to Velban alone may extend survival slightly. This is another regimen that some physicians use in hormone-refractory disease. It is, however, associated with nausea and an increase in thromboembolic events due to the Emcyt, for which most doctors prescribe some anticoagulant.

In my opinion, the most exciting chemotherapeutic advance in the last three decades has been the use of taxane-based chemotherapy in the treatment of hormone-refractory prostate cancer. This treatment can be considered:

- when there is liver or lung metastasis and/or a low PSA (suggesting a small cell variant of prostate cancer)
- rapidly progressive disease
- symptomatic progressive disease
- mitoxantrone and prednisone failure

It can also be used experimentally as front-line therapy in cases where the prognosis is poor (on a clinical trial).

In single-agent studies, both docetaxel (Taxotere) and paclitaxel (Taxol) have been known to have a 40 to 46 percent decline in PSA (greater than 50%) and a 20 to 50 percent measurable response with Taxotere, showing a median survival of 27 months in 35 patients tested. This in itself is fairly unusual, because as stated above, the median survival for hormone-refractory patients is less than 12 months.

When Taxotere was combined with Estramustine, 60 to 90 percent of patients had a PSA decline more than 50 percent, and 25 to 60 percent showed a greater than 75 percent decline, with objective responses of approximately 25 to 75 percent. Improvement in performance status or pain control (greater than 50%) was seen in more than 50 percent of the patients. I suspect that this combination may increase survival time, and there are ongoing randomized controlled trials testing this hypothesis. The results of these trials are eagerly awaited. My personal experience with this combination has been quite positive, as it is easy to administer, relatively free of major side effects, and quite effective in palliating pain and improving quality of life. I believe the Taxotere/Emcyt combination will become the gold standard of chemotherapy in the next several years.

Other modalities used in hormone-refractory patients include external beam radiation and intravenous radiopharmaceuticals, including strontium89 and samarium153.

External beam radiation is used to decrease pain at specific sites and is usually completed in 10 to 15 fractions of radiation treatments. Acute toxicity depends on the site that is irradiated. External beam radiation is especially useful to treat areas of spinal cord compression, and it can be used in conjunction with intravenous radiopharmaceuticals, or bone-seeking agents, which decrease pain in approximately 80 percent of patients. Radiation can compromise bone marrow function; therefore, treatment must be individualized. Usually it is used in patients who have pain in more than one site.

A class of drugs called *bisphosphonates* can inhibit bone resorption and have been shown to reduce fractures and pain from bony metastases. Zoledronate (Zometa) has been shown to be 100 times as potent as the formerly used pamidronate, and it is given over 15 minutes instead of 1.5 hours. This agent should be considered in anyone who has metastatic disease in the bones, especially if they are hormone-refractory, to alleviate pain and avoid skeletal related events. It is increasingly used in patients who are on long-term LHRH-agonist therapy to decrease osteoporosis, a complication of this regimen.

A number of other agents undergoing clinical trials include:

- Atrasentan (ABT-627)
- Provenge vaccine
- thalidomide
- Endothelin-1 (ET-1)
- Iressa (ZD 1839), an EGFR agonist
- Genasense (BCL-2 antisense)
- YM598-ETA receptor antagonist
- 2ME2, a natural derivative of estradiol
- Geldnamysin (17-AAG)
- Bevacizumab (anti-VEGF [vacular endothelial growth factor] antibody)
- Broyostatin (protein kinase C inhibitor)

In summary, the goals of therapy in hormone-refractory patients are to maintain or improve quality of life and, if at all possible, increase survival. The treatment must be individualized according to the patient's needs and ability to take therapy.

Patients who are suffering from prostate cancer today certainly have more hope than at any time in the past, as a number of these therapies are quite exciting for palliating symptoms and possibly improving survival. We anxiously await the results of clinical trials, which will help determine which agents are most useful.

Prescription Drug Alternatives to PC SPES by Stephen Strum, M.D.

If your testosterone level is less than 20 ng/dl and your other indicators of disease are rising, then you probably have androgen-independent prostate cancer (AIPC), or hormonal-refractory disease. In this setting, you have the choice of considering DES, Climara or Estraderm patches, or injectable estrogen such as estradurin or stilphosterol. You could also use high-dose ketoconazole with hydrocortisone (HDK + HC) and/or chemotherapy. The easiest of these therapies are: DES, Climara or Estraderm patches, and HDK + HC. All of these require the care of a physician well-versed in their use of these anti-PC therapies.

Some of you may already be on Lupron or Zoladex with one of the antiandrogens like Eulexin, Casodex, or Nilandron and have problems with a progressively rising PSA. In this case, it is important to first determine your testosterone level. If it is greater than 20 ng/dl, the situation may be brought under control by determining the source of excess testosterone and reducing it. Elevated testosterone may be due to enhanced activity of the adrenal glands, which make "androgen precursors," substances such as DHEA-S and androstenedione, that can be measured in the blood. If these are in the high normal or elevated range, they are a likely cause of the elevated testosterone. In such circumstances, HDK + HC can be used to lower them.

If the testosterone is over 20 ng/dl, the luteinizing hormone (LH) level should also be checked. LH is a substance that is normally suppressed by Lupron or Zoladex. However, some patients may not be receiving these drugs on schedule, may have problems absorbing the drugs, or may have other reasons for not seeing LH suppressed. The LH level of patients on either Lupron or Zoladex should be less than 1.0. Therefore, if the testosterone level is above 20 ng/dl, and the LH is 1.0 or higher, your physician should consider the other drug (Lupron or Zoladex) and/or make sure you are on the proper schedule for receiving the drug. The proper interval could be either every 29, 84, or 112 days, depending on the Lupron or Zoladex formulation you are using.

If the testosterone is less than 20 ng/dl and the PSA level is rising, one of two major scenarios might be operating. First, if you are on a drug like Eulexin, Casodex, or Nilandron, you might have developed what is called a mutation in the androgen receptor. If so, stopping the antiandrogen and looking for antiandrogen withdrawal response (confirmed by a drop in

PSA and/or other markers of prostate cancer) is an appropriate therapy. You can also institute one of the listed therapies for androgen-independent disease.

You could take DES (1 mg, 3 times a day) after first having your blood thinned with an anticoagulant such as Coumadin. The level of anticoagulant is expressed as an International Ratio (INR) and should be between 2.0 and 2.5. Coumadin is the anticoagulant of choice based on the medical literature; aspirin is not.

If you select Climara or Estraderm patches as your choice, the literature indicates that clotting problems should not occur even without the use of Coumadin. The dose of Climara we suggest that your doctor consider is 0.1 mg, using two patches at one time (one placed on the right buttock and one on the left) once a week. New patches are applied each week, and the old patches are removed. The buttocks are used because absorption there is better than the abdomen.

With any estrogenic therapy, the chance of nipple tenderness and breast enlargement is significant. An appropriate way to prevent this is with radiation therapy for 4 days, at 300 cGy per day. For radiation therapy to work most effectively, it must be used prior to starting any estrogenic compound. You would need a referral to a radiation oncologist from your physician to receive prophylactic breast radiation.

IF HDK + HC is chosen, the dose of HDK is 200 mg, 3 times a day, for the first week, and then 400 mg, 3 times a day, thereafter. HDK comes as a 200-mg tablet. HDK is best taken with Diet Coke or Diet Pepsi to enhance absorption. When using HDK, it is important to take hydrocortisone (20 mg) with breakfast and with dinner. After 3 to 4 weeks, if there are no problems with side effects, the evening dose of HC can be reduced to 10 mg while the morning dose is continued.

We are concerned that, since PC SPES is not currently available, prostate cancer patients may not be availing themselves of an effective therapy. If your PSA is rising or you have any other indications that your cancer is progressing, please seek immediate medical assistance. The Prostate Cancer Research Foundation (www.prostate-cancer.org) will make every attempt to refer you to the best prostate cancer specialists in your area. Please call the organization's helpline at 310-743-2116 and ask to speak to one of the helpline staff.

How to Use This Information

Should your disease progress to a hormonally refractory state, your main goal will be to survive as long as possible with a good quality of life.

Keep searching for new drugs and treatments. In doing so, keep the following in mind:

1. Monitor your prostate cancer at least every 3 months by getting a digital rectal examination and a PSA blood test. Remain alert for three consecutive rises.

2. Discuss this chapter with your doctor, and determine if any changes should be made in your treatment plan.

3. Research the therapies mentioned in this chapter. Be aware of the side effects.

4. Attempt to maximize longevity on each treatment phase mentioned in this chapter. For example, before considering treatment for hormonally refractory disease, remain on hormonal therapy as long as possible. Consider intermittent hormonal therapy. Do the same for chemotherapy.

5. Look for alternative treatments that are known to have efficacy to complement your medical treatment plan. Some patients have favorable results with alternative treatments.

Chapter 19

NEUTRON BEAM RADIATION

Neutron beam therapy is a very effective form of external beam radiation. Some medical doctors and literature maintain that certain advanced tumor types are very difficult to kill using conventional radiation therapy. These advanced tumors are referred to as <u>radioresistant</u>. However, neutron beam radiation specializes in inoperable radioresistant tumors appearing in the human body.

Conventional radiation therapies include photon and electron beam radiation, which are available at major clinics and hospitals in the country. Conventional radiation beams are produced by electron accelerators or from radioactive sources such as cobalt. On the other hand, particle radiation therapies include proton beam radiation and neutron beam radiation, which are produced by proton accelerators.

External beam radiation is one of several ways to treat prostate cancer as well as other cancers. The purpose of radiation therapy is to destroy the ability of cancerous cells to divide and grow by destroying their DNA strands. However, in photon, electron, and proton beam radiation, the injury is done primarily by activated free radicals, which are produced from the atomic interactions. These forms of radiation are referred to as low linear energy transfer (low LET) radiation. Neutron radiation's injury is performed by high LET radiation. If a cancerous tumor cell is injured by low LET radiation, it has an excellent chance to repair itself and to continue to grow. With high LET radiation (neutron beam), the probability that an injured tumor cell will repair itself is rather small.

Defining Neutron Beam Radiation

Neutron beam radiation is an approach to external beam radiation that uses the neutron as the particle to deliver energy to destroy DNA. This type of radiation acts directly on the DNA and is defined as a high linear energy transfer (high LET) radiation as opposed to photon, electron, and proton radiation that acts upon DNA (low LET) indirectly via activated hydroxyl radicals.

How Does Neutron Radiation Work?

Neutrons duplicate the same pattern of dose distribution as photons but deposit from 20 to 100 times more ionizing radiation per unit of tissue traversed. Although neutrons cannot be directed or aimed any better than photons, neutrons can deliver improved radiation damage along their path through a variety of ways. The biological impacts of this deposition of energy are numerous.

Cellular sensitivity to neutrons is less affected by certain tumor parameters, which frequently limit photon radiosensitivity. These factors involve slow tumor growth kinetics or inadequate tumor oxygenation. Photon radiosensitivity varies a great deal according to cellular position in the cell cycle. Neutron effectiveness is much less dependent on cell cycle. Slow-growing tumors as well as poorly oxygenated tumors are usually radioresistant to photons. Because neutron effectiveness is independent of cell cycle and oxygenation, repair of damage to tumor DNA is less a problem following neutron radiation than following photon radiation. Therefore, the net result of these differences is that neutrons cause more cell damage than does an equal amount of photon radiation. The biological effectiveness of a dose of neutrons relative to photons will vary depending on the tumor type or organ radiated, and it often varies from proportionality constant of 3 to 8. When specific tumors realize an incrementally greater sensitivity to high LET radiation than to normal surrounding tissues, an important goal has been achieved.

When Is Neutron Beam Radiation Appropriate?

Neutron beam radiation is appropriate for prostate cancer patients who have disease in the following sites, depending on the stage and histology:

- prostate gland
- bladder
- large tumors and metastasis
- neutron-sensitive tumors
- bulky stage T2 and T3 tumors
- tumors in the seminal vesicles
- PSA above 30 ng/ml
- recurrence after surgery
- Gleason score of 7 or higher
- pelvic lymph-node involvement

COMPARATIVE ANALYSIS OF THREE FORMS OF RADIATION

	NEUTRON BEAM	PROTON BEAM	PHOTON BEAM
PSA level	30 ng/ml or higher	20 ng/ml or lower	20 ng/ml or lower
Gleason score	7 or higher	1-7	1-7
Tumor size	Bulky	40 cc	40 cc
Stage	T1 – T4	T1, T2, some T3	T1, T2, some T3
Treatment	4 weeks	5-8 weeks	5-8 weeks
Sites	Lymph-nodes and seminal vesicles	No seminal-vesicle involvement	Seminal vesicles
Dose	20.4 Gy	68 to 84 Gy	68 to 84 Gy

Advantages and Disadvantages of Neutron Beam Therapy

Advantages

Neutron beam therapy offers prostate cancer patients the following advantages:

- It can deposit from 20 to 100 times more ionizing radiation per unit of tissue traversed than can photons.
- There are many biological consequences of this deposition of energy generated by this form of therapy.
- The cellular sensitivity to this therapy is less affected by certain tumor parameters, which limit photon radiosensitivity.
- Slow-growing and poorly oxygenated tumors, typically radioresistant to photons, can be treated with neutrons.
- Injury to tumor DNA is more permanent than it is with photon radiation.
- Neutrons induce cellular injury that is considerably greater than that caused by photons.
- Neutrons can eradicate bulky tumors.
- Five years after treatment, one study found elevated PSA level in 17 percent of neutron-treated patients compared to 45 percent of photon-treated patients.

- In one study, the 5-year actuarial clinical local-regional failure rate was 32 percent for photons but only 11 percent for neutron beam therapy.

Disadvantages

- Only a few treatment facilities offer neutron beam radiation, and patients often have to travel long distances for treatment.

Clinical Trials

Urinary Complications

A study conducted by J.D. Forman et al. involved 273 patients who received conformal neutron and photon irradiation to the prostate seminal vesicles. The researchers collected data on posttreatment urinary complications and examined them in relation to a number of clinical and technical factors. The results revealed that with a median follow-up of 30 months (range: 7-61), the 4-year rate of grade 2 or higher genitourinary complications was 21 percent. Using the univariate analysis, the risk of complication was significantly associated with size of the prostate and neutron beam arrangement. On the multivariate analysis, only the prostate size was significantly associated with the risk of genitourinary complications. In addition, patients whose prostate before radiation was larger than 74 cc had two and a half times the risk of complications that patients with smaller prostate had. The researchers concluded that patients with an enlarged prostate have a higher risk of chronic genitourinary complications than do patients with smaller prostates.

A clinical trial under the auspices of the Radiation Therapy Oncology Group (RTOG) studied 91 prostate cancer patients with stage C and D tumors from 1977 to 1983. The patients were randomized to receive either photon beam radiation or alternating neutrons and photons in a "mixed beam" schedule. Patients on the mixed beam schedule underwent radiation treatment that was approximately 60 percent neutrons for 3 days a week. This combination was chosen due to concerns about the unknown potential for complications using neutrons alone. The photon beam and mixed beam groups were balanced with respect to major prognostic variables. Five- and 10-year actuarial results for clinically assessed local control were 86 percent for the mixed beam group and 61 percent for the photon group. The corresponding 5- and 10-year cancer-specific survival data were 82 percent and 46 percent for the mixed beam group versus 62 percent and 29 percent for the photon group.

Based on these favorable results, a second clinical trial was begun in 1985 in which 172 patients with stage D1, C, and high-grade B2 were randomized and completed treatment. The 5-year actuarial "clinical" local-regional control for patients treated with neutrons or photons was 91 percent and 70 percent, respectively. Combining the results of routine posttreatment prostate biopsies, the resulting "histological" local-regional tumor control rates for neutrons and photons were 82 percent versus 60 percent. By eliminating patients with stage D1 disease, the histological local-regional tumor control rates are the same for both groups, with an actuarial 5-year cancer specific survival of 89 and 92 percent for neutrons and photons, respectively. Because the local-regional tumor control is a determinant of survival, the improved local tumor control achieved by neutrons should realize a survival advantage for the neutron-treated patients when the follow-up data matured.

Accordingly to this study date, complications of treatment were higher for the neutron-treated patients (11% versus 1%). Many of the complications involved the rectum. Rectal complications from neutron treatment were inversely correlated with the degree of neutron beam shaping available at the participating institutions. When neutron beam shaping capabilities allowed conformal radiation fields, severe rectal injury did not occur.

Cost Effectiveness

In another interesting study, R. L. Maughan et al. compared the cost of mixed beam neutron and photon therapy, neutrons alone, and photon therapy in combination with hormone treatment ("The Cost Effectiveness of Mixed Beam Neutron/Photon Radiation Therapy in the Treatment of Adenocarcinoma of The Prostate"). This study indicated that neutron therapy is superior to photon/hormone therapy in achieving local control. The costs for delivering these two different therapies in a large radiation oncology center at Wayne State University were discussed. The cost of a full course of mixed beam therapy was $20,142, compared to $18,871 for the photon/hormone treatment. Although the neutron facility at Wayne State is a state-of-the-art installation, it is also a prototype technology; it is estimated that a modern neutron facility based on the Wayne State design would operate more cost-effectively, thereby reducing the cost of a course of mixed beam therapy to $18,532.

E. Roy Berger, M.D., F.A.C.P. and James Lewis, Jr., Ph.D
Worldwide Experience with Neutrons

A pertinent study by K. L. Lindsley et al. is "Fast Neutrons in Prostatic Adenocarcinomas: Worldwide Clinical Experience." It indicated that clinical local failure rates improved 30 to 40 percent and maybe significantly higher when the result of prostatic biopsy or prostate-specific antigen PSA levels is considered. The low growth rate and cycling fraction of prostate cancer suggest the potential therapeutic advantage of the high linear energy transfer (LET) of neutrons. The Radiation Therapy Oncology trial (RTOG 77-04) compared mixed beam (neutron plus photon) irradiation to conventional photon irradiation for the treatment of locally advanced prostate cancer. A subsequent trial by the Neutron Therapy Collaborative Working Group (NTCWG 85-23) compared pure neutron irradiation to standard photon irradiation. Both randomized trials demonstrated significant improvement in locoregional control with neutron irradiation compared to conventional photon irradiation in the treatment of locally advanced prostate cancer. To date, only the mixed beam trial has shown a significant survival benefit. Future analysis of the larger NTCWG trial at the 10-year point should confirm whether or not improved locoregional control translates into longer survival time.

These findings have significant implications for all local treatment strategies, including dose-escalated conformal photon irradiation, prostate implantation, and neutron radiation. Given the large number of men afflicted with this disease, a positive survival advantage for neutrons or mixed beam therapy would provide a strong incentive for the development of economically feasible clinical neutron facilities.

How to Use This Information

1. If you opt for external beam radiation, consider the neutron approach, particularly if you have been diagnosed with advanced prostate cancer.
2. You may use neutron beam radiation alone or with chemotherapy in treating your prostate cancer.
3. Reserve neutron beam radiation for more advanced prostate cancer patients.
4. The failure rate tends to be more for photon beam radiation than neutron beam radiation.
5. Neutron beam radiation tends to be more appropriate for prostate cancer patients with lymph node involvement than any other form of external beam radiation.

Chapter 20

SEED IMPLANTATION

For more than 10 years, the medical profession relied on three types of treatment for prostate cancer. For early-stage prostate cancer, the gold standard was either radical prostatectomy (removal of the prostate) or external beam radiation. If the disease had spread well beyond the gland, another gold standard known as *bilateral orchiectomy*, or removal of the testicles, was recommended. Any other method, such as external beam radiation or brachytherapy, attempted as a treatment for prostate cancer was frequently discouraged by doctors with comments like, "It is an experimental therapy, and there isn't a five- or ten-year survival study, and therefore, I won't recommend it."

Well, physicians cannot say there is no long-term study to substantiate the treatment we describe next. This treatment was an old unproven one when it was reintroduced by the medical profession in the 1990s, but it has had some excellent results because of improved technology and procedures. What is this treatment? It is *seed implantation*, or *brachytherapy*.

Is seed implantation as effective as radical prostatectomy? Will it become the gold standard for treating prostate cancer patients? It is difficult to say. However, we do know this: many, many radiation oncologists who specialize in external beam radiation have become more proficient in seed implantation, as have many urologists. Although no one has taken a survey of the number of doctors "switching over" to seed implantation, we believe that it is gaining momentum.

A 12-year study done by Dr. Haakon Ragde indicates that seed implantation is "as good or better" than radical prostatectomy. The Northwest Prostate Institute in Seattle has reported on 215 patients treated with brachytherapy and followed for 12 years. The overall control rate was 79 percent, which is equal to or better than the gold standard of 70 percent for radical prostatectomy.

Radiation oncologists in Washington, D.C. (Cancer, July 1, 2000) found that 82 of these patients were considered at high-risk for cancer outside the capsule based on the size of the prostate nodule, Gleason grade, and PSA level; thus, they were treated with both seeds and external beam radiation. Obviously, not all patients should undergo seed implantation only. It appears that only low-risk patients are eligible for this form of treatment. Intermediate- and high-risk patients should get seeds and external beam radiation.

Seed implantation generally has fewer side effects than does radical prostatectomy or cryosurgery. In addition, the recuperation time for most patients treated with brachytherapy is much shorter than with radical prostatectomy, and the procedure is less costly as well.

Understanding the History of Seed Implantation

In the 1970s, Dr. W.F. Whitmore et al. of Memorial Sloan-Kettering Cancer Center in New York performed the first permanent seed implantation using a retropubic approach (abdominal incision above the pubic bone) for inserting iodine-125 (I-125) seeds. This approach required several procedures: (1) removing the lymph nodes for staging purposes, (2) surgically mobilizing the prostate, and (3) freehand inserting of the seeds. During that decade, doctors at Memorial Sloan-Kettering Cancer performed more than a thousand seed implantations, but eventually they abandoned the procedure because of poor results. Unfortunately, their approach proved to be flawed for two reasons: (1) distributing the seeds evenly throughout the cancerous prostate was difficult because of the narrow confines of the pelvis and (2) the poor imaging quality at that time left the physician to more or less insert the seeds "blindly." These two problems, coupled with advances in radical prostatectomy and the refinement of linear accelerators, which improved the effectiveness of external beam radiation, contributed to a waning of interest in the use of seed implantation to treat prostate cancer.

Defining Seed Implantation

Seed implantation is a medical procedure in which a team of physicians (a urologist, radiation oncologist, and radiation physicist) use a radioactive source to irradiate prostate cancer cells, while minimizing radiation to the surrounding tissues. Patients with low to intermediate Gleason scores usually receive I-125 seeds, which have a half-life of 60.2 days; patients with higher Gleason scores usually receive palladium-103 seeds, which have a half-life of 17.0 days. In addition, these higher-risk patients often receive hormonal therapy, external beam radiation, or both. The number of seeds delivered can vary from 50 to 120, depending on the anatomy of the patient and the size of his prostate.

Prostatectomy and Seed Implantation: A Comparison

The following table presents a comparative analysis between radical prostatectomy and seed implantation.

Radical Prostatectomy	Seed Implantation
1. Supported by multiple 10- and 15-year studies.	1. Supported by a 12-year study.
2. Hospital stay of 5-10 days.	2. One-time outpatient or overnight procedure.
3. Cost: $15,000 to $20,000.	3. Cost: $9,000 to $12,000.
4. Suitable for stage A and stage B patients.	4. Suitable for stage A and stage B patients. Stage C patients have been successfully treated in conjunction with external beam radiation
5. Death occurs 1 percent of patients under 75 years of age and 2 percent of patients 75 years and older.	5. No fatalities reported.
6. Some blood loss; occasional transfusion needed.	6. No blood transfusion needed.
7. Lymph nodes, seminal vesicles, and neurovascular bundles are sometimes removed with the prostate.	7. Only in some cases (high-risk patients) are the lymph nodes sampled prior to the procedure Seminal vesicles are sometimes seeded.
8. Not desirable for patients older than 70 or in poor health.	8. Desirable for early-stage disease and works as a boost for high-risk patients. Age is not a factor.
9. General anesthesia is preferred.	9. Spinal or general anesthesia is acceptable.
10. Postoperative patients are usually incontinent for a few weeks to a year, while up to 10 percent of patients suffer long-term incontinence of varying degrees.	10. Incontinence after this procedure is rare.
11. Recurrence rate has been reported to be from 30 to 85 percent within a 10-year period.	11. Recurrence rate is about 21 percent within a 12-year period.

Radical Prostatectomy	Seed Implantation
12. Impotence is reported to occur in 30 to 70 percent of patients.	12. Impotence has been reported to occur in fewer than 20 percent of patients.
13. Usually performed by one or more urologists.	13. Usually performed by a team of a urologist and a radiation oncologist.

Advantages and Disadvantages of Seed Implantation

Although recent studies of seed implantation seem to have reported some excellent advantages, there are also some disadvantages you should be aware of. The advantages are:

- A recent statistical study based on 215 patients followed for 12 years indicates that a higher percentage of implant patients remain free of prostate cancer than with either radical prostatectomy.
- Seed implantation is probably better than surgery for older patients because it is much easier for them to tolerate even when accompanied by external beam radiation.
- A study at the University of California (The Journal of Urology, March 2000) concluded, "At an average of 7.5 months after treatment, the general health related quality of life of patients undergoing brachytherapy with and without pretreatment external beam radiation was similar to age-matched controls."
- Because seeds are inserted directly into the prostate, two or three times more radiation can be concentrated in the site of the disease than can be done with external beam radiation.
- Impotence occurs in fewer than 20 percent of patients under age 70, but more often in patients over 70.
- Side effects are minimal compared to those of radical prostatectomy.
- Postoperative complications are rare and can usually be treated on an outpatient basis.
- It is less costly than either radical prostatectomy or external beam radiation.

The disadvantages are:

- A side effect of seed implantation is frequently burning during urination and sometimes difficulty urinating. However, this subsides after the radiation dose declines. The radiation dose declines for palladium-103 in 3 months and for iodine-125 in 6 to 12 months.
- The size of the tumor must be within an acceptable range; otherwise, CHT, external beam radiation, or both may be needed to shrink the gland and temporarily suppress the growth of the tumor.

Be sure to understand the advantages and disadvantages of seed implantation before you decide on this treatment.

Guidelines for Seed Implantation

Following are some general guidelines for selecting and undergoing seed implantation. These guidelines may vary from one facility to another.

Volume of the Prostate

The patient's prostate should be no bigger than 50 cubic centimeters. If it is larger, then the patient should receive some form of hormonal therapy for 3 months — or until the size of the gland reaches the acceptable level. Once a patient is on CHT, he should remain on it for at least one month after implantation to maximize the radiation dose of the seeds to the entire prostate.

Selection of Treatment

The selection of a treatment is usually based on a patient's stage. Patients with low-grade tumors and stage A, B0, or B1 lesions are usually treated with seed implantation alone. Patients with B2 tumors, high-grade lesions, or a PSA level greater than 10 generally receive external beam radiation and seed implantation usually with hormonal therapy. However, carefully selected stage B2 patients with a well-differentiated lesion confined to one lobe of the prostate may also be suitable for seed implantation alone. Because lymph-node involvement increases with increasing stage and grade, it may be necessary to perform a laparoscopy to assess the lymph nodes, particularly if the PSA level exceeds 20 ng/ml.

Choice of Seeds

The choice of seeds generally depends on the characteristic of the tumor. Patients with a Gleason score of 2 to 6 are usually treated with I-125 because the isotope half-life more closely matches the time it takes the tumor to double in size. Patients with Gleason scores of 7 to 10 usually receive palladium-103. Because of the poor results experienced by patients with poorly differentiated tumors, I-125 is not usually recommended for tumors of Gleason scores above 7. Palladium-103 is preferred for those cases because of its faster initial dose rates. The kill rate of palladium-103 is estimated to be as good as that of I-125. Therefore, the radiation oncologist should choose seeds with this knowledge in mind.

Combination Radiation

Whenever a physician believes that a patient has a larger tumor volume and/or the cancer has probably spread beyond the capsule, he or she may treat the patient with both external beam radiation and seed implantation. In addition, men with PSA levels above 10 ng/ml are candidates for external beam therapy in conjunction with seeds. Usually, patients who have stage B2 or B3 may receive combination radiation treatment. Many doctors also believe that a stage C patient should not receive seed implantation only. Combination radiation therapy consists of moderate doses of external beam radiation (3,000 to 5,000 rads), followed 2 to 4 weeks later with seeds that deliver from 10,000 to 12,000 rads; however, the combined dose of radiation should not exceed 15,000 rads.

Neoadjuvant Combination Hormonal Therapy

Several studies, including those of Fernand Labrie, William Fair, and Mark Soloway, have shown a 25 to 30 percent decrease in margin positivity when hormonal therapy is used for 3 months prior to radical prostatectomy. Adjuvant and neoadjuvant studies by the Radiation Therapy Oncology Group have also shown advantages in terms of PSA-measured freedom from relapse when CHT was used in addition to external beam radiation. These same principles can also be applied to the use of seed implantation therapy as shown by Kenneth R. Blank et al.

Number of Seeds

The number of seeds is determined by the radiation physicist/ oncologist and is usually based on the volume of the gland and the isotope (e.g., palladium-103) selected.

Other Conditions

Patients who have had a transrectal urethral resection of the prostate (TURP) may be at a higher risk for complications after seed implantation. Stage C3 and D patients are usually also undesirable candidates. In addition, patients with severe urinary obstruction due to an enlarged prostate may experience urinary retention following implantation.

Prior to Seed Implantation

There are two techniques available for seed implantation. The preplanned technique requires a study to determine the location and size of the cancer. Using a TRUS, a urologist locates the prostate, and a computer then takes several pictures displaying the location and size of the prostate. These pictures help the radiation physicist determine the number of seeds needed and indicate exactly where they should be placed. The other technique, interactive implantation, relies on ultrasound to facilitate the seed placement and does not require extensive preplanning.

The technique selected by your physician is based upon his or her preferences and training. Sometime prior to implantation, the patient will have a blood test, electrocardiogram (ECG), and a chest X-ray. If he is on CHT, he will be evaluated for any liver dysfunction due to the CHT. A day or two before the operation, the patient will be given instructions about diet. He will also be instructed to take an enema to clear the lower bowel and rectum so that the ultrasound image is optimal. In addition, he will receive an antibiotic right before the implantation.

During the Seed Implant

Seed implantation is performed in the operating room and takes about 1 to 1.5 hours. The patient receives spinal or general anesthesia. In addition, the patient may receive medication intravenously, which will make him feel drowsy. An ultrasound probe is then inserted into the rectum to image the prostate onto a monitor. This helps accurately reproduce the predesigned format for inserting the seeds or allows for their interactive placement. Needles are inserted through the appropriate holes in a template placed on the skin between the scrotum and the rectum. Each needle, containing the specified number of seeds, punctures the skin and is guided using ultrasound to its predetermined position within the prostate with pinpoint accuracy.

One of the chief problems with seed implantation in the 1970s was inaccurate placement and seed migration. This prevented full irradiation of the prostate and thus frequently failed to cure the disease. The addition of ultrasound and new products such as the I-125 Rapid Seed Implant Delivery System eliminates this problem by loading the seeds in straight lines, making them far less likely to migrate.

The Mick Applicator system uses a cartridge and needles. The seed design of the Rapid Seed Implant Delivery System focuses on dose distribution, not necessarily migration. However, the prostate is not shaped like a triangle; therefore, peripheral loading appears to be a desirable method of placement.

Most institutions use a variation of the procedures mentioned: the ultrasound, fluoroscopy-based, and the CT-based with fluoroscopy methods. All of these techniques are capable of producing excellent results.

After the Seed Implant

At the end of the procedure, a catheter is temporarily placed in the patient's bladder to drain urine. The patient is rolled into a recovery room and remains there for about 2 hours until the numbness in his legs subsides. While he is in the recovery room, an ice bag is placed between his legs to reduce swelling of the implant area. The urinary catheter is usually removed when the patient regains sensation in his legs, but sometimes the catheter remains in place overnight.

When the patient is ready to be released from the hospital, he is told not to drive for 12 or more hours and to avoid heavy lifting and strenuous physical activity for 2 or 3 days. Sometimes he is advised not to have intercourse for 2 to 3 weeks. Patients are asked to visit the physician's office in 3 months for a digital rectal examination and a PSA test.

Cure Rate

It is very difficult to effectively compare the success rate of radical prostatectomy with seed implantation because of the array of studies citing conflicting recurrence rates for this treatment. It is difficult to know what or who should be believed. Medicare data indicate that the recurrence rate for radical prostatectomy is 28 percent within 4 years, which would make the cure rate 72 percent in 4 years. Yet, on the other hand, Patrick Walsh, M.D., of Johns Hopkins University, claims he gets a cure rate of 70 percent over 10 years. A. L. Zietman et al. reached a different conclusion. They found that, of the patients with a positive surgical margin or extensive extracapsular disease, 35 to 75 percent will exhibit detectable or increasing PSA levels within 5 years of radical prostatectomy. Some readers may say that the Dr. Ragde et al.12-year seed data may not have included patients with the same extent and grade of tumors. This may or may not be true. However, Dr. Ragde's study also involved stage T1 and T2 patients. Certainly, there are problems comparing one study with another, but the point is that it is difficult, if not impossible, to make definitive statements comparing treatment techniques until randomized controlled studies with enough patients in each treatment arm are followed for a long enough period of time.

A study conducted by Kenneth R. Blank et al. involved 155 prostate cancer patients who underwent ultrasound-guided transperineal implantation of palladium-103 from 1994 to 1998. All patients received at least 3 months of neoadjuvant lutenizing hormone-releasing hormone (LHRH) agonist therapy and were registered in the study. This group of men was compared with 55 men treated with brachytherapy alone from December 1991 to December 1993.

The results showed that men treated with implant alone, men who received LHRH agonist had significantly smaller prostates at the time of the implant (27.7 cc versus 36.3 cc), required fewer seeds (47.9 versus 83.2), and had significantly less radioactively implant (76.3 mCi versus 117 mCi). Genitourinary and gastrointestinal problems in men receiving hormone blockade was minimal, with long-term side effects occurring in only three patients. In addition, potency was preserved in 83 percent.

A study by Haakon Ragde et al. revealed that brachytherapy is at least better than radical prostatectomy. A total of 229 prostate cancer patients (stages T1-T3) underwent transperineal brachytherapy using iodine-125 without hormone blockade. The median Gleason score was 5 (range: 2-10). Of these patients, 147 had a high probability of organ-confined disease and were treated solely with an I-125 implant. The remaining 82 patients were determined to be at increased risk for extracapsular disease and received pelvic external beam radiation in addition to brachytherapy. All patients were followed continuously. Failure was defined as a positive biopsy, radiographic evidence of metastases, or three consecutive rises in PSA level (as defined by the American Society for Therapeutic Radiology and Oncology (ASTRO) consensus article). The results revealed that deaths from intercurrent disease, the median follow-up were 122 months (range: 18-144 months). Fourteen patients were excluded from the analysis due to insufficient follow-up. Adopting the ASTRO definition of failure resulted in minimal change in survival time when compared with Haakon Ragde's previous study, which used a PSA level of greater than 0.5 ng/ml as the failure point. The 10-year disease-free survival for the entire group was 70 percent. In the brachytherapy-only group, the 10-year disease-free survival rate was 66 percent; in patients treated with the addition of external pelvic radiation, it was 79 percent. None of the patients who were followed for the full 12 years had a recurrence between years 10 and 12. Only 25 percent of recurrences occurred more than 5 years after treatment, thus confirming the durability of brachytherapy.

Local cure rate and disease-free successes were determined by PSA testination. At-risk patients also underwent a biopsy and bone scan. Local failures were determined by an abnormal digital rectal examination (DRE), a PSA in excess of 0.4 ng/ml, and a positive biopsy.

Side Effects

When we compare both treatments, seed implantation appears to have fewer side effects than radical prostatectomy.

The side effects of prostatectomy follow:

- Recuperation is longer because of the abdominal incision.
- Infection is possible.
- There is a 60 percent chance of temporary incontinence, and there is a small risk of some degree of permanent incontinence.
- There is a 5 percent chance of cardiopulmonary trouble and rectal or bowel injury.
- There is a possibility of blood loss requiring a transfusion.
- According to Medicare, 1 percent of men in the age group of 65 to 74 who received this treatment died of this procedure, and 2 percent of men aged 75 and older died.
- Recovery may take several to 1/2 years.
- According to Medicare, 31 percent of patients wear pads, adult diapers, or a clamp to deal with urinary incontinence.
- Two years after surgery, 16 percent of patients required follow-up treatment for a recurrence of the disease; 22 percent after 3 years; and 28 percent after 4 years.
- More than 50 percent of patients can have a recurrence due to understaging of the disease.

The side effects of seed implantation follow:

- Fewer than 5 percent of patients will be incontinent.
- Fewer than 15 percent of patients under the age of 70 will be impotent.
- Mild soreness between the legs may last for 1 to 2 days.
- There may be light bleeding or burning beneath the scrotum and blood in the urine for a few days.
- Urination may be frequent or uncomfortable for as long as several months.
- One percent of patients experience proctitis.

How to Use This Information

If you are interested in a less invasive method than radical prostatectomy to treat prostate cancer, consider the following:

1. The names and locations of qualified doctors performing seed implantation are available through the Personal Advisory Service of the Education Center for Prostate Cancer Patients (ECPCP). To contact ECPCP, please call 516-942-5000.
2. Read as much as you can about this treatment; review the research too.
3. Once you have chosen a physician, ask him or her for any materials about seed implantation that are available.
4. Make certain your doctor has performed a minimum of 250 seed implantations.
5. Ask your doctor for the names and telephone numbers of several patients who have had this treatment. Then contact them and ask their opinion of the procedure.
6. Consider undergoing seed implantation if you appear to be a candidate.
7. Choose a doctor who has a wealth of experience using the transrectal ultrasound in analyzing and interpreting prostate cancer tumors.

E. Roy Berger, M.D., F.A.C.P. and James Lewis, Jr., Ph.D

Chapter 21

PROVENGE: A PROSTATE CANCER VACCINE

Although the Almighty gave men a prostate, it does not appear to be a necessary organ. Patients treated with radical prostatectomy or radiation have demonstrated this for many years. Unfortunately, these treatments have the adverse side effects of impotence as well as incontinence. With the advent of gene therapy, scientists and researchers now believe it should be possible to create prostate-targeted vaccines that would cause an immune response to search for, locate, and destroy prostate cancer. One way it might be possible to do this is to combine a prostate-specific agent with an agent that would induce an immune response. Another way could be to combine a prostate-specific antibody with a radiation source or a chemotherapy drug to destroy prostate cancer cells that it is bound to. Regardless of the approach, the result could be a treatment in which no blood is spilled, no radiation burns the body, and no probes freeze and kill tissues.

Describing Provenge

Provenge, also known as APC8015, is a prostate cancer vaccine currently in phase III clinical trials sponsored by the Dendreon Corporation. Dendreon is a biotechnology company in Seattle, Washington, that develops targeted therapy and treatment for cancer. The first one of these phase III trials recently reported results.

APC, or *antigen presenting cells*, are involved in the initiation and expansion of cellular immune responses to carrier and virus-infected cells. Dendritic cells, the most potent APCs, are trained to detect cancer cells by exposure to the target (Valone et al., 2001). Dendritic cells potentiate the effectiveness of the initiation of T-cell and B-cell (lymphocytes) mediated immune responses. Provenge activates these cells to mount a more effective immune response against prostate cancer. APCs do not kill cancer cells; rather, they alert effector cells, like T-cells, to the presence of cancer. T-cells are the immune system's attack cells, and thus they attack and destroy the cancer cells. Provenge consists of autologous (the patient's own) dendritic cells loaded with PA2024, a fusion protein consisting of human prostatic acid phosphatase (PAP) coupled to a targeting molecule, granulocyte-macrophage colony-stimulating factor (GM-CSF). PAP is a tissue-specific antigen that is expressed only by normal prostate cells and in greater than 90 percent of cancer cells of the prostate. GM-CSF is a cytokine, which regulates the survival, proliferation, and differentiation of granulocyte (white blood cells) and macrophage progenitors (cells that destroy other cells by "eating" them) and which are a potent stimulator of dendritic cells (Rini and Small, 2001).

Understanding the Trial

Provenge is a vaccine currently in two randomized double-blind, placebo-controlled trials for patients with asymptomatic metastatic hormone-refractory prostate cancer and patients with rising PSA after prostatectomy but no other signs of disease. Patients in the hormone refractory trial must have a pathology record stating that their original tumor was graded as a Gleason Score of 7 or lower. Patients with Gleason Score 8 or higher tumors are ineligible. Patients are randomized to either the treatment or control group in a 2:1 ratio. In the metastatic trial, approximately 275 patients will be enrolled in approximately 60 sites in the United States. The treatment group receives Provenge, which consists of APCs loaded with prostatic acid phosphatase. The control group receives placebo. At baseline, before the first apheresis (blood filtering for dendritic cells), the patient must undergo screening tests to determine eligibility. At weeks 0, 2, and 4, all patients undergo apheresis followed by an infusion 2 days later with either Provenge or a control. This is the active treatment phase. If a patient's disease progresses after the active treatment phase, further treatment is at the physician's discretion. If the patient is in the control group and progresses, he may have the option to join the open-label salvage protocol (i.e., receive an active vaccine).

Identifying Adverse Effects

Potential adverse effects can occur during the collection of dendritic cell precursors (leukopheresis) and during and after reinfusion of Provenge. During apheresis, patients may experience citrate toxicity (numbness and tingling around the mouth and hands) and, rarely, arrhythmias due to low calcium secondary to anticoagulants used during apheresis. In addition, hypovolemia (decrease in the volume of circulating blood) and low blood pressure may occur, as well as pain, bruising, and infection at the venous catheter site. Reinfusion may be complicated by chills, fevers, muscle ache, pain, and fatigue (Burch et al., 2000). In addition to apheresis or infusion-related incidents, there is the theoretical possibility that patients may experience prostatitis due to the induction of an immune response to PAP; therefore, the PSA may rise without disease progression. Phase I and II trials of Provenge at the University of California at San Francisco and the Mayo Clinic demonstrated that Provenge is generally well tolerated (Valone et al., 2001).

Identifying Patient Eligibility

To be considered for the Provenge trial, patients must have metastatic disease (cancer that has spread outside the prostate), Gleason Score must be 7 or lower, and there must be documented progression of disease while on hormonal therapy. In addition, patients must have no cancer-related pain. There are other eligibility criteria, and your study doctor will determine if you meet all of the criteria (Dendreon Clinical Protocol no. D9902B, 2003). Provenge trial information can also be found on www.clinicaltrials.gov.

Results of the Clinical Trials

In the Mayo Clinic trial, patients received two doses of intravenous Provenge every 4 weeks, followed by three doses of PAP-GM-CSF subcutaneously every 4 weeks. The UCSF trial used Provenge only. Patients in the UCSF study had a higher frequency of antibody responses and higher antibody titers. A substantial number of patients experienced disease stabilization and a longer than expected time to disease progression. Several patients had objective tumor regression on CT scan, and there was decreased PSA in about 20 percent. Both trials supported the efficacy, safety, and tolerability of Provenge in treating hormone-refractory prostate cancer patients.

A double-blind placebo-controlled, randomized, phase III trial was initiated in late 1999 and completed enrollment by mid-2001. A second phase III trial is currently in progress. In late 2002, the Dendreon Corporation announced the results of its first placebo-controlled phase III trial of Provenge: "In addition to delaying the time to disease progression, the investigational cancer vaccine delayed the onset of disease-related pain in patients with hormone-resistant prostate cancer with a Gleason score of 7 or less." For these patients, the probability of remaining free of cancer-related pain while in the study was over 2.5 times higher than for patients treated with placebo. In the same group of patients, median time to disease progression was 9.1 weeks among placebo patients compared to 16.1 weeks in the Provenge-treated group, with a highly significant p value of 0.001 and a treatment effect of 77 percent. In addition, after 6 months of follow-up, the patients receiving Provenge had a progression-free survival nine times that of patients who received placebo (35.9% versus 4%).

In the future, Provenge may be used to delay the need for androgen-deprivation therapy. This is being tested in another trial in patients with hormone-sensitive prostate cancer who have a rising PSA level as the only sign of disease recurrence after radical prostatectomy. Entry into this trial is not restricted on the basis of Gleason Score. In the future, it is hoped that Provenge will be given to prostate cancer patients at high risk of developing a recurrence or at the first detection to enhance the immune system's ability to eradicate cancer cells in the microscopic stage before development of a tumor.

How to Use This Information

Determine your eligibility for the phase III clinical trial. If you are eligible, apply to one of the centers cited in the Resource section at the back of this book.

Chapter 22

TREATING CANCER WITH LIGHT WAVES

In 1903 Niels Finsen won the Nobel prize for pioneering light as an effective treatment for cancer. The first person to be treated with light, who was cured in Germany, had a basal cell carcinoma of the lip. However, with the advent of X-rays and chemotherapy, this light treatment was put on the back burner. Then, in the 1970s, a conscientious doctor in Buffalo, New York, used a substance called HpD (hematoporphyrin derivative) and a visible red light to destroy a malignant tumor. About 10 years later, the Food and Drug Administration (FDA) approved a drug called *photofrin* to be used in the light treatment of various forms of cancer. This FDA-approved treatment has produced some good results throughout the years. In one study, patients with various forms of cancer who had previously failed conventional treatments were administered photofrin-based photodynamic therapy. It has been reported that 70 to 80 percent of the patients responded positively after one light treatment. Unfortunately, this first-generation drug had several serious problems. First, it was not specific to cancer cells, and so it often accumulated in normal tissues, which meant that not only cancerous cells but also normal cells or organs could be damaged. In addition, it did not clear the body rapidly. As a result, whenever patients received photofrin, they had to stay out of the sun for a month or more or experience a serious sunburn. It also became apparent that larger and deep-seated tumors generally could not be treated with photofrin. *Cytoluminescent therapy (CLT)*, an advanced form of photodynamic therapy now used at East Clinic in County Clare, Ireland, appears to eliminate many of these problems. The East Clinic is the only place offering CLT.

Defining Cytoluminescent Therapy (CLT)

CLT is an advanced form of photodynamic therapy that uses light to kill malignant cells of various forms of cancer. It operates on the principle that certain chemicals known as sensitizers are absorbed and can kill cancer cells when they are exposed to a particular type of light. As a result, CLT destroys malignant cancer cells through the use of a fixed-frequency laser light in concert with a sensitizing agent.

How Does It Work?

Initially, the patient receives an intravenous treatment with intensive laser therapy for 30 to 60 minutes. He is then directed to another room where one side of his entire body is given intravenous and oral dosing of a special sensitizing agent called *spirulina* for 90 minutes. He is then rotated to the other side of his body and receives the sensitizing agent for another 90 minutes.

The sensitizing agent can be initiated after only 3 hours and is eliminated from the body after 24 hours, when the patient is sent home. He is given a 4 to 6-month supply of oral capsules of the sensitizing agent and taught how to construct and use an infrared lighting arrangement on a daily basis.

CLT, the sensitizing agent, is injected into the bloodstream of the patient and is absorbed by cells throughout the body. This agent remains in cancerous cells longer than it does in normal cells. When the cancer cells receiving the CLT are exposed to a laser light, the sensitizing agent absorbs the light and creates an active form of oxygen that kills the malignant cells. It is important that the exposed light be carefully timed so that it is given when most of the sensitizing agent has left the healthy cells but is still present in the cancerous cells.

Advantages of CLT

Although CLT is an invasive treatment, it is certainly not as invasive as radical prostatectomy with all of its harsh side effects. Other advantages of CLT over conventional treatment follow:

- It causes minimal damage to healthy tissue.
- Tumors quickly die in a process called *necrosis*.
- Its sensitizing agent can penetrate organs.
- Its sensitizing agent, although not approved by the Federal Drug Administration, tends to be more effective than the first-generation agent.
- Spirulina-based sensitizing agent is reported to be 100 times more effective than the first generation, and an upcoming one is said to be even more powerful.
- It can be used in combination with other treatments.
- It can be used multiple times at the same site.
- The response rates are as good as - or better than - more invasive treatments.

- There are fewer side effects, as well as improved functional and cosmetic outcome.
- The CLT program includes detoxification, immune support, and nutritional guidance, as well as psychotherapy.
- The National Cancer Institute and other institutions are supporting clinical trials.
- New photosensitizing agents may increase CLT effectiveness in cancers located several inches below the skin or inside an organ.
- It does not distinguish between primary and secondary tumors but can treat both with equal effectiveness.
- It is beneficial for most types of cancer.
- It can be applied to almost all areas of the body.
- It works effectively in patients who have had previous conventional treatment.
- Many patients find CLT to be more comfortable and relaxing than other treatments.
- It can be used when surgery is not advisable.

Disadvantages of CLT

The disadvantages of CLT follow:

- The CLT is performed in an outpatient facility or clinic, not a hospital.
- The East Clinic cannot accommodate everyone who wants the therapy.
- Newly treated patients who want to go outdoors need to wear protective clothing, including sunglasses, much of the time.
- It is not possible to predict how many treatments a patient might need or if a particular treatment will achieve lasting benefits.

What Are the Side Effects?

CLT has several side effects:

- Intense malaise.
- Chills and fever.
- Flulike symptoms.
- Night sweats.
- Patients must remain out of direct sunlight for 5 days after treatment.
- Itching is sometimes experienced during the light treatment.

- Patients are sensitive to sunlight for 1 or 2 days.
- Nausea and transient diarrhea.
- Discomfort due to tissue breakdown creating inflammation.
- Minimal to moderate pain.
- Fatigue.
- Where the tumor is near the skin surface, it may slough off, breaking through the skin as the dead cells are eliminated.
- As of mid-2003, the cost of the treatment was not covered by medical insurance.
- All costs for the treatment must be met upfront.
- Children and pregnant women are not eligible.
- Light exposure must be timed carefully so that it occurs when most of the sensitizing agent has left the healthy cells but is still present in the cancer cells.
- The skin and eyes must be shielded from intense light exposure.
- Photosensitivity may cause the skin to become red, swollen, and even blister.
- The procedure can take 3 to 4 months, and tiredness may be experienced.
- Coughing, trouble swallowing, abdominal pain, and painful breathing or shortness of breath.

CLT Is Not for Everyone

CLT can be used to treat many cancers and other ailments. However, the aftereffects can be difficult, so CLT is not for everyone. Patients described in the following are advised not to undergo CLT:

- Those who are bedridden or confined to a wheelchair.
- Patients too ill to travel a long distance.
- Patients suffering from cachexia.
- Those who have had stents implanted because of pancreatic, bile duct, or prostate cancer.
- Those who take supplemental oxygen.
- Those with cancerous tumors of the spinal column.
- Those with a tumor affecting a major blood vessel.
- Depressed patients.
- Those under the age of 18.

Citing Some Results

In a recent study by Timothy R. Nathan of the University College London Hospital and his associates, most patients treated with first-generation photodynamic therapy, whose cancer had returned following external beam radiation, appeared to benefit from light therapy. More than half of the light-treated patients experienced a decrease in their PSA level. In addition, more than a third of the light-treated patients showed no trace of cancer in a posttreatment biopsy.

During the study, the researchers administered light treatment to 14 patients, all of whom had a recurrence of prostate cancer following radiation. After the light treatment, the researchers found that the PSA level decreased in nine patients, reaching an undetectable level in two. Biopsies of five patients revealed that they were tumor-free. Scans showed that light therapy had destroyed up to 91 percent of the cancerous tissue.

Some of the patients experienced side effects. Four had stress incontinence, which improved gradually.

How CLT Is Performed

During the Treatment

There is no advanced preparation for CLT. You will be asked to arrive at the East Clinic early on the morning of the treatment to meet with the director. You should allocate 2 to 5 hours for these meetings. The director will talk with you, ask if you have any questions, and introduce you to a personal attendant who will be with you throughout the day.

Next, you will undergo an ultrasound scan, which will be reviewed by the medical staff. Then you will receive an intravenous infusion of the sensitizing agent and be instructed to rest so that the agent can circulate through your body and accumulate in your cancer cells.

After 2 or 3 hours, the sensitizing agent will have searched, found, and attached to the cancerous cells in your body. At this time, the laser light will be directed to the appropriate area to destroy the cancerous tissue. The laser lights are displayed for only a few minutes. Although the procedure may cause some discomfort, it is usually well controlled by local anesthesia. Any discomfort you experience will be treated with painkillers prescribed by the doctor.

After the Treatment

Within a day or two, if there are no complications, you can go home. You will have to follow up your treatment with your own doctor, who can contact the center if there are any questions. If you wish to return to the center, you may be advised to take an oral agent. Inflammation occurs with CLT as the body deals with the dead cells and eliminates cancerous tissue. Therefore, you may need to take a medication to minimize this problem. You will be supplied with 4 to 6 months of oral capsules of the sensitizing agent and taught how to construct and use an infrared lighting arrangement on a daily basis. You will also be told that carrot juice can aid in the effectiveness of the home infrared treatment. On the final day of your visit to the center, you will see the doctor. You will be asked to remain in contact with the center for the posttreatment consultation.

What You Should Know about the Treatment

1. It costs $21,000. This includes everything associated with the therapy, as well as living arrangements and meals.
2. Most American insurance companies will not cover the cost of this treatment.
3. Few hospitals or clinics in the United States offers this treatment.

How Light Penetrates the Body

Some patients and a few physicians have claimed that CLT is useful for only superficial tumors and cannot get to prostate cancer that has metastasized deep inside the body. This notion is based on faulty and old thinking and perhaps on experience with the FDA-approved photofrin agent. However, spirulina, the sensitizing agent used with CLT is capable of treating deeply embedded cancerous tumors, those that have metastasized throughout the body when the light is applied externally.

The ability of light to penetrate tissues and organs deep inside the body has been confirmed scientifically by Dr. Harry T. Whelan of the Medical College of Wisconsin and NASA's Marshall Space Flight Center in Huntsville, Alabama. Whelan, an expert on the use of light-emitting diodes in medicine, writes that "Spectra taken from the wrist flexor muscles in the human forearm and muscles in the calf of the leg demonstrate that most of the light photons at wavelengths between 630 and 800 nanometers travel 23 centimeters through the surface tissue and muscle between input and exit at the photon detector."

177

Because only 9 inches of light is needed to penetrate most organs of the body, a light photon at wavelengths between 630 and 800 nm is sufficient to reach most parts of the body. This is approximately the absorption range of wavelengths of the photosensitizers.

The Photoflora, the agent used in CLT, is a derivative of chlorin and has an intensive absorption band of 663 nm, as well as an intense fluorescence reaction on cancerous tumors within the range of 658 to 688 nm in which the body could absorb higher wavelengths if necessary.

How to Use This Information

Consider CLT if you meet any of the following criteria:

1. You have undergone surgery, radiation, cryosurgery, but your cancer has recurred.
2. You are hormone-refractory.
3. You experience terrible side effects with chemotherapy.
4. Your doctor says that you have only months to live.
5. You have no more hope.

* * *

An advanced form of photodynamic therapy, photocytolytic therapy developed in Moscow by a team of physicians and physicists working from research conducted originally in the United States in the 1920s, appears to eliminate many of the problems associated with the first-generation sensitizing agent, Photofrin. This form of PDT was first introduced to the West by the East Clinic in Ireland, who trademarked the term cytoluminescent therapy (CLT) to describe it. They also trademarked the term _Photoflora_ to describe the active agent used. The Russians simply call it photodynamic therapy and call the active agent by its generic chemical name, chlorin e6. In the United States, the Aidan Cancer Treatment Center in Tempe, Arizona, uses the term _Spir-Ox_, for oxidized chlorophyll from spirulina platentsis (i.e., chlorin e6). Because _photodynamic therapy_ is an old term indelibly associated in the minds of Western physicians with the problematic Photofrin, and because cytoluminescent therapy is a trademark for one clinic's way of performing the therapy, this section uses the term _photocytolytic therapy_ (PCLT), meaning "light that kills cells," originated but not trademarked by Aidan in the United States.

Defining Photocytolytic Therapy

Photocytolytic therapy, an advanced form of photodynamic therapy, destroys malignant cells through the use of a fixed-frequency light source in concert with a sensitizing agent. The East Clinic in Ireland uses a laser to generate the fixed-frequency light. The Aidan clinic in Arizona prescribes an LED-array (light emitting diode-array) to generate the same fixed-frequency light. Patients of the East Clinic must travel to Ireland for treatment, whereas Aidan patients use the prescribed LED-array at home for as long as they need to. In addition, Aidan can also prescribe a rectal-probe LED-array for illuminating the prostate with the fixed-frequency light directly.

PCLT versus PDT

PCLT uses chlorin e6, an oxidized form of chlorophyll. It is present in virtually all green plants but is usually extracted from spirulina platensis due to its higher concentration there. Green juices or whole spirulina cannot be used for PCLT, because all of the nonoxidized chlorophyll will make it ineffective. Photofrin is essentially hematoporphyrin, a breakdown product of hemoglobin. Hemoglobin is a complex of porphyrin rings around an iron atom; chlorophyll is a complex of porphyrin rings around a magnesium atom. However, this is as far as the similarity goes.

Photofrin does not concentrate well in cancer cells or tumors, and it stays in normal tissue for a very long time. Patients who have been treated with Photofrin must stay out of sunlight for months. Chlorin e6 concentrates in cancer cells or tumors very well and washes out of normal tissues quickly, usually in less than 24 hours. Patients treated with chlorin e6 can usually go out in the sunlight the next day.

Photofrin should not be activated until after all Photofrin in the circulation has completed; otherwise the patient is at risk for severe skin and systemic damage. The theory is that chlorin e6 can be activated while still in circulation, and it will then remain in circulation in its activated state until it collects in tumors. A theory has been formulated by Dr. Charles Knouse at Aidan to explain why deep tumors have been shown in CT scan to regress with PCLT, even though the fixed-frequency light is being shone only on the skin surface. Knouse's theory is this:

1. It is well documented that tumors collect fats from the blood, including cholesterol particles, because tumors are not organized tissue and do not have lymphatic drainage.

2. It has been documented that individual cancer cells avidly uptake fats from the blood, including cholesterol particles, for fatty acid metabolism.

3. It has been documented that oxidized chlorophylls, unlike hematoporphyrin, avidly associate with cholesterol particles in the blood.

4. It is hypothesized, therefore, that by illuminating the skin with fixed-frequency light of the correct frequency at the proper time, cholesterol-chlorin e6 complexes will be activated by the light while circulating in the capillaries of the skin but will not deposit in the skin. That is, they will continue to circulate in some activated state until they deposit and accumulate in tumor tissue as well as individual cancer cells.

In addition, there is literature demonstrating that activated chlorin e6, when it doesn't actually kill a cancer cell, causes the cancer cell to express heat shock proteins. Interestingly, the same literature states that this effect does not happen with Photofrin. The importance of this, to Aidan, is that because heat-shock proteins are intensely stimulating to the immune system, and because heat-shock proteins are "sticky" and tend to carry tumor antigen with them, combining PCLT with immunotherapy is thus a rational idea. Aidan does this, either through a tumor-specific antigen vaccine derived from urine or through live-cell, total killer-cell cultures for reinfusion. Aidan also believes that PCLT can be given in conjunction with chemotherapy instead of immunotherapy in cases where "rescue therapy" is needed. Immunotherapy in combination with PCLT can then be given after the rescue-therapy phase of treatment is completed.

How Is the Treatment Given?

At the East Clinic, the agent (Photoflora) is given intravenously. After about 3 hours, the patient is ushered into the laser room, given eye-protection goggles, and the light is administered. The patient is illuminated from the laser on one side and then the other, and a penlight laser is also used to illuminate selected pinpoint locations. The patient also receives nutritional IVs while at the clinic. Most patients stay at the clinic for 4 days. They are sent home with enough Photoflora capsules to take by mouth for 4 months and told to purchase a heat lamp to use on their skin everyday at home. The East Clinic advises patients to avoid the sun for at least several days after treatment. Serious fatigue, malaise, and lung inflammation have been reported after treatment with the laser and intravenous chlorin e6, and these side effects have been confirmed by the researchers in Moscow.

Seriously ill patients or patients with contraindications are not candidates for PCLT at the East Clinic.

At the Aidan Cancer Treatment Center in Tempe, Arizona, the patient is taught how to administer the treatment at home, and prescriptions are given to the patient for obtaining the Spir-Ox (chlorin e6) and the special LED-array. The patient treats himself at home once a week, taking a moderate dose of the agent by mouth, waiting 4 to 6 hours, and then illuminating the skin areas with the LED-array for several hours. Patients are directed to illuminate the skin overlying tumors as well as the skin surface in general. Probes that can illuminate the prostate are available by prescription. Patients are encouraged to get indirect sunlight starting the day after self-administration of the agent. Side effects are usually minimal with this more moderate treatment. Most commonly reported side effects are mild fatigue the day after treatment, with quick recovery for the rest of the week. No serious episodes of malaise or lung inflammation have been observed. The Aidan Clinic has not had to establish exclusion criteria, due to the mild side effects observed with its way of prescribing PCLT. Indeed, one patient who had been excluded by the East Clinic due to a tumor near a vein was successfully put into remission without side effects, after undergoing PCLT the Aidan way.

How Does It Work?

No matter which light therapy is used, if the agent is concentrated in a tumor and the correct fixed-frequency light is shone on the tumor, reactive oxygen species are generated that are capable of killing cancer cells. When a photon of red light at the correct frequency is absorbed, the chlorin e6 molecule becomes momentarily unstable and releases a singlet oxygen radical, which is perhaps the most reactive species of radical encountered in biological systems. There is little likelihood that a cancer cell can withstand the toxic effect of this kind of radical. Indeed, the Russian researchers believe that cancer cannot become resistant to PCLT.

According to the theory proposed by Aidan, very little chlorin e6 is taken up by normal cells, because normal cells do not take up more than tiny amounts of cholesterol. Cancer cells appear to avidly uptake chlorin e6, however, possibly due to their avid uptake of cholesterol and other fats from the blood. It is interesting that the first sign of cancer is often loss of body fat without dieting. Only after all the body fat is gone does the patient begin to lose protein from muscle (cachexia). This theory would also state that taking the agent orally would be just as effective as intravenously; it is even possible that taking it orally would be more effective than intravenously due to the absorption directly into cholesterol particles from the gastrointestinal tract.

How to Use This Information

1. PCLT costs $14,000; CLT costs $21,000.
2. PCLT is administered the United States.
3. PCLT uses an oral agent.
4. The Aidan Clinic has developed a vaccine for the patient's specific illness.
5. The Aidan Clinic supplies the patient with a light panel, whereas the East Clinic patients must make it themselves.
6. The side effects of PCLT are not as severe as those of CLT.

Chapter 23

HORMONAL BLOCKADE: WHAT'S NEW?

Prostate cancer is the second most frequent cause of cancer death in men in the Western world. Its medicosocial impact is almost similar to that of breast cancer in women. In fact, it has been estimated that 28,900 men in the United States will die from prostate cancer in 2003. As the population ages, the incidence of prostate cancer is expected to increase year by year, with graver consequences and an increased burden on the health system. Thus there is a great need to create methods by which we can dispense therapy to prostate cancer patients. In recent years, attempts have been made to enhance the delivery of medications by administering triple doses and yearly doses for the convenience of both the physician and the patient. In addition, now there is a medication that performs the function of a dual medication by saving the patients not only time but also certain side effects.

FDA Approvals

In the past it took the FDA several years to approve a drug for use, perhaps causing the death of many seriously ill patients. Today, that policy has changed drastically, enabling drugs to be approved within months. The following section discusses some drugs that have benefited from the FDA's policy change in regard to treating prostate cancer with CHT.

Transdermal Patch

The female sex hormone estrogen can be absorbed through the skin, so patches that contain estrogen and can deliver it through the skin were developed. These transdermal estrogen patches are often used to treat women experiencing menopausal symptoms. They have been found to be more effective than estrogen pills because they are less prone to cause blood clots.

Dr. G. Gerber et al. conducted a study to determine the impact of estrogen patches on hot flashes in men undergoing estrogen withdrawal. These physicians used both low-dose (0.05 mg) and high-dose (0.1 mg) patches, which were applied to prostate cancer patients twice a week. Approximately 80 percent of the tested patients experienced improvement in their symptoms.

183

Breast enlargement and tenderness were the major side effects of the patches. They were experienced by 17 percent of the men on the low dose and 40 percent of those men on the high dose. Because this study only involved 12 men, it was too small to accurately assess the other side effects common in patients receiving estrogen treatment for prostate cancer.

Although transdermal estrogen patches appear to be somewhat effective in reducing the severity of hot flashes, it's too early to declare that these patches are as safe for men as they are for women. Additional patients will have to be studied.

In 2001, the FDA approved Trelstar LA, a 3-month controlled-release formulation of triptorelin pamoate, a treatment for advanced stage prostate cancer. In a pivotal clinical trial, this drug was shown to be as effective as the previously approved Trelstar Depot. Patients who received triptorelin pamoate used fewer analgesics after the administration of the drug and gained weight.

Side Effects of Trelstar LA

Side effects of Trelstar LA include:

- fatigue
- nausea
- vomiting
- diarrhea
- decreased blood cell count
- hair loss
- mouth sores
- hot flashes
- loss of sexual drive
- breast tenderness

How Does Trelstar LA Work?

Trelstar LA controls the secretion of gonadotropin when administered continuously in therapeutic doses. In addition, following administration, there is a transient surge in blood levels of luteinizing hormone (LH), follicle-stimulating hormone (FSH), testosterone, and estradiol. After chronic and continuous administration for 2 to 4 weeks, a sustained decrease in LH and FSH secretion and marked reduction of testicular steroidogenesis is observed. A reduction in testosterone levels, tissue, and functions that depend on these hormones for maintenance purposes, these effects are usually reversed after stopping the therapy.

One- and Three-Month LHRH Therapy

In 2002, the FDA approved Eligard (7.5 mg) for the treatment of advanced prostate cancer. Eligard, given in a subcutaneous injection, delivers 7.5 mg of leuprolide acetate at a controlled rate over a 1-month therapeutic period. The product is injected into the body in liquid form, where it solidifies and continuously releases a predetermined dose of leuprolide acetate.

Following are some side effects of Eligard:

- malaise
- fatigue
- dizziness
- hot flashes/sweats
- gastroenteritis
- colitis

In 2002, the FDA also approved another suspension of Eligard (22.5 mg), in injection, to be given every 3 months.

Improving Benefits with Casodex

A study by C.J. Tyrell et al. evaluated the efficacy and tolerability of Casodex monotherapy (150 mg daily) for metastatic and locally advanced prostate cancer. The study involved 1,453 prostate cancer patients with either metastatic or nonmetastatic disease with elevated PSA levels. The men were recruited into one of two identical multicenter, randomized studies to compare Casodex (150 mg/day) with castration. The protocols allowed for combined analysis. At a median follow-up period of approximately 100 weeks for both studies, Casodex was found to be less effective than castration in patients with metastatic disease at entry. With a difference in median survival of 6 weeks in symptomatic metastatic patients, Casodex was associated with a statistically significant improvement in subjective response (70%) compared with castration (58%). Analysis of a quality-of-life questionnaire proved that men on Casodex had more sexual interest and better physical capacity than did those who were castrated. Men taking Casodex had substantially fewer hot flashes (6-13%) compared to the castrated group (39-44%), and the most commonly reported adverse events were those expected for a potent antiandrogen. However, in patients with nonmetastatic disease at entry, the data are still immature, with only 13

185

percent of patients having died. An initial analysis of this immature data suggest that the results in these patients may be different from those in patients with metastatic disease. A further survival analysis in nonmetastatic patients is therefore planned when the data are more mature. The researchers concluded that Casodex (150 mg) is less effective than castration in patients with metastatic disease. However, Casodex was more beneficial than castration in terms of quality of life and subjective response, and it has an acceptable tolerability profile. Thus, Casodex (150 mg) monotherapy is an option for patients with metastatic prostate cancer for whom surgical or medical castration is not indicated or not acceptable.

Another study conducted by a team of European and Australian researchers tracked 480 prostate cancer patients treated with hormone therapy. In the study, 320 patients received 150 mg of Casodex daily, and 138 patients were chemically castrated. After a median follow-up of about six years, median survival time was about 5.5 years in both groups. The disease had progressed in 77 percent of the patients after 6 years, with no statistically significant difference between the two groups.

Because neither treatment option offered a survival advantage over the other, the researchers gauged the extent of side effects. "Quality of life considerations are becoming more important for patients in general and for those with prostate cancer in particular." The most significant difference was in sexual interest. After 12 months, 47 percent of the surgically castrated showed a significant decline in sexual interest, compared to 23 percent of the patients on Casodex.

The benefit of Casodex monotherapy with respect to sexual interest was evident within a month of beginning the study and was maintained throughout.

Although the Casodex group reported fewer hot flashes (13.1% versus 50%), they experienced a higher incidence of breast enlargement and tenderness (49.4% versus 4.4%) and breast pain (40.1% versus 1.9%).

The Casodex group reported a higher quality-of-life, including physical and emotional well-being, vitality, and sexual functioning.

The use of Casodex as a single hormone therapy is not prescribed by many urologists. Yet they should consider it, because patients on Casodex monotherapy feel better and continue to have a libido.

Time Off during Intermittent Hormonal Blockade

A study by Stephen B. Strum et al. treated 255 patients with prostate cancer with androgen deprivation therapy (ADT) using an antiandrogen and an LHRH agonist. Of these men, 216 (85%) achieved an undetectable PSA (<0.05 ng/ml). Ninety-three patients (43%) of 216 patients elected to stop

ADT after maintaining an undetectable PSA for a median of 1 year. Patients were followed off therapy and advised to restart treatment if the PSA level rose above 5.0. Forty-one patients received flutamide as part of intermittent androgen deprivation (IAD) and as maintenance off therapy. These patients were excluded from the study. The remaining 52 patients were assessable for response, either being in the off-phase of IAD for a year or more, or having restarted IAD in the first IAD group. The median duration of the on-phase of IAD was 16 months or a median of 19.0 months (range: 3.6–71 months). The median off-phase was 15.5 months (mean: 24.1 months; range: 3.2-87 months). In 28 patients who maintained an undetectable PSA for a year or more, the median off-phase duration was 29 months (mean: 35.8 months; range: 7.8–87+ months); 9 patients (32%) were still off IAD after a median follow-up of 62 months. Significant independent factors associated with prolonged off-phase duration by multivariate analysis included undetectable PSA on ADT for at least a year, PSA only recurrence after local therapy, and reaching a testosterone level of at least 150 ng/ml in 74 months off ADT. After a median 66 months of follow-up, only 1 or 2 percent of the patients became androgen-independent.

Viadur: A One-Year Implant

In 2000, the FDA approved the Viadur C leuprolide acetate implant as a 1-year implant for the palliative treatment of advanced prostate cancer. The product is the first to deliver 12 months of testosterone-suppression therapy in a single administration.

Side Effects

The most common side effects are as follows:

- vasodilatation (enlargement of blood vessels)
- asthenia (lack or loss of strength)
- gynecomastia
- depression
- sweating

In addition, the insertion and removal of the implant caused bruising and burning in 34.8 and 5.6 percent of the patients, respectively. These reactions lasted for approximately 2 weeks. However, 9.3 percent of patients had bruising and/or burning that persisted, and 10 percent developed reactions beyond the first 2 weeks after insertion.

During the first week of treatment, a transient increase in serum concentrations of testosterone occurs, which may cause pain or bladder outlet obstruction. A total of 4.6 percent of patients experienced these problems.

Treating side effects in hormonal blockade gabapentin may be effective in relieving hot flashes in men who have prostate cancer and are undergoing hormonal blockade.

Results of a Clinical Trial

A 2-year study was conducted of 131 men with advanced prostate cancer who received the Viadur treatment. By the fourth week after insertion of the implant, 99 percent had mean serum testosterone concentrations at desirably lower levels than those previous to the treatment. Furthermore, this testosterone suppression continued throughout the year-long treatment. A total of 118 patients had a second implant inserted for a second year of therapy following the removal of the first implant. None of them had a significant increase in testosterone level after the insertion of a new implant.

Zoladex and Lupron: New Formulations

In the 1990s, the FDA approved new formulations of both Lupron and Zoladex to be used for the palliative treatment of advanced prostate cancer. Before these approvals, only 1-month doses were available for each drug, and a new dose had to be administered every month. In 1995, the FDA approved a 3-month dose of Lupron, and a 3-month dose of Zoladex was approved the next year. Additionally, the FDA approved a 4-month dose of Lupron in 1997. These formulations of Zoladex and Lupron offer greater convenience to patients undergoing treatment with LHRH. Side effects, which include hot flashes and some minimal pain, seem to be similar to those seen with the 1-month injections.

Nilutamide for an Antiandrogen Response

Some physicians fail to include nilutamide on the antiandrogen withdrawal response. Remind your urologist to try Nilandron. Although the antiandrogen withdrawal response will arrest your rising PSA for only a few months, every little bit helps.

Orchiectomy, LHRH Agonists, and Bone Loss

Patients who have osteoporosis and are undergoing treatment for prostate cancer should be aware that less bone loss occurs with LHRH agonists than with orchiectomy. When an orchiectomy is performed, the body reacts to a loss of testosterone by stimulating the pituitary gland to release LH and FSH. Because the high levels of LH and FSH are associated with increased levels of ACTH (adrenocorticotrophic hormone) produced by the pituitary with increased cortisol levels that suppress the osteoblast (the cells that produce the osteoid) to mitiate the formation of new bone. The changes do not occur with an LHRH agonist or treatments involving estrogens. As a result, LH and FSH production are decreased by these agents, and there is no stimulation of the pituitary gland.

Modified Practices in Hormonal Therapy

Using combination hormone therapy to treat prostate cancer is an ever-evolving field. Some physicians who are on the leading edge of prostate cancer treatment have developed creative and effective practices by using either an antiandrogen or an LHRH agonist to deal with the disease. The following section presents some of these practices. They should only be used under the care of a doctor who has had experience with them.

Decreasing the PSA with Casodex after Eulexin Withdrawal

Casodex is an FDA-approved antiandrogen used to treat prostate cancer patients. It is well tolerated when the patient takes the customary dose of 50 mg daily. When either bilateral orchiectomy plus Eulexin - or an LHRH agonist plus Eulexin - was no longer effective (as evidenced by a progressive rise in the PSA level), a triple or quadruple dose (150 or 200 mg) of Casodex resulted in excellent responses in some patients.

In a study involving eight patients, four patients had more than a 50 percent decrease in the PSA level, and two had more than an 80 percent decline. No serious side effects were experienced.

Because this study involved only a small number of patients, a much larger study is necessary to confirm the excellent results demonstrated. It is possible that when Casodex withdrawal takes place, Eulexin may come to the rescue.

Reducing the Dose of Flutamide

Because of the cost and side effects, some oncologists are questioning the merits of patients taking three 250-mg tablets of flutamide every 8 hours. They are considering reducing the dosage to one 125-mg tablet every 8 hours, after patients have been on it 1 or 2 years. In fact, some physicians in Europe have been doing this for years.

Remaining Sexually Active with CHT

Prostate cancer patients who want to remain active sexually can do so by stopping CHT but remaining on flutamide and Proscar. However, this protocol is recommended only for patients with minimal-volume prostate cancer. CHT will probably add more years to their life than will flutamide and Proscar. Clinical trials are now in progress to test this hypothesis.

CHT with Proscar

A few oncologists have added Proscar to CHT to increase its efficacy. The premise behind this is that Proscar blocks 5-alpha reductase, the enzyme that converts testosterone to dihydrotestosterone (DHT); this decreases the amount of DHT available to compete with the antiandrogen for the antiandrogen receptors. There is as yet no available data to verify the effectiveness of this combination. DHT is five times more potent than testosterone in its effects on prostate cancer. Instead of patients receiving 5 mg of Proscar once daily, they receive 5 mg twice daily.

An Expanded Role for Flutamide

In 1996, the FDA approved an expanded role for flutamide, in combination with an LHRH agonist with external beam radiation, in treating locally confined stage B2 and C prostate cancer. Flutamide had already been approved in combination with an LHRH agonist to treat advanced (stage D2) prostate cancer. The latest approval was based on a study conducted by the Radiation Therapy Oncologic Group (RTOG), involving multicenter controlled clinical trials in which 471 patients with stage T2b, T3, and T4 prostate cancer tumors, with no evidence of metastasis, participated.

A total of 456 patients were divided into two groups. Group 1 consisted of 226 patients; group 2 involved 230. Group 1 patients received a 3.6-mg injection of Zoladex every 4 weeks and 250 mg of flutamide orally three times daily for 2 months before and during a course of external beam radiation. In group 2, patients received no CHT but received 1.0 to 2.0 Gy per day of external beam radiation for a total dose of 45 Gy, plus or minus 1 Gy.

With a median potential follow-up of 4.5 years, the cumulative incidence of local progression at 5 years was 46 percent in group 1 compared to 71 percent in group 2. The 5-year incidence of distant metastasis for Arm I patients was 34 percent, compared to 41 percent for group 2. Progression-free survival rates, including normal PSA levels for 396 patients with at least one PSA recorded, were 36 percent in group 1 at 5 years and 15 percent in group 2.

The study found that patients who underwent short-term CHT as well as external beam radiation had a marked increase in local control and disease-free survival compared to patients with locally advanced prostate cancer who received external beam radiation alone. The role of flutamide and an LHRH agonist with external beam radiation seems to be borne out by one of the authors, James Lewis, Jr. who underwent similar treatment prior to the availability of the results of the RTOG study. The Stanford University Medical School group uses a similar protocol for prostatectomy patients whose disease has recurred, both with and without lymph-node involvement.

How to Use This Information

1. If you choose external beam radiation for either early-stage or locally advanced prostate cancer with or without lymph-node involvement, insist on at least 2 or 3 months of CHT prior to radiation and 2 or 3 months of CHT during it.
2. If you are getting a monthly injection of Zoladex, ask your doctor to replace it with a 3-month injection for the sake of convenience. If you are on Eulexin or Casodex and are in excruciating pain, consider substituting Nilandron.
3. If you experience antiandrogen withdrawal, consider taking Casodex if you are on Eulexin, and Eulexin if you are on Casodex. And don't forget Nilandron, which can be used in place of Casodex or Eulexin.
4. If you cannot afford Eulexin or if you have severe side effects from it, ask your doctor to consider lowering the dose to one 125-mg pill every 8 hours if you have been taking it for 1 or 2 years.
5. If your doctor wants you to undergo CHT and you are sexually active, ask your doctor to delay starting you on an LHRH agonist and to prescribe an antiandrogen with Proscar first. However, understand that this therapy has no proven track record.
6. If your doctor wants you to undergo CHT, ask that Proscar be included to possibly improve its efficacy.

7.   Consider using a transdermal estrogen patch to treat hot flashes.
8.   If you are hormonal-resistant, try a triple dose of Casodex.

Chapter 24

QUADRAMET: TREATING MULTIPLE BONE SITES

Bone pain is the most common type of pain caused by prostate cancer. As a result, routine evaluation of each patient complaining of pain is important because the symptoms are often insidious from the onset, and the patient may attribute them to a host of other bone diseases, such as degenerative bone loss, Paget's disease, and arthritis. Such a self-diagnosis may not actually be wrong, but it must not prevent doctors from accurately diagnosing the source of the patient's pain. The description of the pain varies with the individual patient. Different patients may use words that imply different or opposite characteristics, such as *dull/red hot* and *aching/stabbing*. An exaggeration of pain with movement or pressure is often common. Tenderness over a bone may indicate metastasis until proven otherwise. A normal X-ray cannot exclude a bone metastasis, and an isotopic scan is usually much more sensitive. It is believed that a group of substances known as *prostacyclins* are liberated by most tumor deposits in bone, causing both reabsorption of bone around the tumor and sensitivity of nerve endings causing pain. Bone metastases, therefore, can cause pain when they are very small. When metastases enlarge, they can destroy the bone and lead to pathological fracture. Vertebral collapse may lead to nerve-root pain.

Treating Bone Pain

External beam radiation must be carefully considered for patients with bone pain. A solitary metastasis in long bones responds well to a course of external beam radiation. A half-body radiation should be considered for widespread metastases if most of the pain is in either the upper or lower torso. This, however, has been largely replaced by other modalities.

Hemibody Radiation

Spot radiation is effective in palliating bone pain; however, it is not usual for multiple bone metastases to cause pain simultaneously or within a short period of time. If each site of bone pain is irradiated individually, the patient may be inconvenienced by multiple courses of radiation. The hemibody radiation procedure may be a logical alternative for patients who have multiple sites of bone pain. The field and dose of radiation should be delivered to one half of the body. The second half of the body should not be treated simultaneously because the dose that can be given safely to the whole body is much lower than that which can be delivered to half the body. Be aware that the dose for irradiating the total body should not exceed 300 cGy in a single or fractionated dose because of potential lethal side effects. The upper half of the body field usually extends from above the scalp to the navel, and the lower half from the navel to the ankles. Up to 30 minutes is required to do one half of the body. After 4 to 6 weeks, when the blood count has returned to normal, the second half of the body can be treated. Complete pain relief has been reported in 24 to 70 percent of patients and partial pain relief in 24 to 71 percent. The average response time is 6 months, which does not stop additional use of localized therapy if cancer recurs or new symptoms appear. Usually the timetable is commensurate to the majority of the patient's remaining life; therefore, the patient should be grateful that there is a period relatively free of pain because most of the patients will eventually become hormone-resistant.

Side effects of hemibody radiation usually occur immediately and up to 2 weeks after treatment. The symptoms may include nausea, vomiting, elevated temperature and pulse rate, and hypertension. Most radiotherapists agree that 600 cGy is sufficient for the upper half of the body, and 800 cGy is sufficient for the lower half.

An alternative radiotherapy treatment, useful in patients with widespread and painful bone metastases, is the intravenous use of strontium or Quadramet. This therapy should be used to relieve not only localized symptoms in one area, but also for areas of pain distant from the main one. It is usually required when hormonal or other therapy begins to fail, but it is sometimes used if a patient has more than one area of bone pain that does not respond rapidly to systemic treatment. Sometimes, patients live for several years even though they have significantly painful local metastases requiring local radiation. Therefore, radiation must be carefully applied in order to minimize its long-term effects.

In fact, the use of localized external beam radiation and a radiopharmaceutical usually results in a higher response rate and a longer duration of response than either modality alone.

Radiopharmaceuticals for Bone Pain

While hemibody radiation is useful and effective in prostate cancer patients with diffuse and rapidly recurrent pain, it also has significant side effects and is therefore difficult to repeat as a treatment. As a result, an effective and well-tolerated systemic therapy is needed that can go right to the site of pain and that can be repeated. A radiopharmaceutical is a systematic term of radiation that leads to efficient localization at the site of bone metastases. It provides pain relief for 6 months in 80 percent of patients with hormone-refractory disease, while causing minimal side effects. It selectively radiates multiple sites of bone involvement simultaneously. It has also been used occasionally in early-stage prostate cancer before pain occurs in order to delay its onset, and is a reasonable alternative to external beam radiation when it is not easily and readily available.

There are several forms of radionuclide treatments for metastatic bone pain such as strontium-89, rhenium 186, and samarium153 (Quadramet), but only strontium-89 and Quadramet attack both lytic and blastic bone disease. In three different clinical trials of strontium-89 in hormonally refractory patients, a decrease in bone painoccurred in 67 to 80 percent. Pain relief lasted from 3 to 6 months, with 27 percent of the patients becoming pain-free. A temporary increase in pain or flare response was seen in 10 percent of patients. Pain response occurred about 7 to 20 days after strontium-89 was administered.

In a double-blind randomized study, 114 cancer patients with painful bone metastases received a single dose of Quadramet. During the first 4 weeks after administration, patients assessed each day their pain intensity, daytime discomfort, and ability to sleep. During the fourth week, which was considered the primary efficacy point of the study, there was a statistically significant difference in pain relief between the two doses in favor of the 1.0 Cl/Kg dose. These doses should produce tumor regression without injury to the tissue. A single bone metastasis can usually be palliated by doses of 40 cGy in 4 weeks at the rate of 2 cGy per day.

It is very important to assess bone metastases in order to prevent spinal cord compression. Areas of painful involvement in the vertebrae should be treated before structural damage threatens the integrity of the spinal cord. In order to prevent this debilitating complication, the radiation dose must be relatively high, such as 40 to 50 cGy delivered at the rate of 2 cGy a day.

Spot Radiation

If you have pain in a single concentrated area of the body, you should strongly consider undergoing spot radiation. This therapy is similar to hemibody radiation treatment except that the radiation is directed to the specific site of the pain, which usually targets the cancer. The majority of patients (70 to 80%) who receive spot radiation indicate that they receive complete or partial pain relief. Spot radiation usually takes 10 to 20 days to provide relief, which may last 4 to 15 months. The average decrease in platelet count after treatment is 24 to 50 percent.

Bone Damage

Prostate cancer cells spread in the body in two primary ways. The first is through the lymphatic channels that drain the pelvic cavity. As a result, cancerous cells in the pelvic lymph nodes can grow to cause symptomatic metastatic disease. The second way in which prostate cancer spreads is through the venous plexus that drains blood from the pelvic area.

Metastases first affect the surrounding bone tissue by causing certain physiological changes to take place in the bone cells. As a result, chemicals secreted by the metastases stimulate unnatural bone growth and destruction. Usually, abnormal new bone forms as the disease progresses. This new tissue, overly dense and weaker than the normal bone, is referred to as *blastic*. It appears as a whiter area on an X-ray. The blastic outgrowth is in the confined marrow channel, and the actual swelling mass of tumor can produce pressure-causing pain because the surface of the bone has nerve fibers.

A second type of damage is called *lytic* destruction. Bone may become riddled with holes, thus undermining the integrity of the legs, hips, and spine. Lytic change does not appear on a bone scan as prominently as blastic bone change. Therefore, a bone X-ray is an important diagnostic tool if lytic bone change is suspected.

What Patients Say about Quadramet

- "The pain I would get in my back was just like a toothache. It would throb. If I was lying down, it would feel like it [the pain] was raising me up off the bed." - L. R.
- "Tried Darvocet (with no good results), Demerol (no good), time-released morphine (no more pain, but couldn't function from the tired side effect – [I was] listless)... After I had the Quadramet, it was a lot easier to live with me because I wasn't constantly worrying about whether I was in pain or not. I now work part time and am feeling good." - R. S.
- "I'm just very grateful that they came out with the treatment when they did and that we were able to hear of it. The thing that worked for me best was the Quadramet." - L. R.
- "We had been told that there wasn't anything else that the cancer doctors could do for the pain, and then like a godsend, this Quadramet was offered to us as a way of dealing with this

problem... My husband had not felt like visiting with friends or relations, and with the Quadramet he was able to do that again with some degree of comfort." - J. S.

- "I had quite a bit of pain before I had the injections. The pain came mostly at night. I had problems sleeping. After the injection, I was able to sleep again. I was very surprised that I was able to drive 800 miles to my son's house, when I wasn't sure if I would ever be able to make that drive again."

  - M. S.

The Primary Goal for Treating

Multiple Metastatic Bone Pain Sites

The main goal for treating metastatic bone pain is to restore quality of life so that the patient begins to feel good again. Increasing his survival time would certainly be a plus as well.

The following section compares strontium-89 to Quadramet in the treatment of multiple bone pain sites:

1. Relieved the patients with bone pain in the shortest time period. Strontium-89 relieves a greater number of patients with metastatic bone pain compared to Quadramet (67-80 vs. 70-75, respectively). Quadramet relieves patients with bone pain sooner than strontium-89 (1 to 3 weeks vs. 3 to 6 months), with complete response in 25 percent of patients with strontium and about half of the patients on Quadramet.

2. The agent can be used to retreat the patient's bone pain in a short period of time. Retreatment can be performed at intervals of not less than a mean duration of 90 days with strontium-89 and 56 days with Quadramet.

3. A minimum of time should elapse before initial treatment and retreatment. A minimum of 7 days can elapse between treatment and retreatment with Quadramet, and 60 to 90 days with strontium-89.

4. The patient should be able to take other drugs and undergo other treatment in the shortest period of time. While patients undergo strontium-89, other drugs cannot be administered nor other treatment begun before 30 days have elapsed; those on Quadramet can start additional therapy within 7 days.

5. The agent should have a short physical half-life cycle. The short physical half-life of Quadramet is 46.3; of strontium-89 it is 50.5 days.
6. White blood cell count should recover in a short period. White blood cell count rebounds within 4 to 6 weeks in those treated with strontium-89 and within 3 to 5 weeks in those on Quadramet.
7. Platelet count should completely recover during a short period of time. Platelet count recovers in 12 weeks using strontium-89 and the lowest level of 40 to 50 percent of baseline within 3 to 5 weeks.
8. Pain relief should last for the greatest duration. Pain relief lasted for 3 to 6 months with strontium-89, and with Quadramet.
9. The agent should reduce the need for other drugs. Approximately half of the patients reduced opioid usage by the fourth week on Quadramet. No definite figures were available for strontium-89, but it appears to offer a similar benefit.
10. The patient experiencing multiple metastatic bone pain should begin to feel well in the shortest time period. Strontium-89 relieves a greater number of patients with metastatic bone pain compared to Quadramet (67-80% vs. 48-54%, respectively). Quadramet relieves patients with bone pain much sooner than strontium-89 does (3 weeks vs. 3-6 months).

A greater number of patients may be treated for bone pain with strontium-89; however, in the most critical cases Quadramet appears to represent an improvement over strontium-89 in most categories cited in the preceding analysis.

Why Choose This Treatment?

Any patient experiencing multiple metastatic bone pain sites needs a medication that can be administered by a single injection, thus causing pain relief in the shortest period of time, enabling it to attack both lytic and blastic bone disease, having a short physical half-life cycle, so that the patient may undergo another treatment in a short period of time. Quadramet appears to meet many of these criteria.

How to Use This Information

If you have multiple metastatic bone pain sites and wish to use radiopharmaceuticals to relieve your pain, discuss this option with your physician. If another treatment is necessary, wait at least 7 days before instituting that therapy.

Chapter 25

BEFAR FOR ERECTILE DYSFUNCTION

As a result of the success of Viagra, many companies are investigating herbs, vitamins, and drugs to determine if one of them or a combination can effectively eradicate erectile dysfunction (ED), often a side effect of treatment for prostate cancer. Products for the treatment of ED should:

1. Be effective and cheap.
2. Act immediately or within a few minutes.
3. Be easily applied or ingested.
4. Induce a minimum of side effects.
5. Be approved by the FDA.
6. Be satisfactory for your mate.
7. Cause no harm to your mate.
8. Work all the time.
9. Overcome impotence as well as ED.
10. Not have any dangerous side effects.
11. Treat the root cause of impotence.
12. Be administered in one step and be easy to use both physically and psychologically.
13. Not cause cardiovascular complications.
14. Work for at least 80 percent of patients.
15. Help all patients afflicted with serious diseases such as diabetes, hypertension, or poor circulation.

Using these criteria as guides and investigating all of the anti-impotency products, we have discovered that only one product meets most of them. That product, developed by NexMed, Inc. and manufactured in Hong Kong, is known as Befar.

What is Erectile Dysfunction?

Erectile dysfunction is the inability to achieve or maintain an erection sufficient for mutually satisfying sexual intercourse. In essence, the penis has an insufficient or inadequate blood supply due to physiological or psychological factors - or a combination of both.

What Is Befar and How Does It Work?

Befar, a topical ointment that contains the active ingredient alprox-TD, a derivative of Alprostadil, is applied to the tip of the penis to produce an erection. Alprox-TD works by widening the blood vessels in the penis, allowing it to fill with blood. NexMed reports that 83 percent of men with erectile dysfunction were satisfied using Befar.

Alprostadil, approved by the FDA and used for several years around the world, is administered by injection directly into the penis. Users report side effects that include persistent erection, which can both painful and dangerous. Alprostadil itself has been proven to be very effective in restoring potency; however, it is just too powerful to be injected into the penis.

Side Effects of Befar

Users report that the most common side effects are:

- redness at the application site
- some discomfort
- burning sensation for a short period after application
- urinary-tract pain

Advantages of Befar

Befar has several advantages:

1. It has few side effects.
2. It's effective and acts in 10 minutes.
3. It costs less than Viagra.
4. Patients with diabetes and high blood pressure are able to get an erection.
5. Patients with heart problems can use it safely.
6. Alprostadil, the active ingredient in the cream, has already been proven as a treatment for ED.

How Is Befar Applied?

Apply the cream approximately 10 to 15 minutes before engaging in sexual intercourse, as directed below:

1. Remove the cap from the tip of the applicator.

2.   Grasp the tip of the penis and gently open the urethra.
3.   Apply the prescribed dose of Befar.
4.   Hold the penis upright for about 30 seconds to allow the cream to enter the orifice.   The cream does not need to be completely absorbed to be effective.

Befar versus Viagra

Befar	Viagra
In the third phase of a clinical trial in the U.S. FDA approval expected in 2003.	Approved by the FDA.
Takes 10 minutes to act.	Takes 30 to 60 minutes to act.
Comes in cream form.	Comes in tablet form.
Requires one drop.	Requires one or more tablets.
Efficacy is 83 percent.	Efficacy is 82 percent.
No stimulation necessary.	Sexual stimulation needed.
Applied to the urethra	Taken orally.
No deaths have been reported.	About 300 patients have died.
Comes in 100-, 250-, and 1,000-mg doses.	Comes in 25-, 50-, and 100-mg doses.
Effective for men with diabetes, heart disease high blood pressure, high cholesterol, or stress and for men who smoke or who drink too much.	Limited effectiveness for men with diabetes, heart disease (death possible), high blood pressure, high cholesterol, or stress for men who smoke or who drink too much.
Side effects are: -some discomfort -mild burning -some urinary-tract pain	Side effects are: -headache -facial flushing -upset stomach -stuffy nose -bluish vision -blurred vision -urinary-tract infection -diarrhea -sensitivity to light
Price: $15.00 (250 mg) $12.50 (100 mg)	Price: $8 to $9 per tablet

Clinical Trial

The clinical efficacy and safety of Befar cream (250 mg containing 1 mg P6E) were evaluated in four different studies. A total of 356 patients with erectile dysfunction of various causes and intensities were enrolled in the studies. The men using Befar had a statistically significant improvement in success rates for sexual intercourse compared with placebo in various efficacy measurement. In another study, 157 ED patients ages 26 to 75 years with ED etiologies (psychogenic 27%, organic 20%, mixed 53%) and a mean ED history of 5 years were given Befar or a placebo over a 4-week period.

The effectiveness of the medications was evaluated from patient history and patient evaluation questionnaires both before and after the treatment. The researchers used the international index of erectile dysfunction, the sexual encounter profile (SEP), and doctor's and patient's assessment questions. Question 3 (the ability to achieve an erection sufficient for sexual intercourse) and question 4 (the maintenance of erection after penetration) from the International Index of Erectile Function (IIEF) served as primary study end points. The patients addressed each question at both the first and the final visit of the 4-week study. The responses to the questions were graded as follows:

0 = no attempted intercourse,
1 = never or almost never,
2 = a few times,
3 = sometimes,
4 = most times,
5 = almost always.

Questions were also asked about erectile function, orgasm, desire, satisfaction with intercourse, and overall satisfaction. Information about intercourse attempts was also recorded by patients in a diary. In addition, patients were asked a question on improvement in erections.

The evaluation of Befar's efficacy was based on changes in the scores for questions 3 and 4. Befar demonstrated a primary efficacy rating of 68 percent versus 13 percent for the placebo. Clinical benefits, evaluated by physicians based on the patients' diaries, were 74 percent for Befar and 18 percent for placebo, respectively. The frequency of patients reporting improvement of erections indicated the global efficacy of Befar was 75 percent versus 19 percent for placebo. The benefits for the patients with various intensities of ED was also assessed by comparing the number of successful intercourse attempts with total intercourse attempts. In this analysis, the efficacy rates for mild, moderate, and severe ED patients in the Befar group were 90, 65, and 49 percent, compared to 31, 27, and 6 percent for the placebo group.

Dostinex Enhances Befar

In 1996, the FDA approved the sale of Dostinex (cabergoline) tablets for the treatment of hyperprolactinemic disorders. Hyperprolactinemia is caused by a benign tumor on the pituitary gland that results in excess production of prolactin, the hormone that controls lactation. Not only is cabergoline used to treat Parkinson's disease, it also has been found to raise a man's chances of having multiple orgasms.

In clinical trials, cabergoline was prescribed to minimize the effects of the hormone prolactin, which is produced by men at the point of orgasm. The hormone has the effect of reducing a man's desire for more sex by preventing new erections.

Sixty test subjects, all healthy males, between the ages of 22 and 31, needed a break of 19 minutes between orgasms. However, after taking cabergoline, they were able to have several orgasms within a few minutes.

Medical psychologist Manfred Schedlowski, who was involved in the trials at Essen in Germany, said the drug raised the libido to enable the male to reach orgasm again more quickly. He said, "We saw that prolactin rises after orgasm and then thought maybe prolactin is a negative feedback system.

"Men who took this drug had decreased prolactin levels, and reported their orgasm was better and there was a shorter refractory period. We interviewed these subjects and found they were able to have multiple orgasms in very rapid succession. This is sitting very nicely with our hypothesis that orgasms and sexual drive are steered by prolactin and dopamine in the brain."

Men taking cabergoline experienced no side effects during the tests, according to an article to be published in the International Journal of Impotence Research.

One man said, "Dostinex doesn't just make it easy to achieve multiple orgasms. The medication gives the word orgasm a whole new meaning. I have never, not even during my early twenties, felt so engulfed in lovemaking as I do now, at the age of 50, provided I have taken some Dostinex. I have no problem to go on with intercourse for half an hour, and I remain totally focused. And when I reach orgasm, it is with a power that marks the difference between a dribbling ejaculation and a half-a-meter shot."

The standard U.S. price for eight Dostinex tablets (0.5 mg) is $218. This translates into $27.25 per 0.5 mg tablet. But a patient purchases the drug at $1.60 per 0.5 gram (tablet form, not raw material), which is less than 6 percent of the standard U.S. price.

Purchasing Befar

1.   Get a prescription from your medical doctor.
2.   Wire the money to the following bank:
     Bank Name: The Hong Kong & Shanghai Banking Corporation Limited
     Branch Name: Causeway Bay Branch
     Branch Address: 1/F, Causeway Bay Plaza 2, 463-483
                     Lockhart Road, Causeway Bay, Hong Kong
     Beneficiary Name: Drake Pacific Company Limited
     Beneficiary account no.: 495-9-606635 U.S.
3.   Befar is available in two pack sizes:
     a.   0.4% - 100 mg, delivering 300 mcg. of Alprostadil
     b.   0.4% - 250 mg, which can be used as multi-doses for the non-responder
     The 250 mg pack is $15 (U.S.)/tube and the 100 mg is $12.50 (U.S.)/tube. The minimum shipping (FedEx) charge for 1-10 tubes is $50 (U.S.). If the order is larger than 10 tubes, additional shipping will be calculated.
4.   You can fax your prescription and ordering information to 852-28-951-698 or 852-31-109-888. You may also scan and email the information to leolau88@hotmail.com or mail it to the address above.

How to Use This Information

1.   Begin ED treatment by consulting a physician. If you are not supervised by a doctor and you want to begin ED treatment, start with the smallest dose of Befar and work your way up to the highest satisfactory dosage.
2.   Do not mix Befar with other medications.

Chapter 26

COMBATING HORMONE-REFRACTORY PROSTATE CANCERWITH VITAMIN D AND TAXOTERE

Approximately 60 to 70 percent of all men diagnosed with prostate cancer will someday have metastatic disease. As discussed in Chapter 18, when metastatic prostate cancer progresses after initial hormonal therapy, it is referred to as hormone-refractory. Hormone-refractory metastatic prostate cancer is at the present time not curable, and all attempts at therapeutic intervention have been based on palliating the disease and reducing bone pain. Because there is no standard treatment for hormone-refractory disease, new therapeutic strategies are definitely needed. A recent strategy that seems to hold some promise, which is in a phase III clinical trial at the Oregon Health and Science University Cancer Institute in Portland, Oregon, under the leadership of oncologist Tomasz Beer, M.D., is the use of a blend or combination of vitamin D and a chemotherapy drug known as Taxotere (docetaxel).

The intent of this chapter is to cite the therapeutic benefits of vitamin D and Taxotere (docetaxel) and to discuss the results of several clinical studies.

Vitamin D

Researchers and scientists have studied the effect of Calcitriol (vitamin D) on prostate cancer. Their conclusions follow:

- "It's becoming increasingly clear that vitamin D has a host of effects in the body, especially on the growth of tumor cells," said David Feldman, M.D., of Stanford University at a seminar sponsored by the American Institute for Cancer Research in Washington, D.C., in 2002.
- Dr. Feldman and colleagues concluded that "Vitamin D is anti-proliferative and promotes cellular maturation." It seems clear, they add, "that vitamin D must be viewed as an important cellular modulator of growth and differentiation. Vitamin D has the potential to have beneficial actions on various malignancies including prostate cancer."
- 1,25-dihydroxy vitamin D may prove useful in chemoprevention, they say, and/or in differentiation therapy. They maintain an "optimistic

view on the possible use of vitamin D to treat prostate cancer," and say that "further investigation is clearly warranted."

- New forms (analogs) of vitamin D have been developed that have much less effect on calcium metabolism but still retain the vitamin's tumor-inhibiting properties. The action of the vitamin seems to be regulated by a single receptor site, which has the same structure as certain steroid receptors.

- Canadian scientists have reported that in the test tube, cancer-cell proliferation is "strongly inhibited" by both vitamin D and its analogs. In some systems, they say, the analogs (such as EB1089) were 10 to 100 times more potent than the original compound. This activity "predicts their potential usefulness" in animals in inhibiting squamous cancer growth.

- Scientists have concluded that vitamin D metabolism may indeed impact the risk of prostate cancer (Corder, EH, et al., Cancer Epidemiol Biomarkers Prev 1995;4:655-659).

- In one study, serum levels of 1,25-dihydroxy vitamin D (the major circulating form of the vitamin) were significantly lower in 181 men who had been diagnosed with prostate cancer, compared to their age-matched controls. According to the author of that study, Elizabeth Corder, M.D., levels of the vitamin could be used to predict a man's risk for prostate cancer.

- Vitamin D is the principal regulator of calcium homeostasis in the body. It is particularly important in skeletal development and bone mineralization. Vitamin D is a prohormone. That is, it has no hormone activity itself, but it is converted to a molecule that does.

- Vitamin D may have anti-osteoporotic, immunomodulatory, anticarcinogenic, antipsoriatic, antioxidant, and mood-stabilizing activities.

- Very preliminary work suggests that vitamin D may improve glucose tolerance in some diabetics; it may have some favorable effects on spermatogenesis; it may increase seizure threshold in some circumstances; and it might be helpful in bilateral cochlear deafness and in seasonal-related depression. In addition, in one case study vitamin D seemed to obliterate the symptoms of sick sinus syndrome, a heart disorder that is generally treated with antiarrhythmia drugs. Follow-up research is needed.

- Vitamin D may have a role in the treatment or prevention of some cancers. In some nonpreliminary work, it demonstrated a dose-dependent inhibition on cell-proliferation effect on these cells, resulting in potent anticancer activity. Vitamin D and its analogs show significant experimental activity against prostate cancer.

- The anticarcinogenic activity of vitamin D is not fully understood by scientists. Vitamin D has been found to induce apoptosis of cancer cells in vitro and in vivo. It down-regulates the antiapoptotic bcl-2 protein and up-regulates clusterin and cathepsin B.
- Research suggests that a broad range of additional indications may eventually emerge, including uses in cancer.

Taxotere (Docetaxel)

The following list summarizes what researchers and scientists have concluded from studies of Taxotere and its effects on prostate cancer.

- Docetaxel is a semisynthetic chemotherapy drug made from an extract of needles of the yew tree. It is used to treat people with some types of early- and late-stage cancer.
- Many chemotherapy drugs stop cancer cells from dividing by interfering with the cells' DNA, but Taxotere acts quite differently. Taxotere changes microtubules, vital structures involved in cell division.
- Taxotere, one of the most effective anticancer chemotherapy drugs available, is injected into a vein to treat various types of tumors by attacking cancer cells. It is approved by the FDA to treat:

1. locally advanced or metastatic breast cancer that returns after any prior chemotherapy.
2. locally advanced or metastatic non-small cell lung cancer that recurs after prior platinum-based chemotherapy.

Taxotere is given intravenously every 3 weeks, with each treatment lasting about an hour. Taxotere is a drug in the taxoid class of chemotherapy agents, which inhibits cancer-cell division by "freezing" the cell's internal skeleton, which is comprised of microtubules. Microtubules assemble and disassemble during a cell cycle. Taxotere promotes their assembly and blocks their disassembly, thereby preventing cancer cells from dividing and resulting in cancer-cell death.

Taxotere can help destroy cancer cells in the body when cancer is discovered, or recurs, after previous therapy.

Taxotere is part of the taxoid class of chemotherapy, whose original source is the yew tree. Taxanes prevent the growth of cancer by affecting the microtubules.

In worldwide phase II clinical trials, Taxotere demonstrated the highest tumor response rates ever reported for a single agent in men with hormone-resistant disease.

Side Effects of Taxotere

A chronic dosage of 95 micrograms of Taxotere or more in healthy individuals may cause hypercalcaemia – high concentration of calcium in the blood. Symptoms include:

- nausea and vomiting
- weakness
- headache
- somnolence
- dry mouth
- constipation
- metallic taste
- muscle pain
- bone pain
- polyuria (excessive urination)
- polydipsia (abnormal thirst)
- anorexia
- weight loss
- nocturia (nighttime urination)
- conjunctivitis
- pancreatitis
- photophobia (intolerance to light)
- rhinorrhea (excessive nasal mucus)
- itching
- high fever
- decreased libido
- temporary reduction in bone marrow function
- mouth sores and ulcers
- diarrhea
- hair loss
- skin changes
- soreness and redness
- allergic reaction
- fluid retention
- numbness and tingling in hands or feet

- changes in nails
- pain in joints or muscles

How Is Taxotere Administered?

Taxotere is given as an infusion (drip) into a vein through a fine needle (cannula).

Clinical Trial

Calcitriol

In a study conducted by D.C. Smith et al., patients with advanced solid tumors were given calcitriol every other day (QOD). As mentioned, the major side effect of the active form of vitamin D — 1,25-dihydroxycholecalciferol (calcitriol) — is hypercalcemia. Unfortunately, no studies indicate the maximum tolerated dose of calcitriol when administered every other day. Therefore, this trial permitted the ingesting of higher doses of calcitriol, which might have anticancer activity. A total of 36 patients took doses ranging from 2 to 10 mcg QOD; hypercalcemia occurred in three of three patients taking 10 mcg. Hypercalciuria (excess calcium in the urine) occurred at all dose levels. No other side effects were observed. An assessment of serum calcitriol concentrations by an RIA revealed a decrease in concentration time curve. The maximum serum levels occurred at the 10-mg dose. The normal range of calcitriol levels were maintained at near peak concentrations for at least 8 hours following subcutaneous injection. The researchers maintain that substantial doses of calcitriol can be consumed via this route with tolerable side effects. Studies to determine how to ameliorate the hypercalcemia induced by calcitriol and should be conducted.

Calcitriol and Docetaxel

A study is being conducted by Dr. Tomasz M. Beer et al. to determine if the addition of high-dose calcitriol will improve the therapeutic value of docetaxel in androgen-independent prostate cancer (AIPC). Patients in this study followed a reduced calcium diet and also took calcitriol (0.5 mcg/kg) orally on day 1, followed by docetaxel 36 mg/m^2 on day 2. Dexamethasone (8 mg) was given 12 hours prior to and 12 hours after docetaxel infusion. Therapy was repeated weekly for 6 weeks on an 8-week cycle. PSA response (50% reduction confirmed 4 weeks later) was the primary end point. Measurable disease, pain, pain medication consumption, and quality of life were also monitored. Thirty-nine patients were needed to detect a 20 percent absolute increase in PSA level (from 45% expected with docetaxel alone to 65%), with 95 percent confidence and 80 percent power. Thirty patients (77%) achieved a reduction in PSA level. Twenty-three (59% had more than a 75% reduction in PSA level, and nine (23%) reached a PSA level below 4.0 ng/ml. Of the remaining eight patients, the best PSA response was: unconfirmed response, one; stable (under 16 weeks), six; and progression, two. A Kaplan-Meier estimate of the median time to disease progression for all patients was 10.2 months. In 2003, the median survival time had not been reached, and 32 patients (82%) remained alive with a median follow-up of 50 weeks. Grade ¾ treatment-related side effects included: leukopenia, 13 (33%); neutropenia, 7 (18%); hyperglycemia, 10 (26%); gastric ulcer, 2 (5%); duodenal ulcer, 2 (5%); infection, 2 (5%); and one episode each of diarrhea, anemia, anorexia, angina, deep vein thrombosis (DVT), edema, bronchiolitis obliterans organizing pneumonia (BOOP), dyspnea (labored breathing), and aspartate aminotransferase (AST) elevation. These results suggest that high-dose calcitriol may enhance the activity of weekly docetaxel in AIPC without significantly increasing side effects. The PSA response rate of 77% compares favorably with that of 38 (46%) reported in phase II studies of single-agent docetaxel in AIPC. Further study of this regimen is warranted.

Data from another phase II clinical trial suggest that combining docetaxel and calcitriol is as much as twice as effective as using docetaxel alone. The results were so promising that a phase III trial has been launched at 15 sites throughout the United States.

In another study, 31 of 37 patients (81%) treated with calcitriol and Taxotere reduced their PSA level by more than half. In fact, 59 percent of patients reduced their PSA level by more than 75 percent. Studies of docetaxel alone have reported a lowering of PSA level by 42 percent. In addition to PSA response, 8 of 15 men in the study with measurable disease had a significant reduction of their tumors.

How to Use This Information

If you have metastatic hormone refractory disease, this therapy may be of benefit as a palliative treatment.

Chapter 27

COMBINATION RADIATION: WHICH TYPE?

Studies have shown that combination radiation (brachytherapy and external beam radiation) are as good as — or better than — radical prostatectomy. A study discussed in that chapter revealed that combination radiation is better than nerve-sparing radical prostatectomy, radical prostatectomy, and cryosurgery for preserving a man's sexual function.

There are two basic types of combination radiation:

1. seed implant, followed by external beam radiation
2. external beam radiation, followed by seed implant

Because a growing number of prostate cancer patients are opting for combination radiation, it is important that they base their decisions on such relevant factors:

- a review of the various activities involving each of the types as stated by two radiation oncologists who practice their respective forms
- discuss the differences between the two types
- address the unproven comments levied against the radiation oncologists using the seeds-first approach.

As mentioned in Chapter 28, Dr. Frank A. Critz of Radiotherapy Clinics of Georgia (RCOG) is the developer of a treatment known as ProstRcision, in which radioactive seeds are implanted first, followed by external beam radiation. He has been performing this protocol successfully since 1979, though others had difficulty. In contrast with radiation oncologists who discontinued seed implantation when they experienced difficulties, Critz reduced the radiation dose from the I-125 implant and added external beam radiation 21 days later. Since radioactive iodine has a 60 - day half-life, therapeutic radiation was given simultaneously from two separate sources. Because this combination had never been attempted, he used very low radiation doses through 1983, learning how to safely perform the procedure. Two other groups independently attempted this technique in the early 1980s, but they stopped due to complications. After achieving a satisfactory comfort level with combination radiation, in 1984 Critz began using 6,000 to 10,000 cGy of brachytherapy radiation and 4,500 cGy of external beam radiation.

This method of "seeds first" radiation has some skeptics. Dr. Critz's critics accuse him of falsifying the number of patients experiencing serious side effects and the number of long-term recurrences. This is nothing but malicious gossip by jealous doctors. The authors have visited Dr. Critz's facility several times and found him to be open and honest about what he says and publishes. For example, Dr. Critz could inflate his cure rates by calculating outcome with the American Society for Therapeutic Radiology and Oncology (ASTRO) definition of recurrence like all other radiation oncologists do. However, Dr. Critz refuses to calculate with the ASTRO definition and instead calculates with a PSA of 0.2 ng/ml, which produces lower cure rates.

Dr. Critz was able to overcome not only the problems of the early pioneers, but also some of the problems experienced by today's radiation oncologists, solely through his tenacity, ingenuity, and creativity. Take a look at some of his accomplishments:

1. Many radiation oncologists believe that to implant seeds properly in the prostate gland, it should be reduced to 40 cc or less. As a result, many radiation oncologists prescribe combination hormonal therapy to shrink the prostate. Dr. Critz does not believe in doing this unless the gland is exceedingly large. When one of the authors advised a patient with a Gleason score of 10 to consider the seeds-first form of combination radiation, Dr. Critz personally treated him and implanted a whopping 267 seeds. This patient has extensive cancer of the prostate, and a 5-by-5-cm mass extended into the bladder. The accompanying urologist said, "Only Dr. Critz could have done this treatment." The patient experienced routine side effects for a week, and while it is too early to predict his long-term survival rate, his PSA dropped to an astounding 0.2 ng/ml. This man did not receive hormone treatment.

2. Dr. Critz was able to overcome the difficulties encountered by the protocol's of early pioneers by studying their problems and making gradual changes. Sometimes he would decrease the radiation dose, and other times he would increase it, depending on the patient's outcome. Sometimes he would use time as a strategy, delaying or advancing the time given to the two treatments. It took Dr. Critz several years to find the proper dose and time necessary to minimize side effects and to arrive at an acceptable cure rate. The development of other techniques and technologies also helped Dr. Critz perfect the seeds-first approach.

3. Dr. Critz was one of the few radiation oncologists in the United States to implant seeds in failed radical prostatectomy patients with some degree of success.
4. He was the first to maintain, through a peer-review study, that postradiation patients must
5. Achieve a PSA nadir level of 0.2 ng/ml to avoid a recurrence.
6. He has submitted nearly fifty proposals and/or presentations to peer review committees addressing many aspects of the seed-first form of combination radiation. Obviously, if these proposals and/or presentations did not have any merit, they would not have been shared with hundreds of other radiotherapists, sometimes leading to new discoveries and standards of performance to emulate.

The Differences between the Two Treatments

There are several differences between the seeds-first treatment (Dr. Critz's 10-year study), and the external beam radiation-first form of therapy (Dr. Haakon Ragde's 12-year study). They are both described in Table 27-1.

Table 27-1

Proponent/Approach	Ragde/"Beam First"	Critz/"Seeds First"
Period of research	12 years	10 years
Median age	71 years (range: 48-92 yrs)	66 (38-88)
No. patients	229	1,182
Clinical stages	T1-T3	T1, T2
Seeds	Iodine-125	Iodine-125
Median Gleason score	Range: 2-6	6 (2-10)
Low-risk patients (seeds only)	147	--
Intermediate-risk patients (seeds + EBR)	82	--
High-risk patients	--	1,182
Median follow-up	122 months (range: 18-144 months)	84 months (range: 60-126 months)
Failure point	Above 0.5 ng/ml	above 0.2 ng/ml
No. patients failed within 60 months	25%	10%

Table 27-1 (cont)

No. patients failing after 115 months	None	None
Disease-free at 1 year	70%	98%
No. patients with disease progression after 12 years and 10 years	None (12 years)	None (10 years)
No. patients excluded from study	14	None
Survival, Disease-free		
Low-risk patients (10 years)	60%	97%
Intermediate-risk patients (10 years)	79%	
High-risk patients		78%
Percentage of patient failure during 5 years posttreatment	25%	12%

A minor difference in the two studies is the number of patients involved in each. Dr. Critz's study included 953 more patients than did Dr. Ragde's. Another minor difference is that Dr. Ragde's study involved some stage T3 patients, a slight increase in the clinical stage.

How to Use This Information

Perhaps the most significant difference between the two types of combination radiation is the number of patients who failed their respective treatment during 5 years: 25 percent for the external beam radiation-first and only 12 percent for seeds-first. When the failure point is determined as a PSA level of 0.2 ng/ml, the seed-first form of combination radiation and the percentage of patients failing their respective form, it appears that implanting seeds-first has an advantage over giving external beam radiation first. Regardless of the approach you use, consider the experience of your doctor. One who has treated thousands of patients is obviously more qualified to deal with unexpected problems.

Chapter 28

SEEDS FOLLOWED BY EXTERNAL BEAM RADIATION

In order to give prostate cancer patients a glimpse of the many variations of combination radiation, we have asked a radiologist to respond to a series of questions. We hope this information will enable patients to select a therapy appropriate for their needs. One form of combination radiation is practiced by Dr. Frank A. Critz of the Radiotherapy Clinics of Georgia (RCOG) in Decatur, Georgia.

Q.   How do you accommodate those patients who do not remain in Georgia to obtain the external beam radiation phase of your protocol?

A.   Our protocol consists of performing an I-125 seed implant of the prostate followed 3 weeks later by 6 to 7 weeks of external beam irradiation. Many years ago, when we began treating patients beyond the Atlanta region, we sent a few men back to their hometowns for the external beam irradiation component. We also contacted the radiation oncologist in their hometowns, and sent X-rays and detailed recommendations as to how to give the follow-up external beam radiation. All of these men had substantial complications while undergoing linear accelerator irradiation in their hometowns. Most voluntarily returned to Atlanta because of the complications they were experiencing. Consequently, we decided that we will not treat men in our program unless we deliver all treatment: the implant and the follow-up conformal beam irradiation. This policy makes sense. It takes over one year to train a doctor to perform the seed implant and also to integrate the follow-up external beam radiation. Our treatment program is unique for we are giving two sources of radiation at the same time. It is impossible to communicate how to correctly treat someone by a phone call or a few letters to a hometown radiation oncologist. Therefore, men who live long distances from Atlanta have to stay in the Atlanta area during treatment.

The most popular place that men stay is in the Hope Lodge, which is located less than 10 minutes from our main office. The Hope Lodge is a wonderful facility with superb living accommodations, and staying there is free. Additionally, transportation is provided back and forth between the lodge and our facility at no charge. Since so many men and their families stay at the lodge, the lodge is often fully booked. Overflow patients are referred to numerous hotels and motels very close to the clinic, one or two within walking distance. We have negotiated reduced rates at these facilities, and we can arrange transportation for men and their families who do not have a car.

Q.   How do you decide which patients are high risk, intermediate, and low risk?

A.   That determination is based on evaluation of a combination of factors, primarily a man's pretreatment PSA, Gleason score, and clinical stage. We use the Memorial Sloan-Kettering system for determining risk groups. Risk factors are PSA greater than 10.0 ng/ml, Gleason 7 or more, or clinical stage T2b or higher. Men with none of these risk factors are considered low risk; one factor, intermediate risk; and two or more factors, high risk. However, we recognize that defining men by these risk factors is only an educated guess, and these guesses are often wrong. For example, some men with the worst cancers that we have treated have low pretreatment PSA. For example, several years ago, I treated a man with a pretreatment PSA of 0.5 ng/ml who lived only 9 months. He had a Gleason score of 10. Some cancers produce only a low amount of PSA. In fact, we see one or two patients each week who have low PSAs but extensive cancers.

Gleason score based on the biopsy is also an educated guess. Remember, you are sticking very tiny needles into this large prostate. An excellent study was performed several years ago at Johns Hopkins University. They evaluated only men who had Gleason 6 or less by biopsy and then performed a radical prostatectomy. After reviewing the entire radical prostatectomy specimen, one-third of these men were found to have Gleason 7, 8, 9, or 10. In other words, the needles hit the large area of Gleason 6, but the small area of Gleason 8 was missed.

As far as staging is concerned, the Partin Tables have documented that overall 40 to 50 percent of men with stage T1-T2 disease actually have stage T3 disease when the entire specimen is examined under the microscope after radical prostatectomy. There is absolutely no way that you can determine microscopic capsule penetration and that includes endorectal-coil MRI scans, color ultrasound scans, or any other method. In fact, Dr. William Catalona has demonstrated that almost 20 percent of men who have cancer confined to the prostate by microscopic examination of the radical prostatectomy specimen will later develop recurrent prostate cancer. Obviously, these men had cancer cells that had penetrated the prostate capsule and could not even be detected under the microscope when examining the entire specimen. The point of all of this is that classifying men into various risk groups is just an educated guess. I do not believe that cancer should be treated by guesswork.

Therefore, regardless of risk group, for treatment purposes we always assume that men have more advanced disease than what we can determine. We treat all men with an implant first, followed by conformal beam radiation to intensify the radiation dose in the prostate and irradiate around the prostate for cancer that has penetrated the capsule and not been irradiated by the seeds.

However, we do make adjustments with our radiation doses. For example, a man with a Gleason 5 cancer, one needle stick positive, and a PSA of 6 will receive a lower dose of radiation from the seeds by inserting fewer seeds. Additionally, when we deliver conformal beam irradiation, we would give only 4,500 cGy, and the boost field blocks will be drawn tight. In contrast, if we are treating a man with a PSA of 25 and Gleason score 8 and T2b disease, we will insert a lot more seeds, especially concentrating seeds in the area of cancer and will give them a higher implant dose. When we deliver the follow-up conformal beam irradiation, we will treat a larger area through the block and go to a higher dose, typically 5,250 cGy. Also, we implant the seminal vesicles in all men. For men with more extensive cancers, we also give an additional conformal beam boost to the seminal vesicles and base of the prostate. Thus, although in a sense we treat all men the same, the dose from both the implant and the conformal beam irradiation varies tremendously with risk groups.

Q. Why do you use IMRT instead of 3D conformal irradiation?

A. We have been delivering conformal radiation for many years. However, the type of conformal radiation we deliver differs substantially from any other radiation facility. Instead of the typical conformal beam radiation, we use the iodine seeds as a target for ultraprecise conformal beam radiation. This is considerably different from any radiation facility in the United States. The iodine seeds have two uses: (1) to produce irradiation and (2) to be used as a target. You must understand that the prostate gland and cancer cannot be seen on X-rays. However, outlining the cancer and the prostate by insertion of over 100 seeds throughout this organ forms a perfect target for the follow-up radiation because iodine seeds are really a tiny bar of silver with iodine adhered to the bar. The silver metal bar is easily seen on X-rays. Inserting these pieces of metal in the seminal vesicles enables us to treat only the seminal vesicles with high-risk men. Consequently, for years we have treated far less bladder and rectum problems than any facility in the United States because we do not unnecessarily irradiate these tissues. For example, with conformal beam radiation, the margins on the prostate are measured in centimeters. With the seeds in place, supplemented by gold seeds to form an even better target, our margins around the prostate in the area of the bladder and rectum are measured in millimeters, which results in eliminating unnecessary radiation to the bladder, rectum, and sex nerves.

You must also appreciate that with typical conformal beam radiation, the patient is set up with CT scans on the day before treatment begins. The prostate is never seen again throughout the entire course of linear-accelerator external beam radiation. In contrast, with our ultraprecise conformal beam radiation and with the seeds as a target, we make X-ray pictures to aim the machine before treatment each day, and we use laser beams to direct the radiation toward the metallic seeds.

We are now treating men with IMRT after the seed implant, but again, using the seeds as a target for ultraprecise IMRT. The IMRT beams are targeted each day with laser beams at the seeds. Thus, the IMRT we deliver is much more precise than IMRT at other facilities. We hope that this will lower our side effects. As far as I can determine, with conformal beam radiation we already have lower side effects than other facilities. Remember, you cannot deliver ultraprecise conformal beam or ultraprecise IMRT unless you do seed implants first and use those seeds as targets.

Q.   What distinctly separates your technique from others?

A.   The fundamental difference between our program and others is that we perform seed implants with radioactive iodine first and then give follow-up conformal beam irradiation or now IMRT after the implant, using the seeds as a target. To understand this better, we perform an ultrasound-guided, radioactive I-125 seed implant first.

We never use palladium because palladium radiation is given off too rapidly and cannot be mixed with the follow-up linear- accelerator irradiation. It is extremely important to use iodine (60-day half-life) so that you can give both forms of radiation at the same time. Palladium produces radiation over a short period of time (palladium half-life is only 17 days). Thus, palladium burns out too fast and cannot be mixed with follow-up accelerator radiation, which begins 21 days after the implant.

It is also very important to understand how the implant is performed. We place iodine seeds throughout the prostate because we do not know where the cancer cells are located. Dr. Patrick Walsh has performed research on radical prostatectomy specimens and determined that there are an average of seven different areas of cancer in an average prostate cancer patient's instead of the one or two areas found on needle biopsy of the prostate. Additionally, in the areas where we know there is cancer either based on biopsy or palpation, we put extra seeds to increase the seed dose in small areas within the prostate. Some doctors claim that they place seeds outside the prostate. However, since there is no tissue to really hold the seeds, these seeds move around and can float up against the rectum or bladder or can get in the bloodstream and embolize to the lungs. Several reports have been published indicating that up to 20 to 30 percent of men have pulmonary emboli from seeds. The long-term effect of seeds in the lung and other locations outside the prostate is unknown. We do not place seeds outside the prostate because of this problem and also because we are going to treat outside the prostate with the follow-up IMRT. Therefore, it does not make any sense to put seeds outside the prostate.

You also must understand that the urethra, the tube for urination, runs through the middle of the prostate, but it often deviates due to nodules of benign prostate hyperplasia. Thus, it may dip and curve as it traverses the prostate. The importance of all of this is that the urethra cannot take as much irradiation as we would like to give to the cancer. Because of this, we do not place the seeds close to the urethra, which we outline when doing the implant. This has almost eliminated problems with the urethra from irradiation when men are undergoing treatment. We see very little burning from urination caused by irradiation itself while men are being treated. However, prostate cancer cells often touch the urethra and are undertreated from the seeds alone. But just as with cancer cells that have penetrated the capsule, the follow-up IMRT will compensate for the underdosage by the seeds and will provide a curative dose to these cancer cells next to the urethra when combined with the seed irradiation.

Following the seed implant, which is performed on an outpatient basis, men go back to their respective homes for the next three weeks. You must wait three weeks (21 days) on average to let the sudden swelling of the prostate subside. Remember that when we perform the seed implant, we initially insert an average of 25 eight-inch-long hollow needles into the prostate through which we inject the seeds and then remove the needles. These needles cause the prostate to immediately swell about 50 percent in size, which subsequently compresses the urethra, which runs through the middle of the prostate. For example, if a man has a 30-cc prostate, within hours of the implant he suddenly has a 45-cc prostate. This compression of the urethra occurs in every man, but the severity will be dependent upon the degree of urethral compression before the implant. On average, the peak time for swelling is within 24 hours of the implant. By waiting three weeks, much of the swelling subsides before dose intensification begins with follow-up IMRT. Incidentally, since every man develops some degree of compression of the urethra from the prostate swelling, you do not want to add to the urethral problems by placing seeds too close to the urethra, which will give a high dose of radiation to the urethra. That is the other reason we pull seeds back away from the urethra because we know we are going to compress the urethra simply from the needles. On average, you must wait three weeks to let a lot of the swelling subside before you can begin IMRT with the linear accelerator. With radioactive iodine as the seed, this is no problem since the half-life is 60 days. However, if you are using palladium, these seeds will expire in 3 weeks. You cannot mix both forms of radiation at the same time, which is critical to curing prostate cancer.

You should also know that we modify the seed implant from the typical seed-implant method because we are going to provide dose intensification through the follow-up accelerator irradiation.

Thus, the iodine seeds produce irradiation for 60 days following the implant and irradiate cancer cells inside the prostate. These seeds do not give an adequate amount of radiation to irradiate cancer cells outside the prostate, and they do not adequately irradiate cancer cells lying next to the urethra. To compensate for the deficiency of seeds, after waiting three weeks we begin ultraprecise conformal beam irradiation or IMRT. Thus, when we begin the follow-up irradiation, we use those seeds (iodine and gold) as a target to deliver the radiation ultraprecisely guided by laser beams. It is impossible to do this without the seeds throughout the prostate.

We also implant the seminal vesicles, which are organs that are attached to the top (base) of the prostate. Cancer cells, especially if they are in the base of the prostate, can invade into the seminal vesicles. Using the seeds as a target, we can actually radiate only the seminal vesicles, which is what we do in men with high-risk cancer when we give the seminal-vesicle boost. When we give the follow-up radiation, either conformal beam or IMRT, we do it completely different from anyone else. Basically, we use those seeds that we implanted as a target, and also we aim the linear-accelerator irradiation beam every day using a laser beam. By using the seeds as a target, we eliminate this unnecessary irradiation to the bladder, rectum, and sex nerves. We also use the seeds as a target to draw blocks, which block out this unnecessary radiation. Additionally, again using the seeds as a target, we aim the X-ray beam on a daily basis just before giving the radiation to make adjustments as needed. This is not possible without seeds in place.

Besides using the seeds to pinpoint the area to be irradiated, the iodine seeds produce irradiation with a half-life of 60 days. The accelerator radiation is started on day 21. Thus, when we give the follow-up conformal beam or IMRT, the cancer and the normal cells are radiated simultaneously, which causes intensification of the dose. In simplistic terms, instead of 1 plus 1 equals 2, through dose intensification 1 plus 1 may equal 5. Dose intensification is produced throughout the prostate where the cancer cells are located. Additionally, when we pull the seeds back away from the urethra so that we do not burn it from the seed irradiation, the follow-up radiation compensates for lowering the dose in this area. Follow-up irradiation also irradiates all around the prostate in case cancer cells have penetrated the capsule and a man actually has stage T3 disease (remember, location of cancer is really guesswork). Therefore, the follow-up conformal beam radiation produces dose intensification and destroys cancer cells next to the urethra that would be underdosed with seed implant, and it also destroys cancer cells outside the prostate (capsule-penetration cancer cells), always using the metallic iodine seeds as a target.

In other words, all radiation is integrated. If you really think about it, this whole treatment process makes common sense.

Q.   Do you have a special name for your protocol?

A.   Yes, the entire treatment process is called ProstRcision (pronounced – pros-ter-sishun). The letters <u>pros</u> are taken from the word <u>prostate</u>, the capital R is for <u>radiation</u> and the letters cision are from <u>excision</u>. In other words, we are excising the prostate with irradiation in contrast to excising the prostate with a knife. However, unlike actual removal of the prostate with a knife, we leave behind the sex nerves and muscles and only "cut out" the prostate cells, normal and cancerous.

That is why after treatment our goal is to have the PSA fall to 0.2 ng/ml or less. This is the goal for radical prostatectomy when performed by urologists across the country, including Dr. Walsh and Dr. Catalona.

Q.   How many treatments have you and your staff performed?

A.   We treated the first patient with ProstRcision in December 1979. We treated several more men from 1979 through 1983, working out the details of how to integrate both forms of radiation at the same time. After working out the details with the technique, in January 1984, we began a formal study of ProstRcision. The first patient treated was Mr. Adolphus Lester. I recently saw him back for his 19-year checkup. His PSA is 0, and he has had no complications from treatment. Since 1984, we have treated an increasing number of men. Men were implanted by the old-style retropubic or open-implant method whereby we made an incision in the abdomen and implanted the prostate freehand through the open abdomen. All of this occurred before the invention of the ultrasound machine. In August 1992, we began performing ultrasound-guided transperineal seed implants, the modern implant method. The total number of men we have treated is almost 7,000 men, including 6,400 with what we call modern ProstRcision, the ultrasound-guided transperineal method. We currently perform an average 1,200 implants per year.

There are six radiation oncologists in our group who perform seed implants. Two physicians perform seed implants only, and the other four, in addition to performing seed implants, also treat patients with other types of cancers.

Before physicians are allowed to work at RCOG, they must undergo a one-year training program during which I observe them while they perform at least a hundred cases of seed-implant and follow-up accelerator radiation before they are allowed to solo. To monitor all doctors, cure-rate calculations and complication calculations are performed for each physician, in addition to the group as a whole. However, learning about ProstRcision never stops. We have weekly meetings to discuss ways to improve our technique and also to discuss research findings that have been discovered over the past week through evaluation of all the men we have treated.

Some doctors claim that they perform more implants than this. I do not believe this is possible if you accurately treat men and accurately monitor your results both in terms of cure and complications. There are only so many hours in a day.

Q.   Can you identify any side effects from your protocol?

A.   To evaluate side effects, you must first understand how evaluation of complications are performed. Almost all doctors when evaluating complications and side effects do this by performing a retrospective review of patients' charts. The information that goes into charts is typically based on the physician asking patients questions and then writing their own interpretation of what the patient said into the chart. This, of course, is highly subjective. Also, the answers that patients give to questions will depend on how the questions are asked. Of course, patients may want to please the doctor and simply state that they are not having very much in the way of problems, or the doctor may interpret what the patient is saying as not being of any significance. Thus, chart-review evaluation of complications really produces low-ball answers. For example, urologists often report that fewer than 5 percent of patients have urinary incontinence. In sharp contrast, when men have been asked about incontinence using their own questionnaires, urine incontinence rates as high as 40 percent have been recorded in medical journals.

In 1991, we realized the inaccuracy of retrospective chart review to determine the rate of complications. In 1992, we created questionnaires (a total of 42 questions) regarding urinary, rectal, and sexual function. We began giving these questionnaires to men before they were treated, during treatment, and at each follow-up visit. When men could not come back to the clinic, we mailed the questionnaires to them. Since 1992, we have compiled in a computerized database tens of thousands of answers to all these questions regarding urinary, rectal, and sexual function. The answers that we receive from men are entered into a computer database on a daily basis. Doctors have no input into how men answer the questions. Thus, we have gathered complication and side-effect data by prospectively giving men self-reported questionnaires that have been validated. This methodology contrasts sharply with retrospective chart reviews of doctors' interpretation of the complications that men are experiencing. Studies have shown that the methodology we use is far more accurate than asking doctors about the complications.

In recent meetings, we learned that we are the only group in the United States that has a treatment-related morbidity database created in this fashion. Apparently, no one else has ever thought of this methodology, and certainly no one thought about it as early as we did, 1992.

At the present time, I am writing multiple research papers on urinary, rectal, and sexual function to be submitted to medical journals, which hopefully will be published. Because we turn over the copyright to this information to the medical journals when we submit research papers, I would not like to go into a lot of detail. However, I can give information in general terms.

Most men experience some degree of urinary side effects while undergoing treatment. Almost always, the side effects are due to swelling of the prostate from insertion of the hollow needles through which the seeds are injected. We see very few complications from the radiation itself. Swelling compresses the urethra and causes urinary symptoms as a consequence. The degree of complications is directly related to how well a man can urinate before we implant him. For example, a man with a normal-size prostate (25-35 cc) and no urinary side symptoms beforehand on average will have minimal to no urinary side effects. In contrast, a man with a 50 cc prostate (twice the normal size) and already having difficulty with urination will experience a worsening of his preexisting urinary symptoms from the swelling of the prostate. In time, these symptoms decline as the prostate shrinks, but that may take from three to six to twelve months or more depending on the size of the prostate to begin with. Since we pull the seeds back away from the urethra, we see very few complications from irradiation itself.

These urinary side effects are temporary and are mainly more frequent urination, urinating more at night, weak stream (especially in the morning), and more difficulty getting urination started. These symptoms decrease as the prostate shrinks and returns to pretreatment levels. In fact, men with large prostates, since we are destroying both cancer and normal cells within the prostate, usually experience improvement of the urinary symptoms compared to their urinary symptoms before we implanted them. In other words, ProstRcision cannot only cure men of prostate cancer, but in many men it will eventually improve their urinary flow.

Obviously, not every patient experiences the same degree of prostate swelling. A few men have a large amount of swelling and occasionally will need to wear a catheter for a time to let the swelling subside. Each man is different, and you never know exactly what the effects are going to be until men undergo treatment. Of course, this is not unique to ProstRcision but occurs with any seed-implant program.

We see very few rectal side effects in men. This is because we skim a part of the skin inside the rectum because we use the seeds as a target and radiate only through the blocks. Consequently, we see very few rectal symptoms unless men have preexisting problems. For example, if a man has hemorrhoids and he has occasionally seen bleeding, we might irritate those hemorrhoids and cause him to see bleeding. Also, if men are constipated or have firm bowel movements, when the stool is passed it can irritate the irradiated skin inside the rectum and cause some discomfort or blood. However, rectal symptoms are a minor issue, and very few patients require any medication for rectal symptoms.

The ability to preserve sexual function varies with the age of a man at implant and also with his pretreatment sexual function. For example, 95 percent of men aged 50 or less who have normal sex function or some minor problems remain sexually active after ProstRcision. With increasing age the chance of keeping sex function declines. Of course, the normal sex function in men who have never been treated for prostate cancer declines with age. Thus, it is impossible to evaluate sexual function without looking at the decline in sexual ability as men age. You also have to look at other problems such as diabetes and antihypertensive medication, which effects sex function.

Because we have to treat these normal organs around the prostate – sex nerves, rectum, and bladder – in order to get irradiation to the prostate, any man can have some problems with these organs after treatment. When doctors state that they have very few problems or do not have any complications, I do not believe them. They are either giving inaccurate information, or they are keeping very poor records.

Q.   Would you describe your protocol from beginning to end?

A.   When a patient is sent to us by either his urologist or his personal physician or if a patient is self-referred (approximately two-thirds of our patients), we initially gather all of their medical records. This includes all of their PSA records, biopsy reports, description of any other medical problems, and any tests that were performed to determine where the cancer is located including bone scans, etc. Additionally, we request a CT scan of the prostate on all men. We also send men the questionnaires described previously, which they fill out and return. If a patient lives out of state, we have this information sent to us. If a patient lives in Atlanta, we assemble all of this information and then see him in consultation. For patients from out of state, we provide the consultation over the telephone.

After consulting with a man and his family either face-to-face in the clinic or by mail and phone, we then present the case to our weekly prostate cancer tumor board for review by approximately twelve other doctors to see if anyone else has other ideas on management. That tumor board is conducted every Thursday evening.

Following this, we make recommendations to the patient. If he is not a candidate for ProstRcision, we make appropriate referrals for other forms of management. If he is a candidate and wishes to undergo ProstRcision, we schedule him for a seed implant. If he does not have a local urologist from Atlanta, we set up a consultation with one of the urologists with whom we work. It is mandatory that management of prostate cancer patients and performance of the seed implant be performed as a team between urologist and radiation physician. Radiation oncologists are not urologists and should not be performing seed implantation by themselves.

I have heard of radiation oncology groups performing seeds implants alone. This is extremely poor medical practice, and the only reason that radiation oncologists treat patients without urologists is because of monetary greed. A team effort is mandatory.

A patient from out of state comes to our clinic 2 to 3 days before the scheduled implant for direct consultation with us as well as the urologist and anesthesiologist. The seed implant is performed as an outpatient procedure requiring from 30 to 45 minutes. A catheter is inserted at the time of implantation while the patient is under anesthesia, and the patient is discharged and wears the catheter overnight. He comes to our clinic the following day at which time the catheter is removed, a postimplant CT scan is performed, directions are given, questions are answered, and he goes back home.

Three weeks later, the patient returns to our clinic for simulation (mapping out how to give his follow-up radiation), and he begins either conformal beam or IMRT. The linear-accelerator radiation is given Monday through Friday, 5 days per week for 6 to 7 weeks depending on the extent of the cancer. The treatment procedure takes only a few minutes each day, although more time is required to properly align the patient and aim the linear accelerator using the seeds as a target. Getting treatment is similar to having a pelvic X-ray. There are no side effects such as hair loss, nausea, vomiting, etc., nor does the treatment cause diarrhea. The patient may go home weekends.

Throughout the course of stay in Atlanta for the follow-up irradiation, we organize various activities. One of the highlights is the Tuesday night conference in which one of our physicians on staff gives a lecture to men and their families followed by a question-and-answer session. Before the lecture is given, men have supper as a group. This meeting is typically attended by 100 to 200 men and their families. In fact, we encourage all patients just diagnosed with prostate cancer to attend one of these meetings. Not only do they learn about prostate cancer, but it affords them the ability to talk to hundreds of men who are also newly diagnosed. I believe this is the only support group in the United States for men newly diagnosed with prostate cancer. All other support groups are typically for men with incurable or metastatic cancer and mainly on hormones. Our emphasis at this meeting is CURE. We do not talk about anything else.

We also organize field trips such as going to Atlanta Braves games and on museum trips, and we point out vacation spots in Georgia and the surrounding states.

While under linear-accelerator treatment, men are given questionnaires before and after the implant, as described, and weekly throughout the follow-up irradiation. Technique changes in how the irradiation is given are often related to how the questions are answered. Once patients have finished all irradiation, men who live in the region of Atlanta are given clinic follow-ups. Men who live long distances are followed with questionnaires, which are sent out every six months. We follow all men that we have treated, advising them on any problems that might arise; compare their problems with this enormous database that we have created since 1992, and enter the information they send to the database. Consequently our database grows exponentially.

Q.   How long has your center been in existence?

A.   Our first center was built in 1984. All centers are independent of hospitals. This gives us the flexibility to devote all resources to the treatment of prostate cancer and all other malignancies that we treat. We have six centers in the metropolitan Atlanta and nearby areas. We have been given a Certificate of Need to build another cancer treatment center, which will be located in North Georgia (Cumming, Georgia). We spread these cancer centers out to try to alleviate drive time as much as possible.

Q.   What sort of patient would you not accept for treatment?

A.   The only patients we do not recommend ProstRcision for are those patients with distant metastasis. For example, spread of cancer into bone for these men is incurable. However, we have treated a number of men with pelvic lymph-node metastasis in whom we cannot demonstrate distant metastasis. The only other contraindication is men who have severe comorbidity that would either prohibit general or spinal anesthesia.

   On the other hand, we do not refuse to treat patients simply because of the extent of their cancer within the pelvis. We treat a large number of men with very advanced cancer who have been rejected for treatment at other places. For example, we recently treated a man who had seen probably a half dozen physicians, all of whom told him he was not a candidate for any type of treatment. He had a very extensive Gleason 10 cancer with a prostate replaced by disease, which also extended into the bladder. Although follow-up is very short, his PSA is almost at 0.2 ng/ml, despite this extensive disease.

Q.   Will you give some statistics for 5-year and 10-year results?

A.   Based on the treatment of 4,608 men with stage T1-T2 prostate cancer who did not receive pretreatment hormones, our 5-year and 10-year cure rate is 90 percent and 86 percent. This means that of every 100 men whom we treat, 86 have a PSA of 0.2 or less 10 years later. Especially with cure rates described after irradiation, it is extremely important to know how the calculations were performed. In fact, how calculations are performed is just as important as the results that are claimed.

We calculate only with PSA cutpoint 0.2 ng/ml. This means that we do not consider patients free of prostate cancer until their PSA has fallen to 0.2 ng/ml or lower and remains there forever. Failure to cure men is defined by men whose PSA does not fall to 0.2 ng/ml or falls to that level and then rises above it later. Incidentally, this is the identical definition of disease freedom following radical prostatectomy calculated by urologists such as Dr. Patrick Walsh. Since we calculate by the same method, we are able to compare our cure rates apples to apples.

However, and this is extremely important to understand, we are the only radiation group in the United States who calculates with this definition. All other seed-implant doctors and doctors who treat only with linear-accelerator radiation use the so-called ASTRO definition of disease freedom. This definition does not require a specific level to which the PSA must fall (called PSA nadir). The ASTRO definition is based on a guess that cancer will always make the PSA go upward. However, approximately 40 percent of the time that is not correct. Thus, calculation of cure rates with the ASTRO definition are grossly inflated and give extremely misleading information as to how effective a treatment method is or how good the doctors are.

We have written numerous research papers published in peer-reviewed medical journals documenting that radiation results should be calculated the identical way urologists calculate with radical prostatectomy. However, all radiation physicians refuse to calculate by this method.

Therefore, when evaluating cure rates from any program, one must look at: (1) the results themselves and (2) how the results were calculated. As far as can be determined, our 10-year cure rate of 86 percent is the highest of any treatment program in the United States whether radiation, surgery, or anything else.

Additionally, we have never given hormones along with irradiation. We have treated a number of men with ProstRcision who had been placed on hormones before they came to RCOG. Calculation of cure rates of these men versus all the men that we have treated who have never received hormones shows no difference in the cure rates. However, the hormones will artificially lower PSA. Thus, calculation of cure rates in men who have received hormones will be artificially elevated since hormones themselves will make the PSA fall to 0.2 ng/ml or lower. That is why we always subtract the men who received hormones before coming to RCOG from our calculations. Thus, the 86 percent cure rate described previously is in men who never received hormones but were treated only with ProstRcision.

Q. Why do other doctors not treat patients with ProstRcision?

A. Other doctors have tried this with tremendous complications and have written that this cannot be done. It takes a long time to train doctors. This treatment method gives the best results in terms of cure rates and complication rates, but you must know what you are doing. The group in New York City had a 3 percent colostomy rate. We do not recommend this treatment until a doctor has been properly trained and keeps on training. One way you can tell two-day trained doctors is they give radiation first and seed implants second. It's a lot easier to do but not as effective. We are criticized a great deal because we do not go along with the crowd and give irradiation first and seeds second. However, you must remember that we have been doing this longer than anyone in the United States. We believe a lot a criticism is simply due to the fact that doctors often have big egos and they get very jealous of our results. Some doctors have written things about us behind our back. For example, over a year ago one doctor contacted Dr. James Lewis and claimed that we had submitted inaccurate information to medical journals and that he had calculated our data and found that our cure rates were much lower than what we had reported. I have written this doctor several times asking for these calculations in case we did make a mistake. That doctor has refused to show me these calculations. The fact is, he made deliberately false statements about us, which reflects on his integrity.

Chapter 29

EXTERNAL BEAM RADIATION
FOLLOWED BY SEEDS

Although most radiation oncologists in the United States use the external beam radiation first approach, this practice tends to vary among them. The approach indicated in this chapter is one used by a radiologist in the northeast section of the United States. With the use of the IMRT technologies, his results should improve.

Q.   How do you accommodate patients who do not remain in New York to obtain the external beam radiation phase of your protocol?

A.   The patient will be referred to a radiation oncology facility close to the patient's hometown that is familiar with prostate brachytherapy and offers three-dimensional radiation.

Q.   How do you decide whether a patient is low-, intermediate-, or high-risk?

A.   I follow the recommendations of the Department of Radiation Oncology at Mount Sinai School of Medicine, New York, New York pioneered by Dr. Richard Stark and Dr. Nelson Stone with some modifications. Low-risk patients include PSA less than 10, Gleason under 7, and stage T2a or less. High-risk include PSA of 10 or more, Gleason of 7 or more, and stage T3. Generally, the low-risk patients receive a prostate implant alone, while the high-risk patients get combined modality therapy consisting of neoadjuvant and adjuvant hormonal therapy and prostate implant followed by 5 weeks of three-dimensional conformal radiation. The intermediate-risk patients are those which I consider in the gray zone. They can have a Gleason 7, PSA of 10, and T1c or T2a disease. These cases can be treated by implant alone or combined modality therapy, and I make my decision based on other potential prognostic factors such as perineural invasion and the amount of cores that are positive at biopsy. Additionally, a Gleason score of 3 plus 4 equals 7 may result in an implant alone, while a patient with a score of 4 plus 3 equals 7 may receive combined modality therapy. Another factor which influences my treatment plan is a positive

232

seminal-vesicle biopsy, which would result in more aggressive therapy.

Q.   Why do you use IMRT instead of three-dimensional radiation?

A.   IMRT is a more advanced form of three-dimensional conformal radiation that allows for even greater precision in targeting the diseased organ — i.e., prostate gland — while reducing the dose to the surrounding uninvolved organs.   It is a product of more advanced hardware powered by much more sophisticated software. Most centers that have IMRT capabilities would use this modality to treat patients with prostate cancer because of its obvious advantages.

Q.   What distinctly separates your techniques from others?

A.   Our method is based on Mount Sinai's technique of real-time, three-dimensional, ultrasound-guided prostate seed implantation utilizing the Mick Applicator.   The only difference is that we place the internal needles right after placing the peripheral needles, rather than placing them after the perimeter seeds are deposited. This way the central needles are parallel with those in the perimeter and may lead to a more uniform seed distribution. The major downside is crowding of the needles, making hookup to the Mick Applicator difficult.

Q.   Do you have a special name for the protocol?

A.   No.

Q.   How many treatments have you and your staff performed?

A.   Our procedure is done at the J. T. Mather Memorial Hospital in Port Jefferson, New York. Approximately 500 prostate implants have been done since 1996.

Q.   Can you identify any side effects from your protocol?

A.   As of yet, our data has not been analyzed for survival or morbidity. We do see the usual side effects reported with this technique that persists the first 6 to 12 months after implant. This usually includes urinary   morbidity   including   prostatitis,   frequency,   urgency, nocturia, decreased rate of urinary flow, and dribbling. More than half of our patients use alpha-blockers after implant. Symptoms usually resolve spontaneously at one-year after implant. A very small percentage of patients require a transurethral resection of the prostate (TURP) for severe symptoms of bladder outlet obstruction. This is performed at least six months after implant to minimize morbidity from the procedure. Rectal morbidity include rectal proctitis and rectal bleeding. These symptoms usually resolve spontaneously, although a few patients have developed recurring episodes of rectal bleeding requiring consultation with a gastroenterologist or proctologist for management. Its management can be very challenging. Rectal bleeding can start 6 to 8 months after implant, and transfusion is rarely necessary. Impotence is another potential side effect of therapy.

The addition of supplemental external beam irradiation can increase the likelihood of developing any of these symptoms. In our experience the supplemental radiation, acutely, is usually well tolerated and has not dramatically increased the symptoms following the implant and preceding the external radiation. Long-term effects following combined modality therapy, however, still need to be evaluated to see if there is an increased risk of severe complications.

Q.   What living accommodations are available to patients and their families?

A.   Families can stay at the Holiday Inn Express in Setauket, New York. There are other area hotels in the Port Jefferson area.

Q.   What sort of patient would you not accept for treatment?

A.   1. Men with prostates greater than 50 to 60 cc. These patients would be placed on hormonal therapy for cytoreduction. If the glands shrink to less than 50 to 60 cc, then they are candidates for our procedure.
2. Prior to TURP resulting in a large central cavity based on ultrasound or CT evidence.
3. Elderly patients who are medically inoperable.

Chapter 30

HORMONAL THERAPY: A DEFINITIVE TREATMENT?

Hormonal therapy has been a mainstay treatment for prostate cancer since the pioneering work of Charles Huggins and associates more than sixty years ago. However, its role as a primary therapy for early-stage prostate cancer and the timing of its administration in advanced disease have been the subjects of considerable debate. Indeed, since the clinical trials of the Veterans Administration Cooperative Urological Research Group, which was conducted during the 1960s and early 1970s, the concept that early hormonal therapy retarded disease progression but did not prolong survival time has been part of the dogma of prostate cancer therapy. Recently, because of alternative forms of hormonal therapy and the combination of these medications with radiotherapy and cryosurgery, they can be highly effective when applied to relatively small tumors. Therefore, there has been renewed interest in the use of hormonal therapy in the treatment of early-stage prostate cancer.

Identifying the Study Group

Dr. Robert Leibowitz examined the records of 110 consecutive patients who had clinical stage T1 to T3 prostate cancer and were treated from June 1990 to June 1999. All patients' disease was confirmed through a biopsy, which was interpreted at each patient's local hospital. Routine staging was determined with a bone scan, MRI, and CT scan. A ProstaScint scan was not performed. Those patients who had clinical evidence of metastatic cancer were excluded from the study. Patients were not surgically staged to determine if they had T1, T2, and T3 disease. Baseline scans were not routinely used. No patient had received any form of conventional primary treatment. However, all patients had in fact refused local therapy of any kind and were offered triple hormonal therapy consisting of an antiandrogen, an LHRH agonist, and a 5-alpha reductase inhibitor (Proscar). All patients participating in the study were informed of the risks, benefits, and all alternative treatment options prior to the application of triple hormonal therapy.

235

Treatment Highlights

All patients in the study were treated with an LHRH agonist (either 7.5 mg Lupron or 3.6 mg Zoladex every 28 days) and an antiandrogen (either 750 mg Eulexin or 150 mg Casodex daily) plus 5 mg of Proscar daily for a median of 13 months. A maintenance dose of 5 mg of Proscar was also included for an indefinite period.

Success was measured by such factors as the following:

- PSA level
- time to achieve an undetectable PSA level (0.1 or below)
- disease-specific survival

PSA level were measured at 3-month intervals or less during hormonal therapy and at approximately 3-month intervals during maintenance therapy. Blood samples were assayed for PSA at the study site or by local laboratories.

Baseline and follow-up testosterone levels were also measured at 3-month intervals until testosterone levels reached baseline levels or a plateau. Testosterone was also measured during Proscar maintenance to determine androgen recovery.

During most of the patient visits, clinical symptoms and any adverse effects were recorded. Complete blood counts and a comprehensive chemistry panel including liver function tests were performed.

Side Effects

Almost all of the patients in this study experienced the side effects usually associated with hormonal therapy such as hot flashes, loss of libido, loss of potency, and sometimes tender and enlarged breasts. However, these side effects waned when the hormonal therapy was discontinued. Testosterone levels returned to more than 180 ng/dl for all patients who had a normal baseline testosterone level; the median pretreatment testosterone level was 373 ng/dl for 54 patients and the mean testosterone level after treatment was 412 ng/dl range, 9 to 942 ng/dl for 91 patients for those who have been off treatment for more than 12 months.

Demographics of Patients' Baselines

Baseline characteristics of the patients who completed treatment by May 2000 revealed the following:

1. The median age of patients in the study was 67 years (range: 51-86).
2. The mean Gleason score was 6.6 plus or minus 0.1 (range: 4-10).
3. The mean baseline PSA level was 13.2 ng/ml (range: 39-100)
4. The mean baseline serum testosterone level was available for 54 patients, which was 373 ng/dl (range: 154-879).
5. Forty-four percent of the patients had clinical stage T1c, and 40 percent of the patients had clinical stage T2a.
6. Patients with higher stages (T2b and T3) made up 16 percent of the study group.
7. Fifteen percent of patients had Gleason scores of 8 to 10.
8. Eighteen percent of patients had a PSA level of 10 to 20 ng/ml.
9. Twenty patients had a baseline PSA level of over 20 ng/ml.
10. The mean PSA level for patients with a baseline PSA greater than 20 was 35 ng/ml.

Evidence of Remission

The median duration of triple combination hormonal therapy with Proscar was 13 months. All patients in this study achieved an undetectable PSA level of less than 0.1 ng/ml. The median time it took to achieve an undetectable PSA was 3 months (range: 1-10). With a median follow-up of 36 months from the start of hormonal therapy, most of the patients have maintained low PSA levels. The mean PSA level for the entire study group was 1.3 plus or minus 0.1 ng/ml (range: 0-11.0). Eighty-five patients who had been off triple hormonal therapy for more than 12 months had a mean PSA level of 1.6 plus or minus 0.1 ng/ml. These patients continued to receive 5 mg Proscar daily. For the first 57 patients who completed the therapy, the mean PSA level was 1.88 plus or minus .01 ng/ml at a median follow-up of 55 months (range: 38-125). Only 9 of the 110 patients (8%) had a PSA level of more than 4.0 ng/ml. In addition, six of eight patients who were off the therapy for 5 years maintained a stable low PSA without a clinical relapse. As of May 2000, no patients in this study have required further treatment. Disease-specific survival is 100 percent under this triple hormonal therapy protocol. Although 10 patients have died, none of these deaths were due to prostate cancer or a treatment complication. In all cases, prostate cancer was reported by attending local doctors to be controlled or in remission.

Some Claims about Triple Hormonal Therapy

Some interesting claims about this study follow:

- Most importantly, we do not have a large number of patients who have been followed for a long enough time to definitively recommend this treatment. It may be an alternative to watchful waiting or surgery, radiation, and other primary modality.
- Patients with clinically localized or locally advanced prostate cancer can achieve an undetectable PSA level with triple therapy.
- Proscar maintenance prolongs time to relapse.
- The benefit of hormonal therapy appears to be greatest when patients are treated early.
- Patients with small tumors might be expected to have prolonged survival using this form of hormonal therapy.
- A benefit of the protocol is its tolerability.
- Unlike a treatment using only an antiandrogen + 1 Proscar, most patients lose libido and potency and get hot flashes.
- No patient experienced urinary incontinence or leakage.
- A triple dose of Casodex is associated with fewer side effects than is Lupron – for example, hot flashes, lack of sexual interest, and less physical capacity.

Counterclaims by Other Medical Oncologists

For years hormone blockade has been used by many physicians strictly as a palliative treatment for prostate cancer; however, Dr. Robert Leibowitz claims that he has used 13 months of triple hormone blockade followed by Proscar as a definitive primary treatment to control about a hundred of his patients.

We are skeptical of Dr. Leibowitz's protocol since his results have not been reliably reproduced by others. The following summarizes comments by several doubting medical oncologists specializing in prostate cancer:

Dr. Stephen Strum and Dr. Mark Schulz

- They have patients in their practice who have been previously treated by Dr. Leibowitz and who needed to restart hormone blockade after an initial treatment course of 13 months of Proscar, Lupron, and flutamide.

- Their patients have required retreatment after stopping hormone blockade. More than 70 to 80 percent of the patients who had the triple hormonal therapy followed by Proscar had to be restarted on hormonal treatment within five years.

Dr. Stephen Strum

- He has not seen any patients of Dr. Leibowitz that he can recall who have not had progressive disease using his approach.
- He wonders why Dr. Leibowitz is not seeing the PSA recurrence that he's seeing in those men treated with androgen deprivation therapy whose PSAs are undetectable for less than 12 months.
- He is puzzled because both he and Dr. Leibowitz use very similar approaches. He differs with Dr. Leibowitz in the belief that all prostate cancer is systemic at diagnosis.
- He seems amazed that Dr. Leibowitz's data are so much better than his, and he would like to co-joint studies with Dr. Leibowitz using the same protocol to try to answer difficult questions about prostate cancer.

Dr. Charles Myers

- He maintains that the statement "This disease is always systemic" is simply not supported by published data.
- We need to be "cautious in accepting Dr. Leibowitz's conclusions."
- The "various variations in hormonal treatment Dr. Leibowitz has mentioned over the years have been used by a number of other medical oncologists, none of whom can duplicate Dr. Leibowitz's results."
- "I have recently had a chance to review all of the published results on the use of hormonal therapy for localized prostate cancer or cancer that has spread to the lymph nodes. The general pattern is that the patients do quite well for the first four years. Problems begin to develop between the fifth and the tenth year. Dr. Leibowitz has far too few patients out beyond 5 years for us to have confidence that they are doing better than previous studies in terms of disease control."
- "I am a medical oncologist, and part of my salary comes from administering hormonal therapy. Having said that, it is by no means clear to me that hormonal therapy is less toxic than radical prostatectomy or aggressive radiation therapy."

Dr. Labrie Doubts Dr. Leibowitz

Fernand Labrie et al. conducted a study involving 57 patients with localized or locally advanced disease receiving combined androgen blockade (CAB) for periods ranging from 1 to 11 years. Twenty patients with stage B2/T2 prostate cancer were treated for a median duration of 7.2 years (range: 2.8-11.7). They then stopped treatment and were followed up for a median of 4.9 years. Eleven patients with stage B2/T2 also received CAB, but for only 1 year. Twenty-six patients with stage C/T3 disease were treated with continuous CAB for a median of 9.9 years (range: 3.8-11.3); they discontinued treatment with undetectable PSA levels and were followed up for a median of 5.6 years. The median follow-up since diagnosis was 14.6 years for patients with Stage B2/T2 and 16.4 years for patients with stage C/T3 disease.

With a minimum of 5 years of follow-up after cessation of long-term CAB, two PSA rises occurred among 20 patients with stage T2 to T3 cancer who stopped treatment after continuous CAB for more than 6.5 years, for a nonfailure rate of 90 percent. For the 11 patients who had received CAB for 3.5 to 6.5 years, the nonfailure rate was only 36 percent. The serum PSA increased within 1 year in all 11 patients with stage B2/T2 treated with CAB for only 1 year, thus indicating that active cancer remained present after short-term androgen blockade despite undetectable PSA levels. In all patients who had biochemical failure after stopping CAB, the serum PSA level rapidly decreased again to undetectable levels when CAB was restarted and remained at such low levels afterward. Of these patients, only one patient had died of prostate cancer at last follow-up.

The present data suggest that long-term and continuous CAB offers the possibility of long-term control or "possible" cure of localized prostate cancer.

How to Use This Information

Consider the following changes in this protocol:

1. Take 150 mg of Casodex instead of Lupron, and add it upon progression. Have your doctor carefully monitor your disease.
2. If 13 months of triple hormonal therapy does not work for you, switch to intermittent hormonal therapy as long as you remain hormonally sensitive.
3. Remain on the maintenance dose of 5 mg of Proscar during and after the other hormonal treatments.

4. Be very cautious about undergoing this protocol. Perhaps the best group of men to use this therapy are those who have other medical problems, are older than 75, or both.

Chapter 31

PHOTOCOMPOUNDS: A TREATMENT FOR PROSTATE CANCER?

In the first edition of this book, we introduced our readers to an herbal formula called PC SPES in an effort to help realize the vision of one of the authors to enable prostate cancer patients to live longer than they hoped possible. As a result, an estimated 10,000 to 15,000 patients from all over the world, some hormonal naïve and others hormonal refractory, had their lives lengthened or saved.

One prostate cancer patient had a PSA level of 120 ng/ml at the age of 50, an aneuploid tumor, a Gleason score of 9, and disease that spread to his lymph nodes and seminal vesicles. Another man had hormone-refractory metastasized prostate cancer and added Proscar to PC SPES. Both of these patients were supposed to be dead several years ago, but they are still alive today thanks to PC SPES. However, due to poor quality control it was taken off the market.

When this author first mentioned PC SPES, there was the usual number of skeptics. Numerous physicians and probably some patients did not believe in the ability of herbs to treat prostate cancer, but they were proved to be wrong.

Today, this author continues to pursue his vision and so would like to tell the reader about another promising herb called Careseng.

Although the results are early, a small number of patients have gotten some promising results with Careseng. It not only palliates cancer, but it also eradicates cancer cells. This herb seems to be viable not only for prostate cancer, but other cancers as well.

What Are Photocompounds?

Photocompounds are plant-based substances that have medicinal properties formulated to destroy prostate and other cancers. These photocompounds, or *genoids*, are derived from the popular herb ginseng. Ginseng, like most plants, is composed of thousands of compounds. Using these plants in the laboratory, scientists have been able to isolate compounds to arrive at *ginsenosides*. These small subcompounds of ginseng are *glycosides*, or carbohydrate molecules. Each ginsenoside consists of a sugar as well as a nonsugar component. The sugar component (the *anabolic sapogenin*) is used to fuel cell growth. The nonsugar component (the *aglycon sapogenin*) is the main cancer-cell destroyer.

Types of Aglycon Sapogenin

There are many types of aglycon sapogenins, all designated by the capital letter R - for example, Rb1, Rc, Rh1, Rhg, and Rg3. Once in the body, these components are broken down into two substances called *protopanaxadiol (PPD)* and *protopanaxatriol (PPT)*. This breakdown also produces a bacterial metabolite called MI. Researchers believe that these three substances - MI, PPD, and PPT - are the killing force behind this ginsenoside therapy.

How the R-Family Ginsenoside Works

- It may work as an antiangiogenesis agent, blocking the blood supply to the cancer. A Japanese study revealed that ginsenoside Rb2 resulted in a significant inhibition of lung metastases in melanoma in infected mice, compared to the untreated control group. The study suggested that the effects were due to Rb2's ability to block tumor angiogenesis. The effects of antiangiogenesis drugs are one of the brightest fields of study in cancer research.
- It may be able to selectively kill cancer cells. A study conducted at Toyama Medical and Pharmaceutical University in Japan discovered that MI, the metabolic component of PPD, induced cell death in mice melanoma in 24 hours.
- It may be able to reverse precancerous growth during the early stages of the tumors. Researchers from Kanazana Medical University in Japan revealed ginsenosides may be able to stop cancer development at a critical stage. Scientists have also identified five stages in the cell development cycle: G0, G1, S, G2 and M. In this study, the ginsenoside Rh2 effectively froze the development of melanoma cells at the G1 stage, the period immediately following cell division when RNA and proteins are synthesized, putting an end to precancerous growth.
- It may enhance the effects of conventional drugs. A study conducted at the National Defense Medical College in Japan reported that ginsenoside Rh2 improved the effects of the chemotherapy drug cisplatin against ovarian cancer cells. Mice that were injected with ovarian cancer cells were left untreated, or treated with cisplatin alone, ginsenosides alone, or a combination of the two. The cisplatin-ginsenoside group had significantly less

tumor growth and lived significantly longer than any of the other three groups.

Note that in study after study, researchers maintain that ginsenosides did not seem to have any toxic side effects.

Successful Case Studies

- Dr. Jimmy Chan, a naturopathic doctor, biochemist, and a trained practitioner of traditional Chinese medicine, used the treatment on 15 cancer patients in 1999. He reported that 13 of these patients are alive today.
- Since 1999, Dr. Chan has treated more than 300 cancer patients with this therapy.
- Frank Morales, M.D., of Brownsville, Texas, has treated 15 patients with a variety of metastatic cancers.

Some Facts about R-Family Ginsenosides

- Not all ginsenosides have cancer-fighting abilities.
- According to scientists, there are more than 20 different kinds of ginsenosides in ginseng. However, only the R-family seems to have cancer-killing properties.
- Even though a product may contain 90 percent ginsenosides, only those that contain aglycon sapogenins will have the desired results.
- Aglycon sapogenin may be effective against many other kinds of cancers.
- There is evidence that aglycon sapogenin has cancer-prevention properties.
- Patients treated with aglycon sapogenin have less pain and an improved quality of life.
- Aglycon sapogenin goes by such names as Force C, PDB-2131, and no. 372.

Clinical Trial Using No. 372

A mini-pilot clinical trial was initiated by Genetic Services Management, Inc. (GSM), a corporation providing clinical trials to evaluate complementary and alternative medicine approaches to health care. GSM wished to ascertain if any impact might be detected on prostate health through the use of no. 372, a ginseng-based over-the-counter product developed by Pegasus Corporation of Canada. A potentially favorable impact on prostate health would be suggested if the serum PSA level of men with abnormal PSA values changed according to one or more of the following criteria:

1.   previously rising, abnormal PSA values stopped rising and stabilized, and/or
2.   elevated PSA values that were somewhat stabilized began to decline.

Because the trial focused only on the possible contribution of no. 372 to prostate health as reflected by serum PSA level, the candidates did not have to have any prior condition, treatments, or past diagnosis regarding their prostate. For the same reason, abnormal values were subjectively identified by a participant as any value that could aid prostate health.

Enrollment

Five men, recommended by word-of-mouth by other participants, were enlisted to ascertain if there were any reasons to speculate that no. 372 might aid prostate health. A baseline PSA at the start of the trial was obtained, and at least three subsequent PSA values were obtained in the next 3 months after each man started the trial. All started at roughly the beginning of September 2002.

Dosage

To determine a suitable dosage, participant 1 started taking the product approximately 5 months before all the others, taking initially 10 capsules of no. 372 per day, checking his PSA level monthly, and monitoring for any potential side effects. He saw a systematic rise in his PSA level for 5 months. It was hypothesized that perhaps 10 capsules were not enough to induce any signs of prostate health defined by the preceding two criteria. Based on further estimates, the baseline dose was set at 15 capsules per day, and this participant's trial continued, along with the enlistment of four other men who also began taking 15 capsules a day at the onset of the trial. Subsequent anecdotal evidence reinforced the hypothesis that a threshold level was needed to achieve results.

Outcome

Participant 1 saw his PSA decline to 2.73 from 2.97 the first month on 15 capsules, and then decline to 2.15 the second month. In the third month, he suffered a severe but temporary illness, and he took large quantities of painkillers and, later, prescriptions for water retention. The illness abated, and his next PSA level was 2.98; he speculated that the illness and medicines may have affected his overall condition, and we await his next PSA to see what trend, if any, occurs. The patient has identified only one side effect, increased libido, but appears quite happy about it.

Participant 2 began the trial with a PSA value of 4.0, up from 3.2 in December 2001 and 3.9 in June 2002. On no. 372, he had the following monthly PSA level: 3.9, 4.3, 4.3, 4.2. It appeared his rising PSA had stabilized but his latest reading was 4.8.

Participant 3 began with a PSA level of 18.4, up from 13.8 three months prior. His subsequent monthly levels on 15 capsules were 18.9, 17.5, 17.2, 17.5. The small increase of the last value coincides with this participant's significantly increased stress level due to personal issues; this is the third time in three of the five participants that we have observed increased stress coinciding with a rise in PSA. The professional literature suggests that stress can negatively affect this marker, and we may be documenting this fact in this trial. Overall, for this participant, it would appear his PSA may have stabilized. He identifies no side effects.

Participant 4 began with a PSA level of 8.0, and he experienced a jump to 10.5 the first month. Part of the time he took only 10 capsules a day, a dose previously evaluated as possibly being below a useful threshold. Concomitantly, this participant experienced significant stress this first month, which may have negatively affected his PSA. He then decided that we would first bring his PSA down by taking PC SPES before continuing on no. 372. The next month, following the use of PC SPES, his PSA was 7.3, and he felt comfortable terminating the PC SPES. Returning to 15 capsules of no. 372 per day, his next PSA reading was 8.0, a reading with which he was more comfortable. His next month's PSA was 8.4, followed by the 8.0 the next month. He remains quite encouraged, stating that he believes he has achieved stabilization, judging from his 6 years of experience with assisted watchful waiting.

Participant 5 began the trial with a PSA level of 59.85, having had a value of 50.05 the month before. The first month on no. 372 at 15 capsules yielded a PSA value of 70.95, followed by 58.40 the next month. At this juncture, the participant decided to continue with 10 capsules per day, and after one month, the next PSA yielded 51.36. However, the next month the PSA jumped to 73.30, which led to a discussion about dose levels, the discovery of the use of 10 capsules per day, and then the resumption of 15 capsules. The first month at the renewed 15-capsule threshold level yielded a PSA of 73, close to his prior month's value of 73.30, suggesting perhaps he had "started over" and perhaps his PSA might be stabilized. He then reported a PSA level of 72, followed by a PSA of 56. He appears to have stabilized at this point.

Participant 3 was, as hoped, possibly leveling off a potential PSA rise, and then perhaps seeing an apparent modest decline begin. Participant 1, once at threshold, followed this pattern, but the interruption of severe illness may or may not have affected the next value. At the end of the fourth month, his PSA was essentially at the same value as when he started.

Participant 4 might have reflected some prostate health outcome, holding his last PSA to 8.0 from a prior 8.4 and an original 8.0, rather than seeing a rise back to 10.5, which he had 3 months earlier. This may support the hypothesis of potential near-term stabilization.

Participant 5 temporarily confounded the data by switching at the end of his second month to a lower dose, which appears to be below a threshold of impact after he had some noteworthy PSA reductions. Returning to the trial dose of 15 capsules, he had at least stabilized his PSA level.

Participant 2 started off with a stabilization pattern during the first three months, but his fourth value was unexpectedly higher. His last value of 4.5 showed a modest decline again. It will take another reading or two to determine whether this apparent stabilization is verified. Patients 1, 3, 4, and 5 showed the following reductions from their starting values: 20.5, 7.4, 0, and 23.2 percent, while patient 2's PSA level rose by 12.5 percent from his starting value.

Summary

Although a mini-pilot clinical trial of five participants cannot yield statistical "conclusions," nonetheless we offer some cautious observations. All patients seemed to demonstrate PSA stabilization. Two participants (1 and 5) seemed to show that stabilization can arise when the proper dose is taken and no extreme outside conditions are concurrent. Four patients (1, 3, 4, 5) exhibited a reduction from their starting values, and one patient is above his starting value. Combining these observations, we may summarize by noting that: (1) four of five participants (80%) are indicative of possible positive outcomes in terms of stabilizing their PSA levels during the 3 to 4 months of the trial, when an adequate dose level is provided, without adverse events or negative side effects, and (2) there is a possibility of a beginning downturn in some of the PSA values, but more data are needed. Based on these findings, GSM launched a trial in April 2003, encompassing 40 men for four months on the new liquid form of no. 372, which will significantly increase the bio-availability of the supplement. The results of this study should shed more light on the ability of no. 372 to stabilize rising PSA values and possibly initiate long-term decline.

Trial Independence

Neither GSM nor any of its principals and employees have any financial connection to the Pegasus Corporation, nor do they have any corporate affiliation with it or with any of its products under analysis. All data, whatever the outcomes in the next trial, will be reported in full to the public.

How to Use This Information

If you have prostate cancer or any other form of cancer, consider an extract from the ginseng herb as a viable treatment. There are anecdotal reports that many cancer patients have benefited from this herb.

Chapter 32

EXPLORING HIGH-DOSE MONOTHERAPY

Endocrine, or hormonal therapy, which is based on the principle of androgen deprivation, has been the fundamental systemic treatment for prostate cancer for many years. It has been used by numerous patients and reviewed and studied by countless numbers of physicians. In traditional hormonal therapy, it includes surgical castration, diethylstilbestrol (DES), LHRH agonist, and combination hormonal therapy. In nontraditional hormonal therapy, it includes intermittent hormonal therapy, 5-alpha reductase inhibitors, and oral combinations of antiandrogens and 5-alpha reductase inhibitors. The major differences between these forms of hormonal therapy are in their tolerance, convenience, psychological acceptability, cost, reversibility, and compliance. On the basis of these variables, monotherapy with antiandrogens may offer an alternative to established hormonal therapies, although as with all treatments, there are disadvantages as well as possible advantages.

Defining High-Dose Monotherapy

In high-dose monotherapy, patients are treated with an antiandrogen called Casodex (bicalutamide) that significantly reduces the risk of disease progression in men with localized or locally advanced prostate cancer. It is often referred to as "a triple dose of Casodex."

The mechanism by which hormonally sensitive prostate cancer cells multiply and divide is based upon stimulation by testosterone and dihydrotestosterone hooking up to the androgen receptor sites and moving into the nucleus to stimulate protein synthesis. If the androgen-receptor sites are occupied by antiandrogens, the message of protein synthesis and cell multiplication does not get to the nucleus of the cancer cell, and the cells either lie dormant or die by a process called *apoptosis* (programmed cell death).

Clinical Trials

There have been a number of trials conducted using antiandrogens alone to create androgen-receptor blockade. Eulexin (flutamide) was tested against DES in the mid 1970s and was found to be less effective as a single agent. As a result, for a long time there was a lack of interest in exploring the use of monotherapy for treating prostate cancer. However, since Casodex (bicalutamide) was shown to be equivalent to Eulexin when used with an LHRH agonist in the 1990s, there has been a renewed interest in Casodex. In fact, there have been a number of trials investigating Casodex at doses ranging from 50 to 200 mg daily given orally as a single agent.

In a randomized trial of 1,453 patients, 862 were given Casodex (150 mg) and 423 underwent either medical or surgical castration. The proportion of surviving patients who did not have metastatic disease was the same in the Casodex group and the castration group: approximately 35 percent of men in both groups were alive after about seven years. The time to progression of these patients was also approximately the same. Nine quality-of-life indicators were measured in the patients with nonmetastatic prostate cancer, and it was found that physical activity and sexual interest was statistically significant in favor of the Casodex group. Although not statistically significant, the other quality-of-life domains appeared to favor Casodex as far as emotional well-being, vitality, social functioning, pain, activity limitation, and bed disability were concerned. Sixty-four percent of the patients who received Casodex were still interested in sex, compared to 30 percent who had medical or surgical castration. Seventy-one percent who took Casodex continued to feel sexually attractive, compared to 42 percent in the castration group. The adverse events experienced by the Casodex group were gynecomastia and breast pain, which rarely required treatment. It was severe in about only 5 percent of patients. When treatment was required, prophylactic or therapeutic radiation could be given to the breast or Tamoxifen (10 to 20 mg twice a day) could be prescribed for one month, which was found to be helpful in averting these side effects. In addition, it appeared that Casodex preserved bone mineral density better than castration did.

The conclusions of this study were:

1. No overall statistically significant difference in survival or time to progression was noted between the two treatment groups.
2. Quality-of-life benefits (especially physical activity and sexual interest) were improved in the Casodex group.
3. Bone mineral density was preserved.
4. The treatment was well tolerated.
5. There was a potential use for this treatment for adjuvant and immediate hormonal therapy.

Conclusions for metastatic patients in the Casodex group follow:

1. There was a statistically significant difference in time to death (42 days) in favor of castration.
2. Castration was more effective than Casodex for metastatic patients with a high tumor burden.
3. Casodex was superior in measurements of quality of life and subjective response.
4. Both Casodex and castration were well tolerated.

See Table 32-1.

Table 32-1

Antiandrogen Monotherapy					
Trials Comparing Bicalutamide (Casodex) Monotherapy with Castration					
Author	No. Patients	Dose	Stage of Disease	Comparison	Result
G.W. Chodak	486	50 mg	D2	Castration	Longer progression-free with castration
G. Bales	1,037	50 mg	D2	Castration	Longer median survival with castration
C.J. Tyrrell	1,453	150 mg	Metastatic (D2) and locally advanced	Castration	Longer survival in metastatic patients with castration
J.C.O. Boccardo	229	150 mg	Metastatic (D2) and locally advanced	Combined androgen blockade	No difference in progression-free or overall survival
P. Iversen	480	150 mg	Locally advanced	Castration	No difference in survival
Grossfeld et al., <u>Urology</u> 58: Supp 2A, 56, 2001.					

In studies by J.C.O. Boccardo and B.J.U. Chatelain, bicalutamide monotherapy was compared to combination androgen blockade. They found that there was:

1. No difference in disease progression or survival time between the treatment groups.
2. Patients on Casodex maintained greater sexual interest.
3. In terms of quality of life, Casodex was preferable.
4. There was difference in subjective response.

As a result of the preceding studies, Casodex (150 mg) was approved in 53 countries including Canada as of October 2002. It did not, however, receive FDA approval because:

1. The data for the metastatic patients favored castration (a 42-day difference), and castration was more effective than Casodex for metastatic patients with a high tumor burden.
2. The main reason, however, was that the 150-mg dose of Casodex raised serum testosterone levels. (This is an expected result of this therapy, and in the authors' opinion, it should not be a reason to deny approval).

Five trials comparing 50 to 150 mg of Casodex to castration or combined androgen blockade have been conducted. As can be seen in Table 32-1, the low dose Casodex (50 mg) in patients with metastatic disease was inferior to castration; however, the higher dose (150 mg) showed no difference in two of the three trials and only approximately a 1-month difference in favor of castration in patients with metastatic disease.

Table 32-2 presents the pros and cons of Casodex treatment. Data was presented before the FDA at the end of 2002 on the use of 150-mg Casodex for early prostate cancer. However, the FDA voted to reject the 150-mg Casodex dose based upon concerns that it would be administered to thousands of patients who might experience no benefit but still be exposed to the drug's side effects. Unfortunately, the FDA did not seem to consider the side effects and toxicity of the currently approved drugs (LHRH-agonist H-L antiandrogens) for adjuvant use in primary treatment of locally advanced prostate cancer. It was our sincere hope, based upon the data presented, that this dose of Casodex would be approved.

Table 32-2

Pros and Cons of Casodex Treatment

Pros*	Cons†
- Preserves sexual function	- No evidence that early hormone therapy prolongs survival
- Fewer side effects malaise, anemia	- Nipple tenderness/gynecomastia muscle mass, hot flashes
- Less expensive than an LHRH agonist	- More expensive than observation or orchiectomy
- Lowers PSA level lessens anxiety	- Not FDA approved - Not reimbursed reliably

* Crawford, ED: J Urol. 154:1645, 1995 (Editorial).
† Walsh, PC: J Urol. 154:1645, 1995 (Editorial).

An analogy is that of the Early Breast Cancer Trials Collaborative Group of 55 trials including 37,000 women with breast cancer who were followed up to 10 years. Tamoxifen was used as an adjuvant therapy after primary treatment of breast cancer. (Tamoxifen blocks the estrogen receptor of breast cancer patients just like Casodex blocks the androgen receptor in prostate cancer patients.) Five years of Tamoxifen caused a 47 percent reduction in the recurrence of breast cancer compared to the control group, which received no Tamoxifen. Furthermore, there was a 26 percent reduction in deaths when Tamoxifen was taken for 5 years. With this in mind, the underlying question was, Is there a benefit in Casodex therapy for patients with early-stage prostate cancer who received primary therapies or for candidates for watchful waiting?

The Casodex early prostate cancer study is outlined below:

- The program consists of three similarly designed trials:

    o   IL0023: North America
    o   IL0024: Europe, South Africa, Israel, Mexico, Australia
    o   IL0025: Scandinavia (SPCG-6)

- Double-blind, randomized, placebo-controlled
- Early (nonmetastatic) prostate cancer (i.e., with localized or locally advanced prostate cancer)
- Designed and powered for a pooled analysis
- Largest treatment trial reported to date (8,113 patients)

The three trials conducted throughout the world are summarized in Table 32-3. The primary end points for the study were time to objective clinical progression (bone scan, CT, X-ray, MRI, ultrasound, and death) and time to death. Secondary end points were tolerability, time to treatment failure, time to PSA progression, and sexual function/interest by use of a questionnaire (Scandinavian trial only).

Table 32-3

Early Prostate Cancer Trials

Trial No.	No. Patients	Location	Stage	Standard Care	Duration of Therapy	End Points
0023	3292	North America	T1B, T1C, T2, T3, pT4, N0-X, M0	Radical prostat-ectomy, radio-therapy	2 years	1° progress-ion 1° survival
0024	3603	Europe, South Africa, Israel, Mexico, Australia	T1B, T1c, T2, T3, T4, any N, M0	Radical prostat-ectomy, radio-therapy watchful waiting	5+ years	1° pro-gression 2° survival
0025	1218	Scandinavia	T1b, T1c, T2, T3, T4, and N, M0	Radical prostat-ectomy, radio-therapy watchful waiting	Until pro-gression	1° pro-gression 1° survival

N =

M0 = nonmetastatic

N0-X=

PT4 =

The overall demographics as far as patients' age, stage of disease, and nodal status were equivalent in the Casodex group versus the standard care plus placebo group. This was also true of tumor grade, race, and the number of patients who received standard care, which included prostatectomy, radiation, or watchful waiting.

Following are the results of this important trial:

1. The North American trial (0023) showed equivalence of the two groups in objective progression. The other two trials (0024 and 0025) showed a statistically significant improvement in favor of Casodex (150 mg) versus the placebo (trial 0024 trial showed 10.1% progression of the Casodex group vs. 16.2% for the placebo group).
2. The Scandinavian trial (0025) showed a 16.3 percent progression with Casodex, versus 29.3 percent progression with the placebo. Similar results were found favoring Casodex for reducing the risk for bone-scan-confirmed progression. The Casodex group reduced risk for PSA progression by 59 percent after approximately 5 years of follow-up. This was highly statistically significant in all three trials.

Table 32-4 summarizes the survival data. At this point, no conclusions can be drawn about survival because it is too early; however, the lack of difference for non-prostate cancer deaths is reassuring from a long-term safety perspective.

Table 32-4

Summary of Deaths in Early Prostate Cancer Trials

	Casodex	Placebo
No. Patients	4,022	4,031
All deaths	254	267
Prostate cancer deaths	58	69
Non-prostate cancer deaths	196	198

High-Dose Monotherapy with Conventional Treatments

There were improvements in all treatment groups when Casodex was added to radical prostatectomy, radiation therapy, and watchful waiting when compared to the placebo plus the same treatment. Patients' Gleason score, nodal status, and disease stage also improved. Patients who received adjuvant Casodex in addition to undergoing radical prostatectomy had a 37 percent reduction in risk of progression. There was a 41 percent improvement in the risk of PSA progression in patients treated with both

Casodex and radical prostatectomy compared to placebo. There was a clear benefit in patients receiving Casodex plus radical prostatectomy in all subgroups. The greatest benefit in those groups was among those with a relatively poor prognosis.

When Casodex was used in addition to external beam radiation, there was an approximately 30 percent reduction in objective disease progression compared to the placebo group. In addition, PSA progression was reduced approximately 46 percent in patients on Casodex. Again, patients receiving Casodex plus radiation therapy showed a benefit over radiation alone in all subgroups, especially those with a relatively poor prognosis.

It is difficult to understand why data like these did not impress the FDA enough to sanction the use of this drug. After all, Zoladex was approved for use as an adjuvant to external beam radiation therapy when it was shown to decrease objective disease progression. And yet the side effects of Zoladex are considered somewhat worse than those of Casodex (150 mg) by most physicians who treat prostate cancer.

When Casodex was used as immediate therapy versus watchful waiting, there was a 47 percent reduction in the risk of progression favoring the Casodex group. PSA progression was reduced approximately 58 percent when Casodex was compared to placebo at about the 4-year mark. Again, there was a clear benefit for patients receiving immediate Casodex (150 mg) compared to placebo in all subgroups, especially those with a relatively poor prognosis.

In conclusion, at median follow-up of 3 years, the early prostate cancer subgroup analysis showed a significant reduction in the risk of objective disease progression seen with radical prostatectomy, radiation therapy, and watchful waiting. Furthermore, within each form of standard care, the effect in favor of Casodex was irrespective of the standard care, stage, Gleason score, and nodal status. Higher-risk patients derived the most benefit from 150-mg of Casodex in the adjuvant setting. The only subgroup that did not seem to benefit were patients whose PSA was less than 4; they showed equality between the Casodex and placebo groups.

Side effects of Casodex (150 mg) versus placebo are presented in Table 32-5. As noted, the main side effects include gynecomastia and breast pain in the Casodex group. The time to resolution of gynecomastia depended upon the duration of therapy. The longer the therapy, the longer the time to resolution of gynecomastia. Breast pain, however, seemed to resolve once therapy was stopped, no matter the duration of the therapy.

Table 32-5

Side Effects of Casodex (150 mg) vs. Placebo

	Casodex	**Placebo**
Breast pain	73%	7%
Gynecomastia	66%	8%
Asthenia	10%	7%
Impotence	9%	6%
Hot flashes	9%	5%
Back pain	9%	10%
Rash	9%	8%
Constipation	8%	7%
Diarrhea	6%	6%
Alopecia	6%	1%
Weight gain	6%	3%
Incontinence	6%	6%
Hematuria	4%	6%
Loss of libido	4%	1%
Abnormal liver function	3%	2%

Note: These side effects were spontaneously reported regardless of causes.

At this point, survival data are immature, as less than 2 percent of patients in the study have died from prostate cancer. Follow-up regarding mortality will be forthcoming. As already stated, irrespective of standard care, stage, Gleason score, and nodal status, patients on Casodex (150 mg) had an overall 42 percent reduction in objective disease progression as well as a significantly reduced risk of PSA progression. Gynecomastia and breast pain were the most frequently reported adverse effects, which led only about 1 percent of patients to withdraw from the trial.

In summary, Casodex (150 mg) as a single agent has been shown to be an effective adjuvant to radical prostatectomy and external beam radiation therapy and favors its use immediately versus observation. While survival data are pending, the side effects and overall tolerability favoring sexual interest and function, bone mineral density, and quality of life makes this therapy valuable in treating early prostate cancer. Further studies, possibly using Casodex with 5-alpha reductase inhibitors such as Proscar and Avodart, are eagerly awaited, as the latter drugs may in fact add therapeutic benefit. As we go to print, the FDA has not made a favorable ruling on the 150-mg Casodex dose despite its being approved in more than fifty other countries; however, a number of physicians who treat prostate cancer prescribe it based upon the above studies.

High-Dose Monotherapy

The traditional hormonal therapies include bilateral orchiectomy, DES, LHRH agonist, and combination hormonal therapy. The nontraditional hormonal therapies include intermittent androgen blockade, 5-alpha reductase inhibitors, and oral combinations of antiandrogens and 5-alpha reductase inhibitors.

How to Use This Information

1. In situations where an LHRH-A is recommended, discuss with your doctor the possibility of taking 150 mg of Casodex — with or without a 5-alpha reductase inhibitor, (i.e., Proscar or Avodart). These situations include:
   - as a neoadjuvant treatment (i.e., before definitive primary therapy)
   - as an adjuvant treatment (i.e., in addition to primary therapy)
   - when you have failed primary therapy
   - as a form of intermittent androgen deprivation therapy
   - for systemic recurrence of disease

2. If you have a poor quality of life due to the side effects of LHRH-A therapy, ask your doctor about substituting Casodex (150 mg) for the LHRH-A.
3. If you are concerned with remaining potent, consider the above substitution.
4. If you have osteopenia or osteoporosis, ask you doctor about substituting Casodex (150 mg) for the LHRH-A.
5. Casodex (150 mg) is not always as effective as an LHRH-A for patients with metastatic disease, high tumor loads, or both.
6. If breast tenderness or enlargement will significantly affect your quality of life, you should probably not take triple dose Casodex (150 mg) alone.
7. In some cases, Casodex (150 mg) may be a good alternative to watchful-waiting.
8. If you are not in a low-risk group and your PSA level is greater than 4 ng/ml, consider taking Casodex (150 mg).

Just prior to going to print, the following information was released by AstraZeneca, the manufacturer of Casodex. We, therefore, felt that an addendum to Chapter 32 was in order. This information is also available on various Internet sites.

Casodex – Withdrawal of Casodex 150 mg for Localized Prostate Cancer from Canadian and European Markets

Prescribing Information[1]

Casodex tablets 50 mg is indicated for use in combination with a LHRH-A for the treatment of Stage D2 metastatic carcinoma of the prostate.

Background

The use of Casodex 150 mg is not approved in the United States.

The Casodex 150 mg Early Prostate Cancer (EPC) Program is the largest randomized clinical trial program ever conducted in patients with prostate cancer.[2] It includes three prospective, double-blind, placebo-controlled trials that were designed to evaluate whether adding bicalutamide 150 mg to standard care (watchful waiting, radical prostatectomy, or radiotherapy) can reduce the risk of disease progression and improve survival when compared to standard care alone in men with localized or locally advanced prostate cancer (stage T1b-T4, any N, M0). The three studies were conducted in North America (n=3292). Scandinavia (n=1218), and Europe. South Africa, Australia, and Mexico (n=3603). The studies were of similar design, and a planned pooled analysis of all three trials was performed on an intent-to-treat basis.

A second analysis of the EPC program is currently ongoing and is being performed at a median follow-up of 5.4 years.[3] The overall results of this ongoing analysis are similar to the initial findings of the EPC program. In the overall combined analysis benefit a benefit was seen for the primary endpoint of progression free survival across all patient groups with the benefit most evident in those patients with locally advanced disease. No overall survival benefit was seen. Planned subgroup analyses have been undertaken for all three trials within the program. For overall survival some trends were apparent in the subgroup analyses of those patients receiving

Casodex as immediate therapy alone (i.e., the group who had not previously received radical prostatectomy or radiotherapy). Patients with localized disease receiving Casodex alone showed a trend toward decreased survival compared with patients in the placebo group. Patients with locally advanced disease showed a trend toward improved survival with Casodex compared to placebo.

AstraZeneca notified clinical investigators and regulatory authorities including the U.S. Food and Drug Administration, Health Canada, and other international regulatory agencies of these data in June 2003.

In November 2002, AstraZeneca received conditional approval for the monotherapy treatment of localized prostate cancer with Casodex 150 mg in Canada. In August 2003, following the submission of the EPC Second Analysis study results, Health Canada directed AstraZeneca to withdraw the application for this indication.[4] In cooperation with Health Canada, AstraZeneca has written to physicians to recommend that Casodex 150 mg not be administered to localized prostate cancer patients undergoing no other treatment. Patients in Canada are being advised to discuss their treatment with their physicians.

In October 2003, the Committee on Safety of Medicines (CSM; United Kingdom) removed the indication for <u>localized</u> prostate cancer (CSM emphasis) for Casodex 150 mg, citing an unfavorable risk:benefit ratio for this indication based on the second EPC analysis.[5] The CSM reaffirmed the positive risk:benefit ratio for Casodex 150 mg in patients with locally advanced prostate cancer, either as an adjuvant to other treatments (radical prostatectomy or radiotherapy) or alone. The withdrawal of the localized prostate cancer indication does not affect the indication for Casodex 150 mg in the UK for the management of locally advanced, non-metastatic prostate cancer in cases where surgical castration or other interventions may not be appropriate, nor does it affect the indication of Casodex 50 mg for the treatment of advanced prostate cancer when combined with medical castration.

In a "Dear Doctor" letter, the Committee on Safety of Medicines (CSM) said 25.2% of patients given the drug to treat localized prostate cancer were dead after about five years compared with 20.5% of patients on placebo.

"Patients receiving Casodex 150 mg for localized prostate cancer should be reviewed at the earliest opportunity, and Casodex treatment discontinued," the letter said.

The CSM said that the risk-benefit for other licensed uses of the drug, including the treatment of advanced prostate cancer, was not affected by the new data.

Casodex has been approved for the treatment of early stage prostate cancer in more than 40 countries including Canada, Italy, Mexico, Germany, and Australia.

A company spokesman said Austria, Greece, and Portugal were taking similar action to the UK.

He said analysis of the study showed the drug was of benefit in high-risk patients who would otherwise have been managed by watchful waiting, but in low-risk patients there was a small increase in the number of deaths. However there was "no evidence" of a casual link.

References:

1.   Casodex Prescribing Information.
2.   See WA, Wirth MP, McLeod DG, et al. Bicalutamide as immediate therapy either alone or as adjuvant to standard care of patients with localized or locally advanced prostate cancer: first analysis of the Early Prostate Cancer Program. *J Urology 2002;*168:429-435.
3.   Data on file, AstraZeneca Pharmaceuticals LP.
4.   Public Advisory: Important safety information regarding Casodex 150 mg. Health Canada Health Products and Food Branch. 18 August 2003. Accessed 5 November 2003 at
      http://www.hc-sc.gc.ca/hpfb-dgpsa/tpd-dpt/casodex_pub_e.html
5.   Casodex 150 mg (bicalutamide): no longer indicated for treatment of localized prostate cancer. Committee on Safety of Medicines (UK). 28 October 2003. Accessed 31 October 2003 at
      http://medicines.mhra.gov.uk/aboutagency/regframework/csm/
      csmhome.htm

E. Roy Berger, M.D., F.A.C.P. and James Lewis, Jr., Ph.D

Chapter 33

ZOMETA: PREVENTING SKELETAL COMPLICATIONS

Every year approximately 31,000 men die from prostate cancer in the United States. From 85 to 100 percent of these men have bony metastases, primarily osteoblastic in nature. The bony metastases usually are found in the vertebrae, pelvis, and long bones, causing pain, fractures, and spinal cord compression. In a study of 112 men with hormone-refractory disease, the median time to initial skeletal complication was approximately 9.5 months, and bone pain was present in 88 percent of the men.

In 1997, there were nearly one million cases of advanced prostate cancer in the United States and bone metastases were detected in up to 75 percent of those cases. The median survival among prostate cancer patients in whom bone metastases are detected is approximately 3 years.

Defining Zometa

Zometa is an effective treatment for prostate cancer and other cancers that have spread to the bones. It is not chemotherapy but can be used with other cancer treatments such as radiation, hormonal therapy, or chemotherapy.

How Tumors Spread

The mechanism by which a tumor spreads to a bone is somewhat complicated. Generally, new vessel formation needs to occur in the primary malignant neoplasm (e.g., the prostate), allowing tumor cells to invade the blood vessels and aggregates of tumor cells (accompanied by other cells such as lymphocytes and platelets) embolizing into blood vessels and being transported into the capillary bed of the bones. The tumor cells adhere to the blood vessel wall and then migrate out of the blood vessels and into the microenvironment, allowing tumor-cell proliferation and progression of bony metastases.

Bone Metastases: Types and Complications

The primary type of bone metastasis in prostate cancer is osteoblastic — that is, excessive, new, but disorganized bone formation. This bone is weaker than normal bone.

Bone metastases are usually diagnosed by bone scan, plain film, CT scan, and MRI. They usually occur in patients whose PSA level is greater than 10, whose Gleason score is greater than 7, and who have failed primary therapy.

Skeletal–related events (SREs) are serious complications of bone metastases. They are debilitating and painful, and they negatively affect a patient's daily functioning and quality of life. Skeletal–related events include:

1. pathologic fractures
2. spinal-cord compression
3. radiation therapy to areas of bone pain or to treat pathologic fractures or spinal-cord compression
4. surgical procedures to bone
5. change of antineoplastic therapy to treat bone pain
6. hypercalcemia of malignancy

Treating Bone Metastases

Treatment of bone metastases usually involves one or more of the following:

- radiation therapy
- hormonal therapy
- pain management
- orthopedic interventions
- chemotherapy
- bisphosphonates

In this chapter, we will limit the discussion to the use of bisphosphonates, pyrophosphate analogs whose core moiety promotes binding to bone mineral surfaces. Zoledronic acid (Zometa) is the most potent bisphosphonate developed to date. It has been shown to:

- inhibit the number and activity of osteoclasts (the cells that break down bone).
- inhibit tumor - cell invasion and adhesion to bone matrix.

263

- possibly inhibit tumor - cell secretion of growth factors that stimulate osteoblasts (the cells that make bone).
- induce tumor-cell death in certain cancers.
- inhibit invasion and migration of prostate cancer cells.

Zometa is the only bisphosphonate with proven effect in the treatment of bone metastases in prostate cancer patients. It has been approved in over 60 countries for the treatment of hypercalcemia of malignancy and has been used to decrease skeletal-related events.

What the Various Studies Show

Many studies have shown that men treated with androgen-deprivation therapy have an increased incidence and severity of skeletal-related complications. This is usually associated with the duration and intensity of the hormonal therapy given. The indications for hormonal therapy in prostate cancer have been expanding, and they are used earlier in treatment. Previously, they were only used in patients who had failed primary therapy or had metastatic disease. More recently, it has been shown that earlier use of hormonal therapy has been effective (1) in patients who have a rising PSA level, (2) as an adjuvant to external beam radiation therapy, and (3) possibly as an adjuvant to other treatments including radioactive seed implantation, cryosurgery, and even radical prostatectomy. Due to this increased use of hormonal therapy, the risk of bone loss during androgen-deprivation therapy affects many more men than previously.

S. A. Stoch et al. showed that bone mineral density was 17 percent lower in the lateral spine and 10.3 percent lower in the hip in men treated with an LHRH agonist compared to a control group with prostate cancer who were not treated with hormonal therapy. Several studies have shown that LHRH agonist therapy creates a 7 to 10 percent decrease in bone mineral density compared to control. M. R. Smith et al. studied 47 men with advanced or recurrent prostate cancer but no clinical bony metastases. They were randomized to receive leuprolide or leuprolide plus pamidronate (another bisphosphonate), 60 mg, 4 times a day for 12 weeks. Mean trabecular bone mineral density in the lumbar spine decrease 8.5 percent in the men who received leuprolide. There was no change in the men treated with pamidronate plus leuprolide.

This led to an osteoporosis prevention study called Zometa 705. A total of 106 men with recurrent or locally advanced prostate cancer who had negative bone scans were randomized to androgen-deprivation therapy plus 4 mg of Zometa given daily for 3 months compared to androgen-deprivation therapy plus placebo. End points of this study were: (1) change in bone mineral density and (2) incidence of vertebral fractures. Men treated with Zometa had an increase of more than 5 percent in lumbar-spine bone mineral density compared with a decrease in the placebo group ($P < 0.001$). Similar findings were obtained at the hip.

Three randomized, international, parallel, double-blind trials were undertaken involving patients with metastatic prostate cancer, other solid tumors, and multiple myeloma or metastatic breast cancer. As a result of these studies, Zometa was approved in February 2002 for the treatment of patients with multiple myeloma and patients with documented bone metastases from solid tumors in conjunction with standard antineoplastic therapy. It was also approved for patients with prostate cancer who had progressed after treatment with at least one hormonal therapy. It had been previously approved in 2001 for treatment of hypercalcemia of malignancy.

Zometa (4 mg versus placebo) in hormone-refractory prostate cancer patients with metastatic bone lesions was evaluated in 137 centers in 18 countries including the United States and Canada. The inclusion criteria for this protocol are outlined in Table 33-1. The primary study end points included proportion of patients with at least one skeletal-related event, as described above. Secondary end points included those factors in Table 33-2.

Table 33-1

Zometa Phase III Trial: Design Inclusion Criteria

- Prostate carcinoma with documented bone metastases
- Rising PSA level despite hormonal therapy
- Baseline serum testosterone within the castrate range (under 50 ng/dl)
- No opiate analgesics
- Serum creatinine of 3.0 mg/dl (265 µmol/L) or less
- ECOG performance status 0, 1, 2
- Appropriate antineoplastic therapy at study entry

Table 33-2

Zometa Phase III Trial: Secondary Study End Points

- Time to first skeletal-related event
- Time to progression in bone
- Time to overall disease progression
- Pain relief
- Hypercalcemia

- Analgesic use
- Quality of life
- Markers of bone resorption and formation
- Safety profile
- Survival

Patients in this phase 3 trial were equally randomized based upon age, race, performance status, quality of life, time since diagnosis of prostate cancer, and baseline PSA average. There were 214 patients in the Zometa group and 208 patients in the placebo group.

Zometareduced the proportion of patients with SREs compared to placebo by approximately 25 percent. Forty-four percent of the placebo patients versus 33 percent of the Zometa patients had skeletal-related events within approximately 1 year from the beginning of the study. On average, the patients who received Zometa experienced at least 100 more days free of a skeletal-related event compared to the control group. The number of bone complications in 1 year was reduced by almost 50 percent in patients treated with Zometa. Compared with placebo, the mean change from baseline in analgesic pain scores over time was lower at every time point for patients treated with Zometa and reached statistical significance at 3 months. Overall PSA level did not significantly change between the two groups.

The incidence of adverse events (greater than 10 percent) was not statistically significant between the two groups; however, there did appear to be a slight increased tendency for fever, fatigue, myalgia, and bone pain with the initial infusion in the Zometagroup. Renal function was unchanged between the two groups. The patient should be warned of flulike symptoms, which can occur in up to 25 percent of patients; this is usually associated with the first administration of the drug and decreases thereafter. This is characterized by fever, muscle and joint aches, and fatigue. These symptoms can frequently be ameliorated by treatment with Tylenol and/or steroids before, during, or after the infusion. Renal function and serum calcium levels need to be monitored during therapy.

In summary, Zometa is the most potent bisphosphonate available in this country. It is given as a 4-mg intravenous infusion over 15 minutes and is associated with a significant decrease in the occurrence of skeletal-related events, a significant delayed time to the first skeletal-related event, significantly reduced incidence of pathologic fracture, and delayed time to first fracture compared to a control group. Patients who received Zometa reported less pain at every point throughout the course of therapy. It is currently the only treatment approved by the FDA for prostate cancer patients with documented bony metastases who have progressed after treatment with at least one hormonal therapy.

Some states have allowed reimbursement for Zometain any patient with prostate cancer who is receiving hormonal therapy because there are data showing it prevents osteoporosis and osteoporosis-related fractures.

How to Use This Information

If you are currently undergoing hormonal therapy for prostate cancer or have metastatic prostate cancer in the bones, ask your physician about prescribing Zometa in order to decrease bone pain and skeletal-related events.

Chapter 34

ADVANCING THE TREATMENT OF HORMONE-REFRACTORY PATIENTS

The initial treatment for recurring prostate cancer remains hormonal therapy. It has been well known since the 1940s that androgen deprivation achieved remissions in nearly 80 percent of the patients. Unfortunately, despite castrate levels of testosterone, approximately 80 percent of patients progress within 12 to 18 months. Castrate levels of testosterone can be achieved via many means, including surgical removal of both testicles prior to a diagnosis of recurrent prostate cancer. These patients, often referred to as chemical failures, may receive hormonal therapy (androgen deprivation) as well.

Patients receiving their initial hormonal therapy often go into remission and have a marked improvement in their symptoms. It is common for these patients to return to a normal quality life and even resume working. Ultimately, the vast majority of these patients will have a recurrence despite castration levels of testosterone. This recurrence is often referred to as androgen-insensitive, or refractory, disease. This failure to respond to initial hormone manipulation is a serious consequence of the patient's disease. Once the patient develops symptoms of this progression, his survival time can be as short as 12 months.

Although recurrence of prostate cancer may be localized in the area of the prostate itself, the most common site of recurrence is the bone. Patients may experience such symptoms as bone pain, bone fracture, and spinal-cord compression. The patients often suffer from poor appetite with weight loss. Fatigue is a common symptom in patients whether they are receiving chemotherapy or not.

This chapter discusses the increased efficacy of chemotherapy for hormonally refractory prostate cancer, explains second-line manipulation therapy, discusses both estramustine in combination with other drugs and Novantrone in combination with an oral steroid, discusses the improved results that are obtained with Taxotere in combination with other drugs, considers other promising drugs and combinations, and explains why patients should consider chemotherapy.

Making Treatment Decisions

The patient and his clinician will now face a decision regarding the next approach to therapy. Many options exist, including additional hormonal therapy, radiation therapy, and chemotherapy. There have also been recent advances in supportive care of prostate cancer patients, including the development of Zometa (zoledronic acid) (see Chapter 33) for the prevention of skeletal complications. The choice of therapy must be based on several characteristics, including the performance status of the patient, symptoms, other medical problems, and the site of recurrent disease, as well as the patient's ability to attend frequent chemotherapy sessions.

When choosing a therapy, the clinician and patient should have a clear understanding of their mutual expectations. Any intervention should offer a chance of cure, survival prolongation, or improvement in symptoms. Although therapy of hormone-refractory prostate cancer has not been shown to be curative, those patients responding to treatment have lived longer and had fewer symptoms.

Second-Line Hormonal Manipulation

The initial approach after failing initial hormone therapy is often a second line of hormonal manipulation. Those patients being treated with castration alone (surgical or chemical) will often be offered an antiandrogen such as flutamide, bicalutamide, or nilutamide. Those patients already on combined androgen blockade (castration plus antiandrogen) will often be treated by withdrawing the antiandrogen. Responses to addition of antiandrogen occur in up to 40 percent of the patients despite prior hormonal failure. Paradoxically, withdrawing antiandrogens in the setting of combined androgen blockade results in a 20 percent response rate as well. Other options have included the use of high-dose ketoconazole, Megace, and DES (diethylstibesterol). Unfortunately, despite initial benefits in many of these patients, second-line hormonal therapy often has a very short duration of benefit of about 4 months.

Several years ago, the Chinese herbal compound PC SPES gained popularity as a natural product to treat prostate cancer. After initial excitement, this produce was found to be contaminated with several pharmaceuticals and was taken off the market. It appears that PC SPES acted much like DES and had DES-like side effects, including thrombosis, gynecomastia, nausea, and loss of libido.

E. Roy Berger, M.D., F.A.C.P. and James Lewis, Jr., Ph.D

Effectiveness of Chemotherapy

Chemotherapy is an emerging option for patients diagnosed with hormone-refractory disease. Unfortunately, the development of chemotherapy in prostate cancer has trailed many of the advances and successes in other cancers. Prostate cancer patients are often older and have concurrent medical problems (e.g., diabetes, hypertension, heart disease). Recent advances in supportive care and improvement in our understanding of patients and disease have allowed chemotherapy to be given to an increasingly older population. Another impediment to the study of chemotherapy in prostate cancer has been related to how we measure response. Traditionally, a response is defined based on a minimum of a 50 percent reduction in the measurable area of tumor mass. Prostate cancer is often limited to bone involvement, which does not allow easy measurements. There has been increasing use of other markers to define clinical benefit, including PSA decline, time to disease progression, quality of life, and overall survival. The most useful marker appears to be the percentage of treated patients who have a decline in PSA of 50 percent or more. This decline in PSA level has been demonstrated to correlate with longer survival time in clinical trials.

Most prostate cancer patients will be referred to a medical oncologist for consideration of chemotherapy. The urologist will continue to provide the hormonal therapies, as it is common practice to continue androgen suppression even when a man has progressive disease. In addition to hormonal therapy, the patients often continue to receive other therapies, including Zometa. A recent survey of community oncologists revealed that the first suggested therapy in patients failing initial hormonal therapy would be to a second hormonal manipulation. In those patients already failing second-line therapy, chemotherapy should be considered. Although there is an increasing consensus among oncologists, not all of them agree about the role of chemotherapy.

Much of the confusion regarding chemotherapy is a result of changes in practice patterns. Historically, prostate cancer was considered a chemotherapy-insensitive disease. Two large reviews of older chemotherapy regimens, including 43 clinical trials and thousands of patients treated before 1991, demonstrated minimal activity, with an overall response rate of less than 9 percent. Fortunately, there is reason for encouragement for patients and for families whose loved ones have hormone-refractory prostate cancer. The FDA has approved two agents for use in patients with hormone-refractory disease: mitoxantrone and estramustine. In addition, a number of other agents are being studied and at least one, Taxotere (docetaxel), appears to be effective against hormone-refractory prostate cancer.

Estramustine with Other Drugs

Estramustine was the first agent approved by the United States FDA to treat metastatic prostate cancer unresponsive to hormone therapies. This oral therapy is a combination of nitrogen mustard and estradiol. It was hoped that the estradiol would target the prostate cancer cell and the nitrogen mustard kill it. However, estramustine — this drug like many other chemotherapy agents — interferes with mitosis, leading to death of the cancer cell. Single-agent trials of estramustine have demonstrated a response rate of nearly 20 percent. Most exciting are a number of new combinations of chemotherapy drugs, including estramustine, which have demonstrated a response rate of greater than 60 percent. The use of estramustine has been limited due to such side effects as nausea, vomiting, and thrombosis. Researchers are attempting to reduce the side effects by altering the dose and schedule of administration.

Novantrone with an Oral Steroid

Novantrone (mitoxantrone) was approved for use in advanced prostate cancer in the mid-1990s. Novantrone in combination with an oral steroid has become the standard of care across the United States for patients with metastatic prostate cancer failing hormonal therapy. This practice is based on several clinical trials that have demonstrated a benefit in patients with advanced prostate cancer. When compared to the use of a steroid alone, the combination with Novantrone has repeatedly demonstrated a fall in PSA, delay in time to disease progression, and a significant reduction in pain. Although not demonstrating an improvement in overall survival, this combination meets the necessary qualifications for treatment, including delaying progression and improving symptoms. This regimen is tolerated quite well, with less than 10 percent of patients requiring hospitalization for complications of treatment.

Taxotere with Other Drugs

Clinical trials have suggested even more activity for regimens based on Taxotere (docetaxel). This agent is commercially available and is approved in the United States for the treatment of lung and breast cancer. Many oncologists now offer this drug in various combinations as first-line therapy against hormone-refractory prostate cancer. In initial studies as a

271

single agent, Taxotere has demonstrated responses in nearly 50 percent of patients treated. Although Taxotere has significant side effects, studies with a weekly schedule of therapy have demonstrated significant activity and less toxicity.

Taxotere has been combined with estramustine in a number of clinical trials. These combinations have demonstrated the highest activity ever seen from chemotherapy against hormone-refractory prostate cancer. PSA responses have been seen in many patients. As many as 75 percent of patients receiving Taxotere-based combinations have had a 50 percent reduction in PSA, 43 percent have demonstrated a 75 percent reduction, and as many as 20 percent have demonstrated a complete normalization after therapy. In addition, patients receiving Taxotere-based combinations have also had a prolonged period before progression of PSA as well as significantly less pain.

Clinicians today are faced with the dilemma of which regimen to use. A recently concluded clinical trial compared the regimen of Novantrone plus steroids with Taxotere plus estramustine. These results should be available within the next several years. In the meantime, patients and physicians will need to consider the available clinical data and toxicities. From the patient's perspective, there are at least two effective chemotherapy regimens, both of which have shown the ability to delay disease progression and improve the patient's pain. Perhaps the sequential use of both regimens will lead to further improvements and perhaps an improvement in duration of survival as well.

Other Promising Drugs and Combinations

There are a number of promising agents being evaluated in clinical trials. Thalidomide has demonstrated angiogenesis inhibition in prostate cancer and is used in clinical practice in patients who have failed other therapies. Ongoing trials are studying its use in combination with Taxotere. Other exciting agents include Exisulind, an anti-inflammatory agent that leads to cell death for prostate cancer cells, and Provenge, an exciting new vaccine being developed against prostate cancer (see Chapter # 21). The recent clinical successes have led to increased interest in applying many of the newer agents under development against prostate cancer as well.

Changing Your Mind about Chemotherapy

Developing hormone-refractory disease remains a serious complication for patients with prostate cancer. Recent clinical data do suggest a change in how these patients are treated. Prostate cancer is sensitive to chemotherapy with more than 50 percent of patients responding to newer combinations. Although patients with advanced disease have not been observed to live longer, it is reasonable to believe, based on other disease states, that earlier treatment might affect survival. Based on average survival rates of more than 20 months in hormone-refractory prostate cancer patients (whose average survival has historically been about 12 months), we are cautiously optimistic that a survival benefit will be seen in the randomized controlled trials that are being conducted. Ongoing trials are evaluating the role of chemotherapy in asymptomatic patients with increasing PSA level as well as earlier in high-risk patients before or after initial local therapy in patients with hormone-sensitive disease. Available clinical trials do show the following: high response rates, prolonged survival in responders, palliation of pain, reduction in analgesic use, and improvements in quality of life. Although the benefits of chemotherapy in advanced hormone-refractory prostate cancer appear modest, they compare favorably to those documented in breast, lung, colon, and other solid tumors where chemotherapy as part of care is the standard (see Table 34-1).

Table 34-1

Resonse Rate for Major Cancers

	Prostate	Lung	Colon	Breast
	Taxotere Emcyt, and prednisone	Carboplatinum + Taxol	Irinotecan + (CPT-11) 5-fluorouracil + leucovorin (5FU + LV)	Taxotere
Response rate	68%	15.3%	39%	48%
Time to progression	8 months	3.3 months	6.9 months	6 months
1-year survival	More than 60%	31%	70%	60%
Median survival	20 months	7.4 months	15.9 months	15.7 months

Chemotherapy should be considered a valuable asset in the treatment of prostate cancer. Patients should seek referral to a medical oncologist soon after initial failure of hormonal therapy. Although cure of metastatic disease is not yet a reasonable expectation, patients can look forward to therapy that can prolong their lives and reduce their pain.

How to Use This Information

If you have hormonally refractory prostate cancer and have failed second-line hormonal therapy, don't give up. Certain combinations of chemotherapy have been found to be effective with less severe side effects.

Chapter 35

NEWER LHRH AGONISTS

The introduction of LHRH agonists has provided an alternative medical approach to the treatment of both localized and advanced prostate cancer. In localized cancer, they debulk the tumors to facilitate other therapies. In advanced cancer, they palliate the disease by halting the spread of prostate cancer; the earlier LHRH agonists such as Lupron and Zoladex, plus two others, have been used in several other countries for the treatment of prostate cancer. Because they are peptides, they are susceptible to being digested in the stomach or gastrointestinal tract; therefore, other routes of administration were needed to produce a sustained concentration of the LHRH agonists and for a prolonged period of time. Injections, which have to be given daily, and nasal sprays, which must be taken several times a day, are less convenient and less reliable than longer-acting depot preparations. Although LHRH agonists are available in either 3- or 4-month concentrations, there is room on the market for new LHRH agonists, administered differently and for longer periods.

The relationship between prostate cancer and hormone sensitivity was first reported in 1941. In his classic paper, Charles Huggins reported on the beneficial effects of treating prostate cancer by orchiectomy. Orchiectomy, the removal of the testicles, resulted in a marked reduction in the male hormone testosterone, which is produced in the testes, and a consequent improvement in the course of prostate cancer. This discovery, for which he received the Nobel Prize in 1966, ushered in the era of the hormonal treatment of prostate cancer.

In 1971, Andrew V. Schally and Roger Guillemin were able to isolate luteinizing hormone-releasing hormone (LHRH), also known as gonadotropin-releasing hormone. LHRH is a potent brain chemical involved in initiating the production of testosterone. Produced in an area of the brain known as the hypothalamus, its function is to act on another part of the brain, the pituitary gland. This gland controls the production of hormones in the body. The action of LHRH on the pituitary gland in females causes the production of follicle-stimulating hormone (FSH). In males it causes the pituitary to produce luteinizing hormone (LH). FSH acts on the ovaries to produce estrogen, while LH acts on the testes to cause them to produce testosterone. In 1973, Schally and his associates actually created a synthetic form of LHRH, known as an <u>analog</u>.

They were able to determine that when given to men, analogs initially caused the same responses that were seen with naturally occurring LHRH. They caused the pituitary gland to increase the production of LH, and, subsequently, the testicles produced elevated amounts of testosterone. With continued administration of LHRH analogs, however, the pituitary gland began to fatigue from the constant stimulation. As it did, the production of LH all but ceased, as did the testicular production of testosterone. This became a way to use medication to achieve the same beneficial effects on prostate cancer caused by orchiectomy while avoiding surgery. These analogs became known as LHRH agonists and were used in the treatment of prostate cancer for the first time in 1980.

They were introduced into the United States in 1989 when the FDA approved the monthly use of leuprolide acetate, or Lupron. Shortly afterward, the FDA also approved a second agent, goserelin acetate, or Zoladex. Although administered differently, both agents were equally effective in suppressing testosterone production to castrate levels and achieving beneficial effects in prostate cancer. They also had similar side effects. Lupron more comfortably is injected into the buttocks through a smaller needle, while Zoladex is administered subcutaneously into the abdomen through a much larger needle. With the launch of longer-acting, three- and four-month preparations, Lupron and Zoladex almost totally supplanted orchiectomy as the hormonal treatment of choice for advanced prostate cancer.

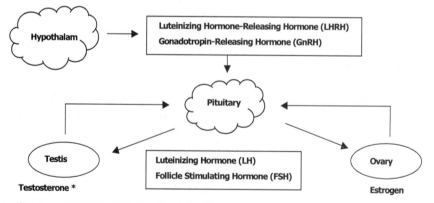

Fig. 35-1

For over a decade, these agents have remained the front-line therapies in hormonal treatment. More recently, three newer agents have been approved by the FDA, giving physicians a wider choice. Two of these, Viadur and Eligard, are formulations of leuprolide acetate, the same LHRH analog used in Lupron, while the third, Trelstar (triptorelin pamoate), is an entirely different analog. While they offer more latitude in selecting a treatment, none of the newer entities has been shown to be more effective than Lupron and Zoladex.

Viadur

Viadur, developed by ALZA Corporation and marketed by Bayer AG, is a leuprolide acetate implant. Approved by the FDA in 2000 for the palliative treatment of advanced prostate cancer, the implant releases leuprolide acetate over a 12-month period. Once released, the leuprolide acetate has the same mechanism of action as other LHRH analogs.

Viadur is placed under the skin of a patient's upper arm during an office visit. The insertion procedure, which can take up to 15 minutes, includes identifying the insertion site, preparing a sterile field, loading the implanter, and administering local anesthesia. After the area is anesthetized, a small incision is made, and a titanium implant is inserted under the skin using the implanter. After the implanter is removed, leaving the implant, the incision is closed using one or two sutures. After 12 months, the implant must be removed. This is done by anesthetizing the area and making a small incision on the upper arm near the implant. Using forceps, the implant is gripped and removed, and the incision closed with sutures. During the removal procedure, a second implant may be inserted for an additional 12 months of treatment.

Local reactions to the insertion or removal procedure included bruising (34.6%) and burning (5.6%). Less frequent reactions included pulling, pressure, itching, redness, pain, swelling, and bleeding. The majority of these reactions resolved within 2 weeks, but they persisted in 9.3% of patients. In a study of 107 patients who received one implant, four developed an infection/inflammation after the procedure, necessitating the use of antibiotics. All of these resolved and therapy continued.

Following implantation, the leuprolide acetate is released in a continuous steady state using an osmotically driven technology. Water from surrounding tissues enters one end of the implant through a semipermeable membrane. This causes a swelling, which pushes a piston toward a compartment in the implant that contains the drug. The drug is then released at a rate equal to the inflow of water. This controlled-release process discharges 120 mcg of leuprolide acetate daily at a rate of less than $1/120^{th}$ of a drop of water over 24 hours.

In a 2-year, 1311 patient study presented the FDA, Viadur, like to other LHRH agonists, caused a transient elevation of testosterone, followed by suppression and decreasing levels. Testosterone was maintained below castrate levels between weeks 2 and 4 in all but one patient; he took 7 months to achieve this level. Once suppressed, testosterone remained well below the castration threshold for the duration of treatment. PSA level also decreased in all patients after insertion. At 6 months, the PSA had decreased by at least 90 percent in 74.2 percent of the patients evaluated. There was no rise in testosterone or PSA after insertion of a second implant.

Viadur is as effective as other LHRH agonists. It has the advantage of acting for a long time without the need for repeated injections. It has been used advantageously in patients who have difficulty getting to the physician's office. It has the disadvantage of requiring a surgical procedure to introduce the medication. Viadur was the second product approved in the United States using leuprolide acetate.

Eligard

Eligard, the newest LHRH agonist, was approved by the FDA in 2002 for the palliative treatment of advanced prostate cancer. Developed by Sanofi-Synthelabo, it is a subcutaneous formulation of leuprolide acetate. Eligard uses a unique delivery system that combines a biodegradable polymer with a liquid carrier and the active pharmaceutical. It can be injected under the skin anywhere in the body. While it is injected as a liquid, it solidifies once it is in the body. The leuprolide acetate is then released as the polymer biodegrades. Eligard is available in both 1-month (7.5 mg.) and 3-month (22.5 mg.) preparations; a 4-month preparation is scheduled to be released in 2003.

Eligard's mechanism of action is similar to that of other LHRH agonists. After the initial dose, there is a transient rise in testosterone levels. This rise, known as the <u>flare phenomenon,</u> resolves in approximately 1 week. As the pituitary fatigues, the level of LH falls, and serum testosterone levels subsequently drop.

In the clinical trials presented to the FDA of both the 1- and 3-month formulations, the mean time for testosterone suppression to reach 50 ng/dl or less was 21 days. Testosterone suppression persisted throughout both trials, and at the end of 6 months testosterone levels averaged 6.1 ng/dl in the 1-month study and 10.1 ng/dl in the 3-month study. Both of these levels are very significant reductions in testosterone levels, which averaged over 360 ng/dl at the beginning of the studies. The actual results could have been even lower, since the measurement instruments could not detect testosterone levels below 3.0 ng/dl. As for the PSA level, the mean PSA reductions were 94 percent in the trial of the 1-month formulation and 98 percent in the 3-month trial. These reductions persisted throughout the 6 months of each trial.

In both studies, testosterone levels were lowered to 50 ng/dl or below in 100 percent of the cases. In fact, with Eligard the levels were 20 ng/dl or below 98 percent of the time with the 1-month formulation, and 94 percent with the 3-month.

These levels are noteworthy because of guidelines published by the National Comprehensive Cancer Network (NCCN). The NCCN is an international organization established in 1995 in alliance with the world's leading cancer centers. Its purpose is to develop practice guidelines for the treatment of cancer using consensus statements from key leaders in urology and oncology. Rather than conducting studies, it uses the recommendations and judgments of experts and authorities in the field. In 2000, the NCCN practice guideline for prostate cancer defined castration levels of testosterone as being less than 20 ng/dl. It suggested that if those levels are not reached, additional therapies should be used.

In the United States, the FDA has always defined castration levels of testosterone as less than 50 ng/dl, and all LHRH agonists had been held to this standard. This was mainly due to the fact that when Lupron, the first LHRH agonist in the United States, was approved, instruments could not measure testosterone levels below 50 ng/dl. Over the years, however, new technologies have refined the ability to measure testosterone levels. While there are no studies that show that a lower testosterone level has any advantages in the treatment of prostate cancer, the NCCN consensus still recommended the lower 20 ng/dl level. More studies will be needed to determine which level is optimal and to test the hypothesis that lower testosterone means improved survival in advanced-state prostate cancer.

There is no current evidence that shows whether older agents such as Lupron or Zoladex achieve this 20 ng/dl level, because studies have not been performed using the newer and more sensitive measurement. Moreover, studies indicate that with all commonly used LHRH agonists, about 5 percent of patients fail to achieve even the FDA testosterone castration levels of 50 ng/dl or less. Eligard was successful in lowering testosterone to 50 ng/dl or less in 100 percent of patients.

Eligard's safety profile was similar to those of other LHRH agonists with regard to the range and severity of side effects. The most common side effect of all of these agents is hot flashes/sweats. This usually occurs in over half of the patients treated and is most likely due to dilatation of the blood vessels resulting from the lowering of testosterone. When asked to grade the severity of the hot flashes/sweats in the Eligard trials, fewer than 1 percent of the patients in the 1-month trial and none of the patients in the 3-month trial rated them as severe. They were overwhelmingly classified as mild and to a lesser extent as moderate. Mild and moderate symptoms required no treatment, and this might be an advantage of the use of Eligard.

Eligard is injected subcutaneously using a small 20-gauge needle. The amount of liquid injected is also small: 0.25 ml for the 1-month dosage and 0.375 ml for the 3-month. Its administration is usually very patient-friendly.

Unlike other LHRH agonists, Eligard requires refrigeration. Prior to use it must be brought to room temperature. If not used, it can be refrigerated again. Patients have reported a stinging sensation if it is injected before it is brought fully to room temperature.

In summary, Eligard offers the proven performance of leuprolide acetate, a very effective degree of testosterone suppression, a comfortable and unique delivery system, and a favorable safety profile with only mild to moderate hot flashes/sweats.

Trelstar

Trelstar (triptorelin pamoate), an LHRH agonist, was approved by the FDA in 2001 for the palliative treatment of advanced prostate cancer. It was the first new analog approved in the United States in over a decade. Available in a 1-month (3.75 mg.) dose as Trelstar Depot and a 3-month (11.25 mg.) dose as Trelstar LA, it was licensed by Pharmacia Upjohn for the American market from Debiopharm of Switzerland. Trelstar has been the second leading LHRH agonist in Europe since 1985 when it was approved. It is available in over 60 countries and has over 2 million patient-months of worldwide use.

Trelstar's mechanism of action is similar to that of other LHRH agonists. In the studies presented to the FDA, 98.7 percent of patients achieved castration levels of testosterone by day 57 with the 1-month formulation and 98.8 percent with the 3-month formulation. Both Trelstar Depot and Trelstar LA were equally effective in maintaining castration levels throughout the 9 months of the study. As would be expected, PSA level decreased as the testosterone levels fell. The mean PSA reduction from baseline levels was 97.1 percent.

The Trelstar submission to the FDA was exceptional because it not only contained data regarding Trelstar, but it also presented a head-to-head comparison between the 1-month formulations of Trelstar and Lupron. This study continued for 9 months. Both preparations showed a characteristic initial rise in testosterone, followed by testosterone reductions. Trelstar had a slower onset of action than Lupron, and by day 29 had achieved castration levels of testosterone in 91.2 percent of patients compared to 99.3 percent with Lupron. By day 57, they were both similar in attaining castration levels in 97.7 percent and 97.1 percent of patients, respectively. From months 2 through 9, however, Lupron maintained castration levels of testosterone in 91.2 percent of patients, while Trelstar maintained them in 96.2 percent. Trelstar, therefore, tended to induce a castration level of testosterone slightly less rapidly but maintained it more effectively.

Interestingly, the 9-month survival rate was significantly longer with Trelstar. The estimate of the probability of longer survival was 97.0 percent for Trelstar, compared with 90.5 percent for Lupron. While this achieved statistical significance, no claims can be made, because a 9-month study is not long enough to reach conclusions regarding survival in prostate cancer, and the primary design of the study was to evaluate only safety and efficacy. With regard to safety, both Trelstar and Lupron were well tolerated and had similar side effects. Hot flashes/sweats, the most common side effect for both preparations, were similar for both, occurring in slightly over 50 percent of patients. There was no difference between the two in analgesic usage or quality of life. Reviewing the data, the FDA concluded that Trelstar is as effective and as safe as Lupron for patients with advanced prostate cancer.

Trelstar, like Lupron, is administered intramuscularly into the buttock, needs no refrigeration, and has a shelf life of 2 years. In its initial FDA submission, Pharmacia Upjohn also received approval for the DebioClip, a closed injection system that allows a vial of Trelstar to be inserted into an injection apparatus without being opened. This avoids contamination and minimizes the potential for needle sticks to health-care personnel. It is likely that it will be introduced in the United States in the latter half of 2003.

Trelstar offers yet another choice in LHRH agents. Despite being new to the United States, it has a long-standing record of safety and efficacy worldwide. It has been shown to be at least comparable to Lupron, with a similar route of administration. Along with Viadur and Eligard, Trelstar is a member of the newer LHRH agonists. As a group they offer greater latitude of choice and should be considered in the hormonal treatment of advanced prostate cancer.

E. Roy Berger, M.D., F.A.C.P. and James Lewis, Jr., Ph.D

How to Use This Information

If you are being treated with either a 1- or a 3-month dose of an LHRH agonist, try one of the LHRH analogs mentioned in this chapter to see if it is an improvement over your current treatment.

Chapter 36

INTERMITTENT HORMONAL THERAPY: MORE EFFECTIVE THAN CONTINUOUS?

Ever since Dr. Fernand Labrie of Laval University in Quebec developed combination hormonal therapy, it has been administered on a continuous basis. CHT includes two hormones: a luteinizing hormone-releasing hormone or LHRH agonist to stop testosterone produced by the testes, and a pure antiandrogen (to be used in combination with the LHRH agonist) to block androgens from attaching to the receptor sites in the prostate cancer cells. The LHRH agonist is administered about once a month by an injection in the buttock, arm, or a muscle in the abdomen. Injections lasting 3 months, 4 months, and even one year are currently available.

LHRH agonists available in the United States include Lupron, Zoladex, Trelstar, Eligard, and Viadur. Antiandrogens that have been approved by the FDA are Eulexin, Casodex, and Nilandron. The latter two are taken once a day. Cyproterone acetate (Androcur) is an antiandrogen that may be available in the United States in the future.

Today, due to the research of several doctors in this country and Canada, continuous CHT is frequently being replaced by intermittent CHT. Most studies have indicated an improved quality of life for patients on the latter regimen. In addition, some studies have shown a longer progression-free survival using this technique.

Experimental studies suggest that intermittent exposure to androgens can suppress certain genes in prostate cancer cells and thus keep them hormone-dependent for longer periods. Animal studies performed in Vancouver using hormone-sensitive tumor models suggest that progression to hormone insensitivity can be delayed for a longer time using intermittent CHT instead of continuous hormonal therapy. In receiving intermittent androgen exposure, the genes are suppressed from mutating to an androgen-insensitive state.

Koichiro Akakura and colleagues of Vancouver used the mouse tumor model to study the effects of hormonal therapy (castration) and tumor regression as well as tumor cell death. To demonstrate the effect of intermittent CHT on cancer, a tumor was transplanted into a succession of male mice. Each of these mice was castrated when the tumor reached a weight of 3 grams. When the tumor regressed to about 30 percent of its original weight, it was transplanted into a noncastrated rat. When it increased to 3 grams, it was then transplanted into another animal, whereupon that animal would be castrated; again, a decrease in tumor size was noted. This cycle of transplantation and castration was repeated successfully four times before the cancerous tumor and the hormonal ablation were no longer effective – that is, the tumor become androgen-independent. This occurred during the fifth cycle.

The effect of intermittent androgen suppression in small groups of patients was reported in 1993. Four stage C3 and stage D patients were treated first with cyprotene acetate (100 mg daily) and diethylstilbestrol (0.1 mg daily). Then they were maintained with cyprotene acetate in combination with 3.4 mpm goserelin acetate (Zoladex) over a month. After 6 or more months of CHT and when the PSA reached the normal range, the treatment was interrupted for 2 to 11 months. Intermittent CHT was reinstated when the PSA level rose to about 20 ng/ml. This cycle was repeated over a period of 4 to 47 months without the prostate cancer cells becoming androgen-independent.

The study revealed several things. Only those patients whose PSA level decreases below 4.0 ng/ml within 5 months by intermittent CHT should be considered for this treatment. Thus far, no obvious unfavorable effects on survival time have been experienced from the intermittent therapy. Pretreatment levels of testosterone return to patients slowly over a period of 8 to 14 weeks when they are off the intermittent therapy. Intermittent CHT appears to have two advantages over continuous CHT: (1) it improves the quality of life with recovery of sexual function, and (2) it reduces the cost of therapy.

Dr. Bob Leibowitz, a pioneer of intermittent combination hormonal therapy in the United States, began using this form of treatment with patients in 1991. He coined the terms *triple androgen blockade (TAB)* or *triple hormone blockade*, which refer to treatment with LHRH-A, Eulexin, and a 5-alpha reductase inhibitor. The two 5-alpha reductase inhibitors available in the United States are Proscar and Avodart. The latter inhibits both 5-alpha reductase, is renzymes while Proscar inhibits 1. There is no data yet using Avodart in prostate cancer, so Proscar has been used to date.

The patient being treated for prostate cancer is given every 8 hours, an LHRH agonist every 28 to 30 days, and finally 5 mg of Proscar once a day. If the PSA falls to an undetectable level between the third and fourth month, the patient continues on TAB for another 9 months, for a total treatment time of 13 months. The antiandrogen is continued for 28 days after the last monthly LHRH-agonist injection. The Proscar is continued throughout the duration of the TAB, and then is maintained at 5 mg once a day (this is called *Proscar maintenance therapy*).

Dr. Leibowitz points out that this treatment is short-term, up-front TAB. The patient is not on intermittent CHT unless retreatment is necessary.

He would retreat the patient if his PSA level rose to about half the pretreatment level. Dr. Leibowitz believes that cure is not necessary for most men with prostate cancer. He also believes that one year of TAB can cause complete disappearance of all prostate cancer cells in many men. A number of other specialists, including the author, are skeptical of Dr. Leibowitz's claims, and they eagerly await a randomized controlled trial before relying on his observations, especially for the treatment of younger men.

So, is intermittent CHT more effective than continuous CHT in lengthening survival time? We just don't know. We need more data to make a sound judgment. We know that about 5 to 10 percent of patients receiving continuous CHT enjoy long-term survival, and some patients even show no evidence of prostate cancer after extensive medical evaluation. We don't know what the long-term survival rates for this 5 to 10 percent would be if they used intermittent CHT. It could be longer, or it could be shorter; however, preliminary data suggest it is unlikely to be shorter. Obviously, these questions could at least be partially answered if there was a study to compare continuous CHT to intermittent CHT over a period of either 5, 10, or 15 years. These studies are currently ongoing.

Jean de Leval and colleagues undertook a small phase III study that compared intermittent versus continuous androgen blockade in the treatment of patients with advanced hormone-naïve prostate cancer. A total of 68 evaluable patients with hormone-naïve advanced or relapsing prostate cancer were randomized to receive combined androgen blockade according to a continuous (33 men) or intermittent (35 men) regimen. Therapeutic monitoring was assessed by use of PSA measurements. Patients in the continuous and intermittent groups were equally stratified for age, biopsy, Gleason score, and baseline PSA level. The outcome variable was the time it took for the tumor to become androgen independent, which was defined as increasing PSA levels despite androgen blockade. Mean follow-up was 30.8 months.

The 35 ISA-treated patients completed 91 cycles, and 19 of them (54.3%) completed at least 3 cycles. Median cycle length and percentage of time off therapy were 9.0 months and 59.5%, respectively. The estimated 3-year progression rate was significantly lower in the intermittent group (7.0% $\pm$ 4.8%) than in the continuous group (38.9% $\pm$ 11.2%, $P = 0.0052$). The data suggest that intermittent androgen deprivation may maintain the androgen-dependent state of advanced human prostate cancer, as assessed by PSA measurements, at least as long as continuous therapy does. Further studies with longer follow-up times and larger patient groups are needed to determine the comparative impacts of complete and intermittent androgen deprivation on survival time.

Benefits of Intermittent CHT

We believe prostate cancer patients <u>can</u> benefit from intermittent CHT. You can use it:

1. when other primary therapies have failed,
2. as a way of possibly maintaining a hormone-sensitive state,
3. as a therapy to improve your quality of life.

The following questions may assist you in making a decision:

1. How important is your quality of life? If you are on or have been on hormonal therapy in the past, how did it affect you?
2. What is the probability of putting your disease into complete remission?
3. Are you willing to take a risk with intermittent CHT?
4. How far advanced is your disease? Which therapy would prolong your life?

These are difficult questions to answer. Your responses may depend upon whether you are:

1. a new patient and have recently been put on CHT
2. in good health and have more than 10 years to live
3. currently on CHT and enjoying a long-term survival
4. having bothersome or intolerable side effects from CHT
5. are willing to undertake a treatment that has not yet been proven to be more effective that conventional hormonal therapy. What stage your cancer is and what therapeutic option you have are also considerations.

S. Larry Goldenberg, M.D., et al. studied 47 patients who underwent intermittent hormonal therapy. There were 14 stage D2, 10 stage D1, 19 stage C, 2 stage B2, and 2 stage A2 patients with a mean follow-up time of 125 weeks. CHT was administered for a minimum of 6 months until the lowest PSA level was attained. Then hormones were withheld until the PSA level increased to a mean value of 10 to 20 ng/ml. This intermittent combination hormonal cycle of treatment was repeated until the PSA level did not respond to the hormones. Cycles 1 and 2 were tested for 23 and 25 weeks, respectively, with a mean period of therapy of 30 and 33 weeks, respectively, and an overall percentage time on therapy of 41 and 45 percent, respectively. The mean time needed to achieve the lowest PSA level was 20 weeks for cycle 1 and 18 weeks for cycle 2. When the cycle was halted, the testosterone level returned to normal within 8 weeks (range: 1 to 26). Patients reported that during the off-treatment phase in both cycles, they experienced an improved sense of well-being, recovery of libido, and restoration of potency and normal activity. In 7 patients with stage D2 disease, prostate cancer progressed to a level in which the median time off hormones was no longer effective after a mean of 20 weeks in cycle 1 and 108 weeks in cycle 2. Several patients in the study died, one from cancer-related illness, with a mean and median overall survival time of 210 weeks for cycle 1 and 166 for cycle 2, respectively.

The data from this study indicate that patients can be cycled on and off therapy and can achieve several regressions and remissions in response to hormonal therapy. As in other reports, the patients reported an upgrade in their quality of life. However, whether intermittent CHT is more effective in improving survival time than continuous CHT remains to be seen.

Goldenberg's study illustrates that intermittent CHT can relieve the side effects of hormonal therapy and allow for an improvement in a patient's quality of life while off therapy. Whether it prolongs the time to hormone independence, or may actually be harmful, will have to await phase III randomized studies that are being initiated by Southwest Oncology Group and others.

Akakura and colleagues in Vancouver strongly believe that intermittent CHT should be considered experimental, and that the gold standard of therapy for advanced prostate cancer remains CHT. Intermittent CHT should only be used by experienced urologists and oncologists until there is a better understanding of which patients may be helped or harmed by it.

How to Use This Information

1. Although intermittent CHT has been effective in animal studies, we do not have enough knowledge about how effective it is with human prostate cancer. We believe that more experience with this mode of therapy may lead to beneficial results for prostate cancer patients in the long run, not only to improve the quality of their lives, but also in terms of overall prolonged symptom-free survival.

2. Treatment decisions should be made under the guidance of an experienced urologist or oncologist.

3. If you are currently on continuous CHT and are willing to take a risk (although the risk may be small), find a urologist or an

oncologist who is interested in or has some experience with intermittent CHT and proceed with this therapy.

4. If you are older than 70 and have been diagnosed with very early stage prostate cancer, you might want to consider intermittent CHT. Start with a year on the hormones, and have your disease monitored carefully. After a year, stop the hormones, but continue the Proscar and monitor your PSA carefully. You may be one of the 10 percent who experience long-term survival on CHT. If your PSA begins to rise, you and your physician must decide when to restart CHT and if other treatment is necessary.

5. If you are on intermittent CHT, the following should take place:

6. During your first cycle, stay on continuous CHT for either 6, 9, or 12 months.

7. If your PSA reaches an undetectable level within 3 or 4 months, you are then eligible to go on intermittent CHT.

8. If you have completed your first cycle, stop continuous CHT and watch your PSA. If it should rise to an unacceptable level, go back on continuous CHT, and repeat the cycle as many times as possible.

9. Consider including Proscar or Avodart with CHT; remain on Proscar or Avodart as maintenance therapy when you stop the hormones.

Chapter 37

PROSTATE CANCER AND HEART DISEASE

Many patients make the mistake of focusing just on the fact that they have prostate cancer. However, of all men diagnosed with prostate cancer, just under 40 percent will die of the disease, while close to 30 percent will die of other causes, largely complications of cardiovascular disease, such as high blood pressure and atherosclerosis, or diabetes mellitus. Diet and lifestyle choices that lead to cardiovascular disease also increase the risk of metastatic prostate cancer. These disease processes are all favored by a diet rich in red meat, dairy fat, and egg yolks as well as a stressful lifestyle and lack of exercise.

One of the best examples of how these disease processes are liked is the recent clinic trial by Saxe and colleagues. This study looked at men whose cancer had recurred following radical prostatectomy. Their cancers were rather rapidly growing, with a median PSA doubling time of 6.4 months. After these men were placed on a heart-healthy diet and taught stress-reduction techniques, their PSA doubling time lengthened to 17.7 months. Apparently, the same diet and lifestyle changes needed to reduce the risk of cardiovascular disease also markedly slowed the progression of metastatic prostate cancer.

If you have been diagnosed with prostate cancer, you should take a health inventory to assess your risk of cardiovascular disease. You should then formulate a comprehensive plan designed to optimize treatment of prostate cancer and to treat or prevent cardiovascular disease. Proper nutrition is a key part of this process.

Animal Fats

The Western European and American diet that is rich in animal protein and fats has been associated with an increased risk of prostate cancer as well as heart disease. There a number of different factors linking this diet with cancer. The act of browning meats, especially broiling or frying them under high temperature, creates cancer-causing chemicals. Boiling or steaming meat reduces this problem.

A second problem appears to exist with a special kind of fat found in animal, but not plant, products called <u>arachidonic acid</u>. This omega-6 fatty acid has been shown to have profound effects on cancer cells. Arachidonic acid is converted by the body into a series of powerful hormones that stimulate the growth and spread of cancer cells. Other arachidonic acid products suppress the immune system by killing natural-killer cells and cytotoxic T cells that might otherwise slow the progress of the cancer.

Prostaglandin E2 is one of the products of arachidonic acid that prostate cancer cells produce in abundance. This stimulates the formation of new blood vessels to support the growth of the cancer. Additionally, prostaglandin E2 is toxic to the cells of the immune system. Nonsteroidal anti-inflammatory drugs, like ibuprofen, aspirin, and Celebrex, all relieve pain and inflammation because they block the formation of prostaglandin E2. Interestingly, chronic ingestion of these drugs is associated with a decreased risk of prostate cancer, presumably reflecting the importance of prostaglandin E2 in the development of prostate cancer. While these drugs are useful, however, they are not without problems, including gastric distress and bleeding, diarrhea, and occasionally temporary loss of kidney function. Thus we believe it is far safer to reduce the amount of arachidonic acid in the diet by substituting plants for animals as a protein source.

Arachidonic acid can also be converted into lipoxygenase products. One, 12-HETE, plays a major role in the ability of prostate cancer to spread throughout the body, and it also promotes the formation of new blood vessels that support the growth of the cancer. A second lipoxygenase product, 5-HETE, promotes the survival of prostate cancer cells in the absence of the male sex hormone, testosterone, as well as in promoting cancer growth. Drugs are available that block the formation of these lipoxygenase products, but dietary reduction of arachidonic acid is again a far safer way to limit this process.

How are you going to obtain enough protein for good health if you reduce your intake of meat, dairy fat, and egg yolks? Most will find this easy. First, a combination of whole grains and legumes provides a very healthy and tasty alternative. Most traditional cuisines contain recipes that fit this description: succotash, red beans, and rice from the US; pasta, beans, and minestrone from Italy; and soy-and-rice combinations from much of Asia are all good examples. Ocean fish, which are rich in the omega-3 fats EPA and DHA, are also heart- and prostate-healthy sources of protein. Eggwhite is superior to any meat product in terms of protein quality and is fat-free. Nonfat dairy products lack arachidonic acid, but may interfere with your body's ability to activate vitamin D.

Healthy Fats

In the recent past, low-fat diets were recommended as optimal for health, but it is now clear that some fats promote health. The Mediterranean diet is rich in olive oil, with up to 40 percent of the calories coming from this source. Yet, this diet is associated with a reduced risk of both heart disease and many forms of cancer. This may partly be due to the properties of olive oil, which is largely composed of monounsaturated fats and is low in both saturated fat as well as polyunsaturated fats that might undergo conversion to arachidonic acid. Additionally, olive oil is also rich in some of the same polyphenols found in green tea. Finally, olive oil contains phytosterols that can diminish the absorption of cholesterol from the gastrointestinal tract. Both polyphenols and phytosterols have been reported to slow or block the growth of human prostate cancer cells in the laboratory.

There are other sources of fat similar to that found in the olive. Almonds, filberts, macadamia nuts, pistachios, and cashews all contain levels of monounsaturated fat similar to that found in olive oil. Additionally, almonds are also a rich source of phytosterols. These nuts combine well with grains to help provide a quality source of protein.

As mentioned, ocean fish, particularly those from cold water, are rich in the omega-3 fats EPA and DHA. Epidemiologic studies show a reduced risk of prostate cancer in men who have several servings of fish per week. Additionally, these omega-3 fats appear to play an important role in the function of both the brain and the eye as well as reduce the risk of heart disease. Wild-caught salmon, tuna, sardines, herring, haddock, cod, halibut, and artic char all fit these requirements.

The Case for Antioxidants

There is a strong case for the role of antioxidants in the prevention of prostate cancer. In addition, antioxidants may slow the progression of existing prostate cancer.

In order to understand the role of antioxidants, you need to know the role that oxidative damage plays in the development and progression of prostate cancer. When human prostate cancer cells are exposed to the male sex hormone, testosterone, these cells produce a surge of hydrogen peroxide and other strong oxidants. These oxidants then cause damage to the genetic material (DNA) and other components of the cell. This oxidative damage can be diminished by the addition of antioxidants, such as vitamin C and vitamin E.

The above experiments were conducted in the laboratory. How do we know whether these results are relevant to what happens in men? One recent study examined the prostates of men, either at autopsy or during a radical prostatectomy, for oxidative damage to the DNA in the gland. Researchers found that beginning with puberty the amount of oxidative damage to the genetic material in prostate tissue increased steadily with age.

Furthermore, when the amount of oxidative damage exceeded a threshold, the risk of prostate cancer increased rapidly. This threshold was generally exceeded somewhere between 40 and 60 years of age. Thus, this study documents a tight association between oxidative damage to the DNA and the risk of prostate cancer.

The ultimate test of whether a treatment is useful is to compare it with no treatment in a randomized controlled clinical trial. Selenium was the first antioxidant tested in this way. One of the major actions of selenium is that it converts the oxidant hydrogen peroxide to water. The clinical trial that tested selenium used selenium-yeast at a dose of 200 mcg per day. This form and dose is widely available and costs about 10 cents a day. After 10 years of follow-up involving more than 1,000 subjects, the group that received selenium had a 50 percent reduction in overall cancer deaths. Prostate cancer deaths were decreased by 64 percent. If the men had a normal PSA when they entered the trial, prostate cancer deaths were reduced by 75 percent. Selenium at this dose caused no side effects. Selenium is now available in a wide range of forms, but only selenium-yeast has been subjected to extensive clinical testing.

Vitamin E is the second antioxidant that was subjected to a randomized controlled clinical trial. In this study, more than 20,000 subjects were randomly assigned to one of four groups: no treatment, beta-carotene, vitamin E, and vitamin E plus beta-carotene. The form of vitamin E used was artificial alpha-tocopherol and the dose was only 50 IU. The men receiving vitamin E experienced a 40 percent drop in deaths due to prostate cancer compared to the no-treatment group. Interestingly, those receiving beta-carotene alone did less well than those who received nothing. Subsequent laboratory studies have suggested that gamma- or delta-tocopherol may well be more active than alpha-tocopherol. Furthermore, doses much larger than 50 IU have proven to be safe and have been used in other studies.

The third antioxidant to be tested is *lycopene*, the red pigment in tomatoes. Men were randomized to 30 mg of lycopene or no treatment for 2 months prior to radical prostatectomy. At the time of surgery, those receiving lycopene had less extensive cancer. Lycopene appears to be very safe, and doses much higher than 30 mg a day may well prove to be quite safe.

Some of the most interesting and promising antioxidants have not yet been subjected to appropriate clinical testing. For example, there are water-soluble compounds found in a wide range of plants that have impressive antioxidant activity. These include the polyphenols found in green tea, chocolate, olives, and many fruits. In the laboratory, polyphenols have impressive anticancer activity. Green tea polyphenols are able to cause the shrinkage of human prostate tumors growing in mice.

The anthocyanins are another group of water-soluble plant pigments with antioxidant activity. These chemicals are red to purple in color and account for the intense color of the red beet as well as many of the red to purple berries, such as elderberries and blueberries.

Members of the cabbage family, including broccoli, kale, mustard greens, and turnips, contain a range of chemicals that suppress the progression of cancer. One group of chemicals, best represented by sulforaphane found in broccoli, triggers a master switch in cells that causes a dramatic increase in a wide range of antioxidant defenses. These plants also contain lutein, an antioxidant similar to lycopene that appears to have similar health benefits. In addition, these plants also contain indole-3-carbinol, a chemical that can inhibit bcl2, a protein that plays an important role in helping cancer cells survive hormonal therapy.

These various antioxidants act together in an antioxidant defense network. For optimal suppression of oxidant injury, the various antioxidants should be present in the proper proportions. Administering large doses of a single antioxidant out of proportion to other antioxidants can cause problems. For example, vitamin C can cause oxidative damage if administered in too large a dose.

There are some situations where antioxidants need to be used with caution. Radiation therapy kills cancer cells by causing an overwhelming amount of oxidative damage. In the laboratory, antioxidants have been shown to lessen the damage caused by radiation. Similarly, the chemotherapy drug doxorubicin has been shown to act as a strong oxidant. This plays a role in the heart damage caused by this drug, but it also may be involved in its anticancer activity. For this reason, you should check with your oncologist about taking antioxidants if you are being treated with radiation or chemotherapy.

Table 37-1

A Sample Antioxidant Program

Selenium-yeast	200 mcg a day
Vitamin E (mixed tocopherols or gamma- and delta-enriched)	200–400 IU
Lycopene	30 mg a day
Vitamin C	500 mg (time-release form) twice a day
Green tea	4–10 cups a day
Cabbage family	one or more servings each day
Sulfur (in the form of taurine, N-acetylcysteine, or glutathione)	
Red–purple fruits and vegetables	daily

Vitamin D

The common form of vitamin D you will encounter in drug or health food stores is vitamin D-3. This is also the form of vitamin D you make when your skin is exposed to the sun. Vitamin D-3 must undergo conversion to 25-hydroxy-vitamin D-3 in the liver. The latter is then converted to 1, 25-dihydroxy vitamin D-3 by the kidney. Calcitriol is another name for 1, 25-dihydroxyvitamin D3. Calcitriol suppresses the growth and spread of prostate cancer. As a result, the risk of developing prostate cancer increases significantly if your blood levels of calcitriol are below 40 pg/ml. Furthermore, high doses of calcitriol have been reported to slow the growth of prostate cancer in humans as well as markedly improve their response to Taxotere chemotherapy.

Many men with prostate cancer have low levels of calcitriol. Lack of exposure to sunlight, especially during winter, can lead to low vitamin D-3 levels, resulting in less formation of calcitriol. Additionally, many people over the age of 50 have reduced capacity to convert dietary vitamin D-3 to calcitriol. Finally, a diet high in calcium can block the formation of calcitriol. One solution is to adhere to a low-calcium diet and either take vitamin D supplements or get plenty of sun exposure. For many patients, the most practical solution is to take calcitriol capsules. This prescription drug is typically taken in doses of 0.25 to 0.5 mcg a day.

Sugar

In the United States, we are experiencing an unprecedented increase in obesity and diabetes mellitus. These problems are exacerbated by the consumption of large amounts of sugar and carbohydrates that rapidly release glucose into the bloodstream. Some patients have a particularly dangerous form of diabetes mellitus called <u>syndrome X</u>. In addition to diabetes, they exhibit abdominal obesity, high blood pressure, and elevated blood lipids. These patients experience accelerated atherosclerosis, leading to an increased risk of heart attack, stroke, and other vascular complications. Because of these observations, many patients are concerned about their sugar consumption and question whether this might also worsen their prostate cancer.

Investigators at the Harvard School of Public Health examined the link between sugar consumption and the risk of prostate cancer and obtained a surprising result. Increased sugar consumption <u>reduced</u> the risk of prostate cancer. Apparently, the ingestion of sugar increases the activation of vitamin D-3 to calcitriol, thus suppressing the progression of prostate cancer. This conclusion is further supported by the observation that diabetics have a lower risk of developing prostate cancer.

These findings have important implications. Modest consumption of sweets may not be a problem for prostate cancer patients who are not at risk for diabetes, high blood pressure, or atherosclerosis. This is important because fruits, while sweet, are full of antioxidants and other chemicals that have many health benefits.

How to Change Your Diet and Lifestyle

Over the past 8 years, many men have tried to alter their diet and lifestyle. In 1999, Charles Myers, M.D. a medical oncologist with a subspecialty in prostate cancer was diagnosed with prostate cancer and was forced to make these changes in his own life. As a result, he have found that certain things help, and I suggest the following guidelines:

1. A list of foods that are healthy does not help you create a cuisine that is tasty and attractive. The cuisines that have reached international popularity reflect thousands of years of experimentation by whole nations devoted to the task of eating well. It is foolish to think you can match this performance on your own. The cuisines of Italy, India, China, Japan, and Thailand have all found wide acceptance in other countries. Each of these cuisines can easily be modified to make them adhere to the dietary guidelines of

this chapter. You are much more likely to be successful if you choose a cuisine you like and can get excited about eating than you are if you just go out and boil up some brown rice. My wife and I selected Italian and Mediterranean cuisines as the basis for our cooking and have found the result to be very satisfactory.

2. Do not make the change gradually. If you make a rapid and complete changeover, you will be amazed at how well you will feel compared to how you felt on the average American diet. Also, the full impact of diet on prostate cancer becomes obvious within 8 to 10 weeks. If you make a complete changeover, you will be able to quickly assess how sensitive your cancer is to your new diet. I have seen everything from complete arrest of tumor progression to no benefit at all. If you are not going to benefit at all, it is useful to find this out as quickly as possible.

3. Diet is not a religion. If you are in a situation where it is not possible to adhere to your diet, life will not end if you compromise. Also, if you must cheat on the diet in order to make life acceptable, the world will not end. You should just pick yourself up and try again. Remember, you are in a battle that will span many years, and you have to pace yourself.

    I have found it valuable to know about treats that are "safe." For example, dark sweet chocolate (without milk or butter fat) is delicious. It is a very rich source of polyphenolic antioxidants similar to those found in green tea. Additionally, the fat in dark chocolate is cocoa butter that is rich in fatty acids that kill prostate cancer cells in tissue culture. One of my favorites is a dark chocolate bar filled with raspberry preserve.

4. It can be difficult to adhere to these recommendations if you travel. If you do travel, try to eat in Italian or Asian restaurants. Most of these will have at least one dish that fits your requirements. I carry almonds and dried fruit with me. For long trips, I might take a small electric steamer along with brown rice and other grains. I have found that lentils and dried green peas can be steamed with brown rice and spices to make a meal when no other options exist.

How to Use This Information

Find a diet for maintaining a healthy heart, one that will foster the principles mentioned in this chapter. Such diets are available in books, on the Internet, and from your doctor.

Chapter 38

MANAGING PROSTATE CANCER PAIN

At stage D3/T3 of your prostate cancer, you will most likely begin to worry about how your life will end and to think about who you can talk to about this. You can talk to family, friends, clergy, your doctor, and other health professionals. Most advanced prostate cancer patients worry more about the possible pain and suffering associated with their final days than about the death itself. It's only normal to be afraid of the pain you may have to endure and to be concerned about the burden you may impose on your family and friends. Almost all family members and "real" friends will want to do their utmost to help you attain maximum comfort. By all means, talk with them. Tell them how much you love them and will miss them. Listen to them. It's okay to cry; crying will help you to vent any pent-up emotions. Tears are the "safety valves of the heart." It may help to bring you and your friends closer together.

If it is too much for you to have a final gathering, try to write out some of your thoughts, feelings, or desires or to videotape them. Be open and honest. The pain accompanying metastatic prostate cancer can be greatly alleviated by multiple therapeutic maneuvers. Concentrating on forgiving and loving everyone close to you may help you to relieve the emotional pain associated with your disease.

Pain in Prostate Cancer Patients

Pain can be described as a sensation that hurts. It can cause discomfort, distress, or agony. It may come as a steady or throbbing sensation. It may be stabbing, aching, or pinching. Because individual patients feel pain differently, only you can define it. One patient who had metastatic prostate cancer described his pain as "a sensation of ten continuous and severe toothaches."

Prostate cancer pain can be acute or chronic. Acute pain is severe and usually lasts for a short duration. It usually indicates that body tissue is being damaged in some manner, and the pain disappears when the injured tissue heals. On the other hand, chronic pain may range from mild to severe, and it usually remains for a long duration.The pain problems that prostate cancer patients had in previous years were frequently contributed to by doctors. Many physicians were not prescribing sufficient dosages of drugs to fully and continuously relieve patients of pain. The <u>National Cancer Report</u>

in August 1991 stated, "The undertreatment of pain is a serious and neglected public health problem resulting in unnecessary suffering for many patients and their families." The National Coalition for Cancer Pain has stepped into the picture and identified a national program to promote pain prevention and relief as components of an individual patient's plan of care. It has also established the patient's right to pain relief and pain control. If you are experiencing pain, your doctor has a responsibility to develop an effective pain-relieving plan for you. Your doctor should also take your medical history. Some of the most common parameters to include in the plan are:

- type of pain
- intensity
- duration
- time of occurrence and frequency
- precipitating and alleviating factors
- psychological factors
- somatic symptoms

Causes of Prostate Cancer Pain

Prostate cancer patients may have pain for two reasons: pain may be due to the tumor itself, or it could result from the treatment received by the patient. For example, after a radical prostatectomy, a patient will feel pain as a result of the operation. Some doctors give the patient pain-relieving medication before he wakes up after the operation. However, after the medication wears off, the patient may begin to feel the pain again.

Prostate cancer pain may depend on the stage of your disease and on your tolerance for pain. Prostate cancer pain that lasts for more than a few days may be associated with one or more of the following:

- poor blood circulation because prostate cancer has blocked blood vessels
- blockage of an organ or tube in the body
- pressure on organs or bones in the body
- infection or inflammation
- side effects from chemotherapy, radiation therapy, radical prostatectomy, cryosurgery, or some other treatment
- stiffness from inactivity
- psychological responses, such as tension, stress, depression, or anxiety

Relief from Prostate Cancer Pain

Several physicians indicate that few of their advanced prostate cancer patients suffer seriously with pain. Why? Because medicine and other treatments can usually relieve the pain. Patients need to tell their doctor or nurse as soon as the pain begins.

When experiencing pain, tell your doctor or nurse the following:

- all of the places it hurts
- the intensity of the pain
- what aggravates the pain
- what lessens the pain
- how much relief you are getting from the medication
- Don't be reluctant to ask the following:
- What medication can give me the most relief?
- How and when should I take the medication? For how long?
- What side effects can I experience? What should I do if they occur?
- Should I try nondrug methods to relieve pain, such as relaxation or massage?

Treatment for Prostate Cancer Pain

The following is a brief description of the multiple ways in which prostate cancer pain may be treated:

- *Drugs*: Pain medication administered orally (via pill or liquid), transmucosally (absorbed through the mucous membrane in the mouth via highly concentrated liquid or lollipop), transdermally (via skin patch), rectally (via suppository), by subcutaneous injection (under the skin), or intravenous injection (into the vein).
- *Adjuvant drugs*: Medications that enhance the effectiveness of pain control when given in addition to pain medications.
- *Nonmedical methods*: Relaxation techniques.
- *Hypnosis:* Person is put in a state of intense concentration.
- *Biofeedback*: Patient learns how to control inner function of body through mind control and electronic survey. Usually for mild and/or functional pain such as migraine headache.
- *Acupuncture*

- *Transcutaneous nerve stimulation* (TENS or TNS): Electrical impulses are sent through pads applied to the skin in the affected areas.
- *Epidural dorsal column stimulator:* Electrodes are surgically implanted over the spinal cord. Patient controls electrical impulses.
- *Infusion pump:* A self-contained ambulatory device used to deliver a constant flow of medication into the bloodstream to relieve pain. Newer versions are programmed to provide patient-controlled analgesia.
- *Implanted intrathecal catheter pump:* An implanted pump that delivers medication into the spinal cord area.
- *Nerve block*: Anesthesia or alcohol is injected at a point in the nerve fibers.
- *Cordotomy*: Precise area in the spinal cord where bundles of nerves are located is cut.
- *Nerve-root clipping*: Nerve roots, responsible for carrying the pain, are clipped.
- *Rhizotomy*: Pain nerve is cut where it enters the spinal cord.

Drugs for Prostate Cancer Pain

It makes good sense to treat each patient's level and kind of pain according to his individual need. Drugs that relieve pain are called *analgesics*. These drugs act on the nervous system to relieve pain without loss of consciousness. Although analgesics provide relief from pain, they do not affect the *cause* of pain.

Two Types of Analgesics:

- Nonprescription or over-the-counter pain relievers, which are suitable for mild to moderate pain.
- Prescription pain relievers used for moderate to severe pain.

Nonprescription Drugs

Nonprescription pain relievers are analgesics that can be bought without a doctor's prescription. They are effective for relief of mild to moderate pain. Although many of these nonprescription pain relievers have different names, nearly all contain one of three medicines. They are aspirin (Bufferin, Ascriptin, Ecotrin), acetaminophen (Anacin-3, Tylenol), and ibuprofen (Advil, Motrin, Nuprin). Recently, Naproxen, a nonsteroidal anti-inflammatory analgesic, has also been approved for over-the-counter sales.

Prescription Drugs

For many years, the most widely used prescription pain relievers have been narcotics. Narcotics are drugs that relieve pain and cause drowsiness or sleep. In addition, they all have similar side effects like nausea, vomiting, constipation, itching, and muscle twitching. Historically, these drugs, also called *opioids* or *opiates*, came from the opium poppy. Today, many narcotics are synthetic; that is, they are chemicals manufactured by drug companies.

Frequently used opioid pain relievers include:

- codeine
- hydromorphone (Dilaudid)
- levorphanol (Levo-Dromoran)
- methadone (Dolophine)
- morphine
- oxycodone (in Percodan)
- oxymorphone (Numorphone)
- fentanyl (available in transdermal and transmucosal forms)
- A new class of drugs called *bisphosphonates* (Aredia, Zometa) has been shown to be effective in alleviating pain, lowering elevated calcium in the bloodstream, and sometimes stabilizing the strength of the bones involved with metastases.

You can get these pain relievers only with a doctor's written prescription. They may be taken by mouth, by injection (intramuscularly or intravenously), or by rectal suppository. There are also other methods of giving pain medicines for more continuous pain relief.

Another group of prescription pain relievers is similar to ibuprofen (in large doses, ibuprofen requires a prescription). They are called *nonsteroidal anti-inflammatory drugs (NSAIDs)*. Included in this group are ibuprofen, Nalfon, and Trilisate. Useful for mild to moderate pain, they may be especially helpful in treating the pain of bone metastases. Because NSAIDs are not narcotics, their use does not result in drug tolerance or physical dependence.

These drugs are used alone or with prescription pain relievers to treat moderate to severe pain. Some are more effective than others in relieving moderate pain.

The World Health Organization has developed a Cancer Pain Relief Program to serve as a guide for the use of analgesics to relieve cancer pain. There are three steps to the program:

1.   A nonnarcotic alone or with a NSAID is recommended for mild pain.
2.   A weak opioid is recommended with or without a NSAID for persisting or increasing pain.
3.   A strong opioid with or without a NSAID is recommended.

Adjuvant Drugs

Adjuvant drugs are prescription medications that can enhance the effectiveness of opioids and NSAIDs in pain management. Some of these drugs have independent analgesic effects as well. This group of drugs comes from several categories.

- psychotropic drugs
- antidepressants (amitriptyline, Prozac)
- antipsychotics (haloperidol)
- antianxiety (lorazepam)
- stimulants (dexedrine)
- antiseizure drugs (Neurontin, Tegretol)
- local anesthetics (Mexiletine, lidocaine)
- steroids (prednisone)

Complications of Prostate Cancer Pain

There are basically five complications associated with prostate cancer pain:

(1) Spinal Cord Compression

Approximately 20 percent of prostate cancer patients with metastasis may experience spinal cord compression, a very serious complication that will affect the patients' quality of life. Spinal cord compression occurs when cancer cells expand from a vertebrae body pressing into the spinal cord, eventuating in the loss of function of the spinal cord below the point of compression. The symptoms associated with spinal cord compression are as follows:

- severe pain in the back

- tingling and numbness, usually in the lower extremities
- loss of sensation
- leg weakness
- difficulty walking
- constipation
- urinary retention

If you have any of these symptoms, notify your doctor immediately. An MRI scan can often show early signs of cord compression. If spinal cord compression is evidenced by the MRI scan, it means that your prostate cancer has invaded the dura, the membrane surrounding the spinal cord.

Stated previously, spinal cord compression is an extremely serious problem. If your doctor reports that you are heading for, or have, spinal cord compression, he or she will most likely treat you with large doses of a drug called *Decadron* (a corticosteroid). Your doctor will follow up your treatment with spot radiation to the spine or will ease the pressure on the spinal cord with an operation called *nerve decompression*. If you have not been treated with either orchiectomy plus Eulexin or Casodex (CHT), your doctor may prescribe this treatment. Untreated, spinal cord compression usually causes paralysis with loss of bowel and bladder function.

(2) Bone Fracture

When prostate cancer invades bones, they become brittle and may break. As a result, patients with metastatic prostate cancer are prone to broken bones. Those bones most susceptible are those that support the body: the hips and the thighs. Sometimes, your doctor may want to put pins in the hipbones. Or you might have to use crutches or a wheelchair to transport yourself. Radiation to the areas in danger of fracturing can sometimes avert this complication and alleviate the pain associated with the local tumor.

(3) Urinary-Tract Obstruction

If you are experiencing weak urine flow, hesitancy in beginning urination, a need to push or strain to get your urine to flow, intermittent urine stream, difficulty in stopping your urine, dribbling after urination, a sense of not being able to empty your bladder, or not being able to urinate at all, your prostate cancer may have become extensive enough to block your urinary tract. A TURP is one of several treatments that can eliminate urinary-tract obstruction. Local radiation is another.

(4) Constipation

Constipation is a problem for prostate cancer patients who take strong painkillers, such as morphine, which sedate the digestive tract. To counteract this problem, some doctors prescribe mild laxatives or stool softeners along with the painkiller. Another way to alleviate constipation is to add high-fiber supplements to the diet.

(5) Weight Loss

When you lose weight, it means you are losing your strength. As a result, your body is losing its ability to fight illness. To counteract this problem, it's better to have several small nutritious meals each day rather than adhere to a traditional breakfast, lunch, and dinner. Avoid junk food. Stay with recommended diets. Make each calorie count, and consider trying calorie-packed liquid nutrition supplements like Ensure or Sustecal.

Managing Pain

Localized prostate cancer (within the capsule) is generally considered asymptomatic unless it is obstructing the urinary tract. As the tumor grows and perforates the prostate capsule (stage C), the organs, nerves, and bones in the pelvic area may become involved, resulting in pain.

If you are affected with locally advanced cancer, you may experience symptoms such as difficulty and pain while urinating, bloody urine, or (rarely) pain upon ejaculation. The tumors can block the ureters and cause painful hydronephrosis. This usually presents as unilateral flank pain. The spreading tumor may also cause vascular or lymphatic blockage, resulting in painful or swollen legs. The scrotum also may become edematous and enlarged. Involvement of pelvic nerves can result in pelvic pain, which can be radicular, extending down one or both lower extremities.

To manage your pain if you are affected with locally advanced prostate cancer, the treatment should be focused on treating the cause of the pain — the cancer itself — whenever possible. Stage C disease is frequently treated with full-dose radiation directed to the prostate and sometimes to the pelvic lymph nodes. If radiotherapy is successful, you can expect partial pain relief within a few weeks after treatment commences. Full pain relief may not occur until 2 to 3 weeks after radiotherapy is completed. Combination hormonal therapy, if not previously used, can frequently alleviate the pain by causing a decrease in the size of the local tumor. Often CHT can be initiated and then followed by radiation therapy.

For pain that persists during radiotherapy, analgesics should be prescribed according to the severity of the pain. For mild to moderate pain, such oral nonnarcotics as aspirin or acetaminophen (Tylenol) are appropriate first choices. Propoxyphene (Darvon), codeine, and hydrocodone (Vicodin) or oxycodone (Percocet) may be prescribed for pain that does not respond to these milder analgesics. Dosage schedules should take into account the duration and plasma half-life of the medication and, when necessary, be timed to anticipate the cyclical nature of your pain. For example, if your pain occurs on a 3.5-hour cycle, analgesics should be taken every 3 hours to prevent the pain from reaching its peak when it is more difficult to control. Pain is better controlled before it becomes severe and persistent; "nipping it in the bud" is usually the most effective therapy.

Pain in Stage C and D Patients

Pain and Widespread Disease

Eighty percent of patients with widespread prostate cancer will have metastases to the bone and resultant pain. The ribs and spine are most frequently involved, as are the long bones. The pain usually is described as a constant ache, varying in intensity, and is generally well localized.

LHRH Analogs plus Antiandrogens

Because prostate cancer is a hormonally sensitive disease, pain at stage D can be effectively managed by systemic hormone therapy, which is designed to cut off the supply of androgens and thus inhibit the growth of prostate cancer. Reduction of bone pain in response to hormonal manipulation can be dramatic. This can be accomplished via bilateral orchiectomy, estrogen therapy, or treatment with LHRH agonists (Lupron, Zoladex) to inhibit gonadotropin and its resultant testicular testosterone production. Approximately 80 percent of patients will experience a decrease in tumor mass, both local and systemic, resulting in a decrease in pain over a period of hours to a few days.

In addition, studies initiated by Dr. Fernand Labrie — and confirmed in this country by the Intergroup and several other studies — have demonstrated that CHT with Lupron or Zoladex plus Eulexin or Casodex achieves maximal androgen deprivation, inhibits prostate cancer growth, and is effective in palliating the pain of advanced prostate cancer. (CHT also has been shown to increase median survival time by about 7 months over those patients receiving Lupron alone.) Eulexin or Casodex should be given at the same time as Lupron to prevent the painful "flare-up" that can occur with Lupron or Zoladex (there is an initial unopposed release of testosterone for about a week).

Spot Radiation

Spot radiation therapy can be extremely effective in palliating pain by reducing the tumor and thereby relieving pressure on nerves and the spinal cord — in fact, it is the treatment of choice for spinal cord compression. It is also frequently used for localized pain, particularly bony metastases. Side effects are few, and relief is relatively swift.

In addition, radiation therapy is very useful as a prophylactic treatment to prevent fracture of weight-bearing bones. The indication for radiation in this situation is pain or cortical involvement or both, especially if more than one-third of the transverse diameter of the long bone is involved.

Spinal Cord Compression

When prostate cancer infiltrates the spinal column, as it frequently does, the pain can be severe. Spinal cord compression is an oncological emergency with severe consequences, which can result in paralysis and both urinary and fecal incontinence. Physicians should be alert to the possibility of spinal cord compression in men with prostate cancer and be aggressive in confirming and treating the diagnosis, even in the absence of corroborative findings. The pain accompanying spinal cord compression may be difficult to control. Physicians should have a high index of suspicion and conduct appropriate diagnostic tests, such as MRI, CT scan, or myelography, to arrive at a definitive diagnosis, so that the problem can be treated promptly and the neurological deficits avoided.

Symptoms of compression can develop and worsen abruptly over the course of a few weeks or more slowly. They begin with neck or back pain or bilateral radicular pain (usually around the sides). Other symptoms include numbness, tingling, and other paraesthesias, weakness in the legs, difficulty controlling bowel and bladder, and electric-shock sensations, especially with moving the head up and down (l'Hermitte's sign).

Treatment for spinal cord compression usually consists of the administration of dexamethasone (Decadron) with radiation therapy. Occasionally, nerve decompression surgery may be necessary. Usually, 10 mg of dexamethasone is given intravenously, followed by 4 mg every 6 hours (IV or by mouth). The edema around the area of cord compression is thereby decreased, and patients sometimes notice improved neurologic function and less pain shortly after receiving the dexamethasone.

Nevertheless, radiation therapy should be started immediately so that tumor cells will be destroyed, thereby helping to restore normal cord function.

Pain in Hormonally Refractory Patients

If you are in the terminal stages of your illness and have failed systemic hormonal therapy, you may require substantial pain palliation as the disease progresses. At this stage, your comfort is paramount. Treatment options include:

Analgesics

Analgesics, either nonnarcotic, narcotic, or a combination of both, will play a central role. The complexities of pain modulation in the cancer patient mean that there is no standard pharmacological treatment of choice. Rather, guidelines for pain management at this stage emphasize a thorough understanding of the pharmacology of the drugs to be prescribed and a willingness to adjust therapy (including route of administration) as side effects occur or tolerance is achieved.

When oral analgesics are no longer effective, then subcutaneous, intravenous, or intramuscular narcotic infusions can be considered. Fentanyl (Duragesic patch) is a synthetic narcotic analgesic that is delivered through the skin (transdermally). This patch can frequently obviate the need for injectable analgesics.

Intravenous infusions of narcotics are frequently used to treat bed-confined terminal patients, but they may also be delivered to ambulatory patients through a venous access device (Port-a-Cath) using a portable infusion pump. Patient-controlled analgesic (PCA) systems are now available using specially programmed pumps. Studies of postoperative patients have shown that they use appropriate amounts of drug to maintain adequate pain control and do not overdose themselves. However, PCA use on an ambulatory-care basis remains controversial. PCA systems have not often been used for cancer pain, since such pain is usually best controlled by fixed-schedule dosing to prevent pain recurrence. Intrathecal (direct injection around the spinal cord) administration is also a consideration in certain circumstances.

Bisphosphonates

The bisphosphonates, a group of drugs that inhibit bone resorption and mineralization, have some therapeutic efficacy in the control of pain from bone metastases in general and in prostate cancer specifically. These drugs may be particularly helpful for patients with a life expectancy of several months for whom rapidly escalating narcotic treatment may inhibit quality of life. As of 2003, the FDA had approved three drugs in this group: etidronate (Didronel), pamidronate (Aredia), and zolendroic acid (Zometa).

Steroids

The pain of metastatic prostate cancer has been treated successfully with steroids such as low-dose prednisone. Prednisone, which inhibits the secretion of adrenocorticotropic hormone, has been shown to improve symptoms in approximately 30 percent of patients studied. Response, however, usually is transient, although a few patients have experienced prolonged pain relief. Prednisone must be used with discretion, especially in ambulatory patients, because they can develop proximal myopathy (muscle weakness), leaving them unable to get up from a bed or chair.

Hemibody radiation

Hemibody radiation is extremely effective in ameliorating pain and can avert the need for large doses of narcotics. For example, all 10 patients in a study by Unyime Nseyo, M.D., and colleagues reported pain relief within 48 to 96 hours after therapy. Other studies have reported an 80-percent response rate. The average response lasted 4 months.

The drawback of hemibody radiation is the risk of toxicity associated with high dosages, including bone marrow depression. In the Nseyo study, however, radiation reactions were relatively minor (flulike symptoms and muscular aches and pains in two patients) compared to the relief the therapy provided. Despite its drawbacks, hemibody radiation used judiciously can be considered a viable option for many patients for whom other treatments have been ineffective.

Radioactive isotopes

Radioactive phosphorous and other systemic radionuclides have successfully palliated diffuse skeletal pain. This modality is limited to patients who do not suffer from severe bone-marrow failure.

Strontium-89

A new treatment for dealing with prostate cancer bone pain is strontium-89. It is a radioactive isotope that is injected into the body during an outpatient procedure. Similar to calcium, strontium-89 is absorbed immediately by the bones. An exceptional feature of this isotope is that it actually searches for and treats the metastatic bone disease. More specifically, strontium-89 is absorbed by the tumor in the bone, instead of by bone marrow, by a ratio of 10 to 1. Studies have reported relief from pain in 50 to 80 percent of patients.

A trial study by A. T. Porter and colleagues is probably the premier study on strontium-89. This controlled trial was performed in eight Canadian cancer centers in order to determine the effectiveness of strontium-89 as an adjunct to local external beam radiation. Hormonally refractory metastatic prostate cancer patients received local external beam radiation and either one injection of strontium-89 or a placebo.

A total of 126 patients were recruited for the study. No significant differences in survival or in relief of pain at the index site were noted. Intake of analgesics over time demonstrated a significant reduction of pain in the patients with strontium-89. Progression of pain, as measured by new pain sites or by the requirement for external beam radiation, showed a statistically significant benefit in the patients who received strontium-89. Patients receiving strontium-89 experienced a reduction in PSA, PAP, and alkaline phosphatase. A quality-of-life analysis was performed as a multivariate dataset and demonstrated an overall superiority of strontium-89, with alleviation of pain and improvement in physical activity being statistically significant. In addition, an evaluation of side effects demonstrated increased hematological problems in the group receiving strontium-89.

In summary, this trial demonstrated that the addition of strontium-89 is an effective adjuvant therapy to local external beam radiation. It found that strontium-89 reduces the progression of metastatic prostate cancer, as evidenced by new sites of pain; reduces the need for further external beam radiation; improves quality of life; and lessens the need for analgesic support.

Strontium-89 has a half-life of 51 days in the body. One dose has proved to be effective in relieving prostate cancer bone pain for an average of 3 to 6 months. An advantage of strontium-89 over spot radiation is that it also acts on new sites of metastasis that crop up while it is in the body. It is effective - and indeed indicated - when there are two or more painful metastatic sites.

In a few studies, doctors found that when strontium-89 was combined with local spot radiation, progression of pain was delayed 7 months longer than when radiation was used alone.

The side effects of strontium-89 are as follows:

- There is a potential for bone marrow damage, indicated primarily by a decrease in platelets.
- Some patients have reported a mild increase in pain a couple of days after receiving the compound.
- Because strontium-89 is radioactive and is excreted in the urine for the first 48 hours, patients must urinate into a special container, not the toilet. The doctor will advise the patient on how to dispose of the contaminated urine.

Questions and Answers about Strontium-89

Following are some of the most frequently asked questions about treatment with strontium-89:

Q: How is strontium-89 administered?

A: Strontium-89 is administered on an outpatient basis. The patient will receive a single dose, which is slowly injected into the body through a vein over 1 to 2 minutes. Its effects usually last for 6 months. Additional doses are given at intervals of 90 days if necessary.

Q: I understand strontium-89 is effective in about 80 percent of patients. How will I know that it is helping me?

A: Initially, you will feel no effect whatsoever. In fact, you may feel a slight increase in pain for 2 to 3 days after the injection. After about 1 to 2 weeks, sometimes a little longer, you will notice that your pain is diminishing. This decrease in pain will continue, and the effect should continue for several months. You may find that your need for analgesics decreases. If, after 3 or 4 weeks, you notice no improvement in your condition, see your doctor so that he or she can prescribe another treatment for your pain.

Q: What are the side effects of strontium-89?

A: The possible side effects are as follows:

- Some patients may experience a mild facial flushing immediately after the injection.
- As indicated, some patients report a temporary increase in pain, lasting 2 to 3 days after the injection.

310

- The patient's platelet and white blood cell levels may be depressed by about 30 and 20 percent, respectively.

Q: What is the cost of strontium-89? Is it covered by Medicare?

A: The strontium-89 treatment costs about $1,850. It is covered by most insurance companies and by Medicare.

Q: Can my family doctor give me the treatment?

A: Probably not, unless he or she is qualified in the safe use and handling of radioisotopes and has been licensed by the appropriate government agency to use them according to state regulations.

Q: What precautions must I take if I take strontium-89?

A: The precautions consist of the following:

- Wash your hands thoroughly after using the toilet.
- Immediately wash any linens or clothes that have been stained with urine or blood. Wash them separately from other clothes, and rinse them thoroughly.
- If you should cut yourself, wash away any spilled blood.
- Avoid leaking urine or blood on the linens and other areas of the environment.

Q: What should I do if my pain comes back?

A: Consider another injection of strontium-89. In a study by Ediven Smith, M.D., and colleagues, 20 patients with advanced metastatic prostate cancer received a total of 28 doses of strontium-89 in order to evaluate its palliative and toxic effects. Criteria for participating in the study included failed conventional therapy and the presence of bone pain. Baseline data included age, alkaline phosphatase, white blood count, platelets, and bone scan, all correlated with pain assessment. These baselines were followed up for a minimum of 3 months at monthly intervals after the patients received strontium-89. The results of the study are cited as follows:

- Alkaline phosphatase decreased from 5.4 to 3.7 and then increased at 12 months to 4.3.
- Platelets decreased from a mean of 198 to 148.

- Pain improved in 54 percent of patients, remained unchanged in 36 percent, and was worse in 20 percent.
- Performance status of patients improved in 64 percent, remained unchanged in 14 percent, and worsened in 18 percent.
- Analgesic requirements decreased in 43 percent of patients, remained unchanged in 36 percent, and were worse in 21 percent.
- The mean duration of response to strontium-89 was 3 months.
- The study proved that a favorable response to strontium-89 was achieved in 64 percent of patients with advanced prostate cancer. This treatment may have greater benefits in patients with bone pain and less advanced disease.

Samarium-153 (Quadramet) is a new radioisotope used to treat bone pain due to metastatic disease. Like calcium and strontium-89, it seeks out areas of new bone formation and therefore becomes localized near metastases. This radioactive isotope, like Strontium-89, irradiates and kills tumor cells near it, thereby reducing pain. The advantage of samarium-153 over strontium-89 is that it spares more of the bone marrow, allowing better blood counts. This may allow your doctor to add or continue chemotherapy and avoid the problems associated with low blood counts such as infections, transfusions, or bleeding.

Samarium-153 is injected in the same way as strontium-89 and can also occasionally cause a slight increase in pain during the 72 hours after administration. Pain relief is often noted within a week and reaches a maximum at 3 to 4 weeks after injection and often lasts for 3 to 6 months.

The precautions that need to be taken after treatment with strontium-89 also apply to samarium-153 as given. However, because samarium-153 is eliminated from the body more quickly, precautions are only required for 12 hours after injection.

Spot radiation

Spot radiation is a localized external beam, usually from a cobalt or linear accelerator machine that is targeted at one or several areas of bony metastases. It generally helps to ease prostate cancer pain in the sites being treated. Spot radiation usually provides several months of pain relief in prostate cancer patients. It also helps to prevent or alleviate spinal cord compression. In several studies, 55 percent of prostate cancer patients received complete relief from pain, 33 percent had partial relief, and only 12 percent experienced either little or no relief.

Chemotherapy

Chemotherapy, either by a single drug or in combination, has some therapeutic effect on prostate cancer, and some patients have reported pain palliation following such therapy. Overall, however, clinical reports on this modality are mixed. Chemotherapy has a limited impact on the systemic control of the disease and, therefore, on its pain-alleviating ability. It should be considered, however, in patients who suffer from generalized progressive disease. Although survival figures have not been improved, oncologists have seen good pain palliation. However, there have been studies indicating an improvement in quality of life and pain palliation using chemotherapy.

Neurosurgical procedures

Neurosurgical procedures are invasive measures used to relieve pain. They should be considered for patients whose pain is not responding to any of the modalities discussed and/or for whom the side effects of analgesic therapy are excessive.

Intrathecal morphine infusion

Intrathecal morphine infusion is the preferred procedure for cases in which there is pain in the pelvis and lower extremities. Either a portable or implantable pump is placed on the body, and a catheter leading to the subarachnoid space is tunneled subcutaneously. Morphine can then be given by continuous infusion and titrated to the patient's pain. Obviously, this procedure requires physicians who are thoroughly familiar with its use.

Patients can develop opioid tolerance, however, thus limiting the procedure's long-term usefulness. Respiratory depression is a serious potential side effect. Another obstacle to the use of neuropharmacologic delivery systems in the elderly and medically indigent is that these devices are expensive and may not be reimbursed by Medicaid or Medicare.

Percutaneous cordotomy may be useful for patients who suffer with unilateral pain, usually below the T8-T10 vertebrae. Rhizotomy is rarely indicated unless the patient is not ambulatory and has not responded to other modalities.

Guidelines for Physicians: Narcotic Analgesics in Pain Management

1.   Start with a specific drug for a specific type of pain.
2.   Know the pharmacology of the drug prescribed, including:
        a. duration of the analgesic effect

b. pharmacokinetic properties of the drug

c. equianalgesic doses for the drug and its route of administration

3. Adjust the route of administration to the patient's needs.

4. Administer the analgesic on a regular basis after initial titration of the dose.

5. Use drug combinations to provide additional analgesia and reduce side effects — for example, nonsteroidal anti-inflammatory drugs, antihistamines (hydroxyzine), and amphetamines (dexedrine).

6. Try to avoid drug combinations that increase sedation without enhancing analgesia — for example, benzodiazepine (diazepam) and phenothiazine (chloropromazine).

7. Anticipate and treat side effects such as:

a. sedation

b. respiratory depression

c. nausea and vomiting

d. constipation

8. Watch for the development of tolerance.

a. Switch to an alternative narcotic analgesic.

b. Start with one-half the equianalgesic dose, and titrate the dose for efficacy.

9. Prevent acute withdrawal.

a. Taper drugs slowly.

b. Use diluted doses of naloxone (0.4 mg in 10 ml of saline) to reverse respiratory depression in the physically dependent patient, and administer cautiously.

10. Do not use placebos to assess the nature of pain.

11. Anticipate and manage complications.

a. overdose

b. muscle twitching

c. seizures

Prostate Cancer Pain: Questions and Answers

The following are common questions that prostate cancer patients pose to their doctors, nurses, relatives, and friends.

Q: Will I become addicted to pain medication such as morphine?

A: When pain medication is given and taken in the right way, patients rarely become addicted. However, it's best to ask your doctor, nurse, or pharmacist how to use pain medication correctly and safely. Some patients will need the pain medication for only a short period - that is, until the pain goes away. On the other hand, if your pain is severe, the last thing that should be on your mind will be whether or not you will become addicted to the medication.

Q: Will I lose control of my senses while I am on pain medication?

A: Most patients do not get either "high" or lose control when they take medication as prescribed. True, you may feel sleepy when you first take the pain medication, but this feeling will eventually go away. A few patients get dizzy or feel confused when they take the medication. If this should happen to you, tell your doctor or nurse. Changing either the dose or type of medicine will usually solve this problem.

Q: Will prostate cancer pain cause other problems?

A: Yes, prostate cancer pain can cause one or more of the following:

- tiredness
- depression
- anger
- worry
- loneliness
- stress
- feeling sorry for yourself

Q: Can prostate cancer pain interfere with my daily activities?

A: Yes, it is possible. Depending on how severe it is, prostate cancer pain can impact or interrupt your:

- sleeping routine
- quality of life
- sex life
- eating habits
- attitude toward friends and family
- interest in work and hobbies

Q: When I asked my doctor about my pain, he did not give me a satisfactory explanation.
What should I do?

A: You have a right to ask your doctor about how you can be relieved of prostate cancer pain. In fact, all patients should insist that their doctor answer all of their questions about pain, its origin, and its treatment, including side effects. The sooner you speak your mind, the better. It's usually better to control pain in its early stages, before it becomes severe. If you feel uneasy with your current doctor or nurse, get another doctor or ask for a nurse who is more compassionate .

The FDA has approved the marketing of a treatment-delivery device for chronic pain management in those prostate cancer patients who do not respond to conventional treatment regimens. Patients can experience the benefits of daily pain-management therapy with improved mental acuity and reduced drug side effects. This device, the Infusaid model 400 single-catheter implantable pump, is manufactured by Strato/Infusaid, a subsidiary of Pfizer.

Until now, the only implantable pumps for pain control have required periodic surgical exploration due to battery depletion. With its inexhaustible power supply, the Infusaid implantable pump does not require surgery due to battery depletion, and its constant-flow feature requires lower drug doses, thus limiting the sedation, nausea, and vomiting that often result from high dosages of systematic narcotics.

With its approval for the intrathecal infusion of Infumorph (preservative-free morphine) for malignant and nonmalignant pain control, the Model 400 Pump would be a noteworthy example of current trends in pain management.

Assessing Prostate Cancer Pain

Communicating with your doctor about the frequency, intensity, and duration of your prostate cancer pain is the key to treating it effectively. One way in which you can do this is by taking a pain inventory similar to the one following, which was adapted from one developed by Pain Research Group, Department of Neurology, University of Wisconsin-Madison.

Date:_____

Name:_____

1. Throughout your life, you have probably experienced pain from time to time (such as minor headaches, sprains, and toothaches). Have you had pain other than these everyday kinds of pain today?

    1.   Yes   2. No

2. Please rate your worst pain by circling the one number that best describes your pain at its WORST in the past 24 hours.

    0   1   2   3   4   5   6   7   8   9   10

    Least Pain   Worst Pain

3. Please rate your pain by circling the one number that best describes your pain at its LEAST in the past 24 hours.

    0   1   2   3   4   5   6   7   8   9   10

    Least Pain   Worst Pain

4. Please rate your pain by circling the one number that best describes your pain on an AVERAGE day.

    0   1   2   3   4   5   6   7   8   9   10

    Least Pain   Worst Pain

5. Please rate your pain by circling the one number that tells how much pain you are experiencing at this moment.

    0   1   2   3   4   5   6   7   8   9   10

    Least Pain   Worst Pain

6. What treatments or medications are you currently receiving for your pain?

    _____

7. In the past 24 hours, how much relief has pain treatment or medication provided? Please circle the one percentage that shows how much relief you have received from your pain.

    0% 10% 20% 30% 40% 50% 60% 70% 80% 90% 100%

    No Reief   Complete Relief

8. Circle the one number that describes how, during the past 24 hours, pain has interfered with your:

Daily Activities

0	1	2	3	4	5	6	7	8	9	10

Does not interfere   Completely interferes

General mood

0	1	2	3	4	5	6	7	8	9	10

Does not interfere   Completely interferes

Walking ability

0	1	2	3	4	5	6	7	8	9	10

Does not interfere   Completely interferes

Normal Work-includes both outside the home and housework

0	1	2	3	4	5	6	7	8	9	10

Does not interfere   Completely interferes

Relations with family members, friends and acquaintances

0	1	2	3	4	5	6	7	8	9	10

Does not interfere   Completely interferes

Sleep

0	1	2	3	4	5	6	7	8	9	10

Does not interfere   Completely interferes

Quality of Life

0	1	2	3	4	5	6	7	8	9	10

Does not interfere   Completely interferes

How to Use This Information

1. Describe your pain accurately so you can tell your doctor where the pain is located.
2. Ask your doctor how you can be relieved of prostate cancer pain and what the various side effects of these treatments are.

3. Investigate the various nonmedical treatments for prostate cancer pain, and engage in one or more of them to supplement your pain treatment.

4. Avoid taking more of the drugs than prescribed. Talk to your pharmacist if you have any doubts.

5. Know the complications associated with prostate cancer pain, and report them to your doctor as soon as they occur.

6. Stay informed about how your doctor manages your prostate cancer pain, and get another opinion if you are not satisfied with your pain relief after working with your doctor for an adequate period of time.

7. Use the pain inventory in this chapter to discuss your prostate cancer pain with your doctor.

PART IV PROSTATE CANCER INFORMATION

Chapter 39

CANCER CARE AND HEALTH INSURANCE

Although it has been estimated that over 80 percent of physicians in the United States participate in some form of managed care, more doctors are expected to sign on. Many hospitals encourage their doctors to sign with as many different insurance plans as possible in to attract-or avoid losing-potential patients. Managed care is a growing business. It enrolls about 33 percent of the people in this country. More than 80 percent of employees are in some form of managed care. In fact, a physician who does not join a managed-care network could see very few patients. The main factors to focus on when assessing most health plans are availability of resources and limitations in terms of where you can go to receive treatment. For example, a prostate cancer patient with advanced disease may need to go out of state to receive neutron beam radiation instead of photon beam radiation.

How to Deal with Your Health Insurer

The rising cost of medical care and the resulting pressure on premiums have made health insurance a top priority for people who want their medical expenses covered at a reasonable cost. The health insurance system is quite complex and constantly changing. When people speak of their health insurance, they usually mean insurance that protects them not only against all or part of the costs of medical care but also includes issues related to access and quality. Traditional commercial insurance programs that allow patients to be seen by a doctor or hospital of their choice and then pay the full amount of the bill have all but disappeared.

With the support and involvement of government, business, and the insurance industry, managed care has become a key strategy for containing rising health care costs. Although managed care differs from traditional insurance, they both cover an array of medical, surgical and hospital expenses. Many may also have pharmacy benefits.

More than half of all Americans have some kind of managed-care plan. There are various managed-care plans that work differently but can be generally put into two categories: health maintenance organizations (HMOs) and preferred provider organizations (PPOs). These plans typically provide comprehensive health services to their members and offer them financial incentives to use providers that participate in the managed-care network.

321

HMOs offer a wide range of health services to subscribers. For a fixed monthly premium in advance of any treatment, subscribers are entitled to the services of certain physicians and hospitals contracted to work with the HMO. Unlike commercial insurers, HMOs are distinct because they provide financing of health care plus the health care itself. HMOs stress preventative health care, early diagnosis, and treatment in the least costly setting. HMOs can use (1) an open-panel network of physicians who work out of their own private offices and participate on a part-time basis or (2) a closed panel, in which salaried employees of the HMO work out of its facilities. Many HMOs use a gatekeeper model that requires the patient's primary care physician's authorization before specialty services are delivered. Some HMOs offer open access and permit patients to visit specialists without permission from the primary-care doctor. Although pure HMOs do not provide reimbursement for in-area, out-of-network care, point-of-service plans do provide a benefit, albeit lower than for in-network care.

HMOs may also have a closed or restrictive formulary that may limit your access or increase your cost for certain drugs. Subscribers are given incentives to use generic drugs over name brands. Oftentimes there is only a benefit for generic drugs, and the patient must pay the full cost for the brand name. Some HMOs are instituting reimbursement programs for drugs that are creating problems for patients to access their physician. They are either trying to pay the physician for drugs and chemotherapy agents at such a low rate, or having someone else provide the drug, that many physicians are electing to not see their patients. Many HMOs have limits on off-label use of drugs. In some cancers, physicians and patients want to use a drug for a purpose other than the one the FDA approved the drug for. Plans make a case-by-case decision on whether to cover off-label use of the drug, and they may deem some off-label use experimental if they believe there are insufficient scientific data.

Access to new tests and treatments is another restriction imposed by some HMOs under the guise of experimental. As medical technology produces new services for cancer patients, managed-care plans evaluate these services in order to decide what they will cover. They review published medical studies of the new test or procedure, review government approvals, and consult with leading experts. If the plan believes that a new test or procedure has not been sufficiently studied or its effectiveness is uncertain, the plan may designate the service as experimental. For example, some plans will not cover positron emission tomography (PET) because they consider its use with some cancers to be experimental.

HMOs provide members with a grievance and appeals process to address complaints and concerns. A *grievance* concerns misconduct that may or may not deal with denial of benefits. A grievance may deal with issues such as physician incompetence, quality-of-care concerns, balance billing, and redirection to a treatment or diagnostic facility that is not the site recommended by the treating physician. An *appeal* deals only with denial of benefits.

The grievance process begins when a member lodges a complaint with the member - service department of the managed-care plan. If it cannot be resolved at that level, the member may file a formal written grievance or complete a special grievance form. The nature of the problem, what has been done to solve it, and the member's opinion of how the problem should be resolved need to be included in the written complaint. The committee members, composed of representatives of various departments of the health plan, meet periodically to review written grievances. The committee may find in favor of the member or uphold the original actions of the plan. If the member is not satisfied with the committee's decision, he or she can request in writing a hearing. Another committee will review the facts of the case and issue its decision. Some plans may have even higher levels of appeal. Check your policy to see if further recourse is available.

The appeals process involves problems with payment for medical services and benefit decisions. When the plan denies a request for specific medical services or refuses to pay for them, the member may appeal the decision through the written appeals process. The member will need to address why the service should be covered and submit any medical records or documentation to support the position. A written statement from the physician recommending the denied services can be used to offer a professional medical opinion as further support of your appeal.

If the plan does not resolve your complaint satisfactorily, then contact the state agencies that oversee managed-care plans where you live. These include the state health and insurance departments and attorney general. The phone numbers for these state agencies are in the state government listing in the phone book. File your complaint in writing, and document events as carefully as possible. Ask your physician to advocate for you, and provide the plan and state agencies with medical studies or expert opinion that supports your case. In some cases, consumers may need to seek legal help and may consider filing a lawsuit to get the care they need.

Medicare subscribers have the ability to enroll in HMOs and receive enhanced benefits in exchange for adhering to provider restrictions and compliance with medical management programs. Although Medicare subscribers give up many of their rights when they join an HMO, they do receive a wider array of covered services at a lower cost. The federal government still provides oversight to its HMO members through regulations that emphasize access to care, patient protection, and financial stability. Not all Medicare HMOs use draconian cost-containment measures, but overall membership in Medicare HMOs has been declining over the past few years. If you are a Medicare member who is satisfied with the service provided by your HMO, then you should consider remaining enrolled and take advantage of the increased benefits.

A PPO is a collection of health providers who offer their services to certain groups at prearranged prices. In exchange, the group refers its members to the participating providers for health care services. Unlike HMOs, PPOs operate on a fee-for-service basis, not on a prepaid basis. Members of the PPO select from among the preferred providers for needed services. Also, in contrast to HMOs, PPO health care providers are normally in private practice. They have agreed to offer their services to the group and its members at fees less than what they normally charge. Groups that contract with PPOs are very often employers, insurance companies, or health-insurance benefit providers. Medicare currently is experimenting with a PPO model to augment the HMO. In a PPO, a member is not mandated to use participating providers; however, a reduced benefit is typical if they do not. For instance, individuals may pay a $100 deductible if they use PPO services and a $500 deductible if they go outside the PPO.

To fully understand your health insurance, you need to examine your evidence of coverage, which is a detailed description of the medical benefits available to a member of a managed-care plan, most often provided to members after they enroll in the plan. In reviewing the policy's terms or conditions, you can identify covered services, maximum limits of coverage, maximum out-of-pocket expenses, deductible and co-insurance amounts, and preexisting-condition time limits. If you are choosing an HMO, it is important to review the participating panel to ensure there is an adequate number of physicians in the plan or that your personal physician is a participating provider.

Cost Management Programs

Managed-care plans offer varying levels of medical cost management programs in their insurance offering. There are four general approaches insurers use for cost control. A policy may require a mandatory second opinion, precertification, ambulatory surgery, and case management.

Mandatory Second Opinions

In an effort to reduce unnecessary surgery, many health polices contain a provision requiring the insured to obtain a second opinion from another physician before undergoing non-life-threatening surgery. Benefits may be reduced if a second opinion is not obtained. You should be notified of the second-opinion requirement during the precertification process.

Precertification Review

To control expenses, many policies require policy owners to obtain approval from their health plan before entering a hospital on a nonemergency basis or receiving an expensive outpatient service. Even if the admission is on an emergency basis, most policies with this type of provision require the insured to notify the health plan within a short time, usually 24 hours after being admitted. The health plan then determines how much of the hospital stay it will cover. If the insured wants to stay longer, the additional expense is the responsibility of the insured. However, most plans have an appeal process, which allows the member to have the denial of coverage reevaluated. Most managed-care plans have a member services department that can assist members with the appeal process. If this appeal does not yield the results the member believes is warranted, he or she can always file a complaint with the state's department of insurance, which investigates complaints filed against HMOs.

Ambulatory Surgery

Where once an overnight stay was required, advances in medicine now permit many surgical procedures to be performed on an outpatient basis. To encourage insureds to use less expensive outpatient care, many polices offer some sort of inducement. For example, a policy may waive the deductible or coinsurance if the policy owner elects to be treated on an outpatient basis rather than as an admitted patient.

Case Management

Case management, as referred to here, involves a specialist within an insurance company, such as a registered nurse, who reviews a potentially large claim as it develops to discuss treatment alternatives with the insured. For example, the insured's policy may require that chemotherapy be performed only at a hospital. However, if it makes economic sense to the health plan-and practical sense to the insured-to have treatments conducted at a physician's office or in the patient's home, the insurance company, through its representative, might agree, as long as certain conditions are met. The purpose of case management is to allow the health plan an active role in managing what could potentially become a very expensive claim. However, the physician and patient still have the right to ensure care is delivered in a safe and efficacious manner.

Some managed-care plans may use a much more sophisticated approach to an illness by furnishing a disease-management program. Under a disease-management program, the patient is often directed to receive care from an organization that provides the full array of services for a specific disease. It may also include a limited number of facilities identified as a center of excellence. HMOs may consider allowing a patient to receive care from the local provider rather than at a regional center of excellence if cost and care are not compromised.

How to Pick a Health Plan

It is crucial that you understand your health insurance options and select the one that best fits your needs. Since managed-care plans save money by aggressively controlling how, where, and when health-care services are provided, it is critical that you know exactly what is covered before selecting such a plan. Services you and your family need and want should be compared to what the plan is offering. You may choose to pay more for the availability of desired or needed services.

Here are some questions you should ask when considering health insurance.

1. **How affordable is the cost of care?**

   - What is the monthly premium?
   - Should I try to insure most of my medical expenses or just the large ones?
   - What deductibles will I have to pay out-of-pocket before the plan starts to reimburse me?
   - After I've met my deductible, what percentage of my medical expenses are reimbursed?
   - How much less am I reimbursed if I use doctors outside the insurance company's network?

2. **Does the insurance plan cover the services I am likely to use?**

   - Are the doctors, hospitals, laboratories, and other medical providers that I use in the insurance company's network?
   - If I want to use a doctor outside the network, will the plan permit it?
   - How easily can I change my primary-care physician?

- Do I need to get permission before I see a specialist?
- What are the procedures for getting care and being reimbursed in an emergency, both at home or out of town?
- If I have a preexisting condition, will the plan cover it?
- If I have a chronic condition such as cancer or arthritis, how will the plan treat it?
- Are the prescription medicines I use covered by the plan?
- Will the plan pay for complementary medical therapies such as acupuncture or chiropractic?

3. What is the quality of the insurance plan?

- How have independent government and nongovernment organizations rated the plan? For example, the National Committee for Quality Assurance (NCQA) uses a Consumer Assessment of Health Plans (CHPS) report for every medical plan and facility.
- What kind of accreditation has the plan received from groups such as the NCQA or the Joint Commission on Accreditation of Healthcare Organizations (JCAHO)?
- How many patient complaints were filed against the plan last year? How many were upheld by state insurance commission or the state medical licensing board?
- How many members drop out of the plan each year? State insurance departments keep track of disenrollment rates.
- Do the doctors, pharmacies, and other services provide convenient hours and locations?
- Does the plan pay for preventive health care such as nutritional counseling, immunizations, and health screenings?
- What do my friends and colleagues say about their experiences with the plan?
- What does my doctor say about his or her experience with the plan?

4. Can I buy an individual policy?

If you are unemployed, return to school, or are self-employed, you may need to buy an individual health insurance policy. The following are a number of options that you may consider:

1. Ask your insurance company if you can convert its group policy to an individual policy. You will pay a higher rate than you did before,

and your benefits may be limited, but the terms will still probably be better than if you buy your own policy.

2.   If you are married, see if your spouse's employer will add you to its group plan.

3.   Join a group health plan offering reasonable rates through a trade association, alumni group, or professional association.

4.   As a last resort, you can buy an individual policy. The rates will be high and coverage limited, but it is important to be protected against financial ruin if you or your family are hit with a major illness or injury. If you are self-employed, most of your health insurance premium will be tax-deductible.

To find the best policy, ask a health insurance agent or broker to help you find the contract that gives you the most for your money while meeting your medical needs.

5.   If I change jobs or become unemployed, can I continue my coverage?

If you switch employers, you have the right to carry your group health insurance for up to 18 months under the Congressional Budget Reconciliation Act (COBRA) . You must pay the full premium but at group rates far cheaper than the individual rates you would pay for similar coverage. Health insurance under COBRA is available if you are in one of these situations:

1.   You leave a company and become unemployed or self-employed for up to 18 months.

2.   You are a widow, widower, or child of an employee who dies while working for the same company for 3 years or more.

3.   You are the ex-spouse or child of an employee who has left the company where he or she was employed at for at least 3 years.

4.   You are the child of an employee who left a job and have not yet reached age 23.

5.   Please note that if you want COBRA benefits, you must apply through your employer's benefits department within 60 days of leaving your job. Otherwise, you may be denied coverage.

6.   Where can I get more information on health insurance?

If you have specific questions about your health insurance coverage, contact your health plan's member services department or speak to the benefits administrator where you work. For information on Medicare, call the agency at 800-638-6833, or log onto www.medicare.gov.

Consumer information on the various health insurance plans is available from three leading insurance trade associations:

- American Association of Health Plans
  1129 20th St., NW–Ste. 600
  Washington, DC 20036
  www.aahp.org

- Life and Health Foundation for Education
  2175 K St., NW-Ste. 250
  Washington, DC 20037
  www.life-line.org

- Health Insurance Association of America
  555 13th St., NW–Ste. 600 East
  Washington, DC 20004
  www.hiaa.org

How to Use This Information

Don't give up without a fight.   You may need to take some aggressive steps to get some HMOs to approve a benefit.

Chapter 40

JOINING SUPPORT GROUPS TO LENGTHEN YOUR LIFE

In a study of 86 women with breast cancer, David Spiegel, M.D., professor of psychiatry at Stanford University School of Medicine, discovered that those who participated in weekly support-group sessions lived an average of 18 months longer than those who did not. In fact, the study also revealed that the more frequently a woman attended these sessions, the more she benefited. For example, the average survival time for women who attended from one to ten sessions was 36.2 months. This figure rose to 41.5 months for women who attended more than ten sessions.

Although we have not been able to find a similar study for men with prostate cancer, we believe that participation in prostate cancer support groups would probably extend a man's life. Support groups have a positive effect on a patient's psychological state because they provide a buffer against stress and anxiety, thereby cushioning the body from the consequences of stress hormones. As a result, the body's immune system is able to counteract the effects of prostate cancer more efficiently.

Living with prostate cancer will be difficult for you as well as for those who care for you. Everyone involved faces a multitude of problems, challenges, and decisions. It is easier to deal with these difficulties when people with similar needs get together to share information and support each other. This process helps you realize that you are not alone with your problems.

Support Groups for Prostate Cancer

Four main prostate cancer support groups have been established in the United States in addition to a number of smaller local groups. The main groups are presented here in order of the size of their membership:

US TOO

According to its president and CEO John A. Page, US TOO has more than 100,000 participants in 500 chapters worldwide. US TOO's mission is to help survivors of prostate cancer and their families lead healthy and productive lives—physically, mentally, and spiritually—by offering fellowship, shared counseling, discussions about medical options, and a positive mental outlook.

US TOO is a not-for-profit organization that provides information, counseling, and educational meetings to assist men with prostate cancer in making decisions about their treatment with confidence and support. US TOO was founded by and is run by prostate cancer survivors.

US TOO is made up of independent chapters, which form a network under the aegis of the parent group, US TOO International. Each chapter holds regular meetings for prostate cancer survivors and their families. The meetings provide information by specialists in various fields related to prostate cancer, including surgery, radiation, medication, nutrition, and psychology. Meetings are free and are open to family members, friends, and health care professionals who are interested in prostate disease.

US TOO offers the following benefits:

- The help and support of various medical disciplines, which is needed for the survival of its members.
- A clearinghouse for audiovisual and printed materials for members. The US TOO International library on prostate cancer is available to chapter leaders for use in planning meetings that will appeal to new members and meet the needs of current members.
- A quarterly newsletter, the US TOO Prostate Cancer Communicator, developed and written by volunteers.
- Fellowship, peer counseling, education about treatment options, and discussion of medical alternatives without bias. One goal of US TOO is to foster public awareness of prostate disease.
- Care, concern, acceptance, and understanding while acknowledging the special needs of prostate cancer patients.
- A forum for medical experts to inform group members about treatment options, after-treatment counseling, an opportunity for questions and answers, as well as discussions with these experts.
- Support and reinforcement through rap sessions. Family members are encouraged to attend and can benefit from support and sharing at group meetings.

For more information, you may contact US TOO:

US TOO International, Inc.
930 North York Rd., Ste. 50

E. Roy Berger, M.D., F.A.C.P. and James Lewis, Jr., Ph.D

Hinsdale, IL 60521-2993
800-80-US-TOO (800-808-7866)

Patient Advocates for Advanced Cancer Treatments (PAACT)

PAACT has over 30,000 members worldwide. It is led by a champion, Lloyd Ney, who looked death squarely in the eye in 1982 when he had 32 cancer lesions throughout his skeleton. His doctor gave him 6 months to live. Ney did not pity himself, nor did he give up. Instead, he became stubborn. He was going to beat this terrible disease using knowledge and information as his weapons, and he did. Using a combination of Lupron and Eulexin, Ney is alive today without a trace of prostate cancer.

In 1984, PAACT was formed, based on the belief that combination hormonal therapy should be the first choice of treatment for prostate cancer. PAACT was instrumental in securing FDA approval of Eulexin (flutamide) in the United States and in pioneering the acceptance of combination hormonal therapy. PAACT recognized the significance of the PSA level, recommending its use as early as 1989, for a more accurate diagnosis of prostate cancer and as a monitoring biomarker of activity and progression.

PAACT continues to stay in touch with the FDA to secure the controlled release of drugs approved by foreign countries. It also maintains contact with many members of Congress to assure that proper attention is given to prostate cancer. PAACT has advocated a review by Congress of the regulatory procedures of the FDA. Apparently, PAACT believes it is time to take a closer look at the criteria and personnel used to evaluate the efficacy of new drugs, to expand and broaden participation in Investigation of New Drugs (INDs), and to accelerate the approval of New Drug Applications (NDAs). The regulatory procedures for the approval of new drugs by the FDA have been reviewed by the President's Cancer Panel ad hoc committee, and PAACT is proud that it was asked to testify before this committee at the request of the National Cancer Institute.

PAACT offers the following benefits:

- Extensive research and investigations. PAACT has shared the results of its efforts with both patients and physicians.
- Education for the patient so he is aware of all of the treatment options available. As a result, he can exert his right to select a treatment based on his informed judgment.
- An information electronic mailbox available 24-hours a day, 7 days a week. Patients can use it to request information on a variety of diagnostic and treatment options.

- The <u>Cancer Communication</u> newsletter, which enables members to stay abreast of the latest techniques, products, and medical briefs.
- A questionnaire on some aspect of prostate cancer is sent to PAACTs 30,000 members, and PAACT publishes the results.
- Information on new developments in the detection, diagnosis, evaluation, and treatment of prostate cancer. New developments occur almost daily.
- Help for semi-indigent patients in acquiring financial support so they can get medication.
- Resources on the Internet. PAACTs website address is: www.osz.com/paact.

For more information, contact PAACT at:

> Patient Advocates for Advanced Cancer Treatments
> 1143 Parmelee, NW
> Grand Rapids, MI 49504
> 616-453-1477

Man-to-Man

Man-to-Man is an American Cancer Society program that offers group education, discussion, and support for men with prostate cancer. The organization has chapters in many states and an estimated 15,000 to 20,000 members nationwide. The original program was founded in Sarasota, Florida, by our departed colleague Jim Mullen.

Volunteer coordinators invite speakers, publicize meeting schedules, and make arrangements for monthly meetings. The speakers are usually therapists. Wives and partners of members are invited to the Man-to-Man meeting held the first month of each quarter. The other eight months they meet separately in a group called Side-by-Side.

The Man-to-Man program developed as a natural response to the desire of men faced with prostate cancer to make informed choices about their treatment and to share their collective wisdom. It is an ideal vehicle for meeting a man's need for knowledge through an exchange of information, trust, and respect. This partnership of the American Cancer Society with volunteer health professionals and survivors has proved to be a valued service for all involved.

Man-to-Man offers the following benefits:

- Group education and support: a forum for men to learn about diagnosis and treatment options through presentations, written materials, and videos. Specialists in various fields related to prostate cancer share information on medical topics and quality-of-life issues. A comfortable and confidential meeting environment encourages men and their families to discuss their concerns openly and honestly and to share solutions to common problems. No medical advice is offered.

- Personal visits and telephone support: one-on-one support from specially trained prostate cancer survivors.
- The <u>Man-to-Man Newsletter</u>, which provides news and information about prostate cancer, including research and treatment, messages from men living with prostate cancer, and Man-to-Man activities.
- A Web site (www.cancer.org) designed to create awareness of prostate cancer issues and to provide links to more specific information about the detection and treatment of prostate cancer.
- Public awareness of prostate cancer issues. Man-to-Man promotes opportunities for greater public understanding of prostate cancer, particularly the importance of early detection and treatment.

For more information, contact Man-to-Man at:

> Man-to-Man
> c/o American Cancer Society
> 1599 Clinton Rd., NE
> Atlanta, GA 30329
> 800-ACS-2345 (800-227-2345)

Education Center for Prostate Cancer Patients (ECPCP)

ECPCP was founded in 1996 by three prostate cancer survivors, James Lewis, Jr., Ph.D., Frederick N. Mills, Jr., and Ralph Alterowitz, two of whom are former assistant directors of PAACT. Lewis is the organization's executive director, and Mills is president of the board of trustees, a dedicated group consisting of men and women. ECPCP is also guided by a medical advisory board consisting of world reknown urologists and medical oncologists specializing in prostate cancer. ECPCP has over 3,000 members from all across the country. In addition, the Center has several thousand subscribers to its critically acclaimed newsletter, the <u>Prostate Cancer Exchange</u>.

ECPCP's mission is a little different from that of the other groups mentioned. It is not a traditional support group, where people come together and meet. Rather ECPCP is known as a national leader in providing education to prostate cancer patients and their families. ECPCP searches the world in order to investigate and report on the latest medical research on prostate cancer. It focuses on both conventional and alternative treatments, and it reports on every latest trend and development, both in the United States and abroad. ECPCP's mission is to help save or lengthen the lives of prostate cancer patients, to help improve their quality of life, and to enable them to make effective diagnostic and treatment decisions by offering them education, advice, counseling, and the latest research.

ECPCP offers the following benefits:

- All members have free, unlimited access to ECPCP's Personal Advisory Service. Prostate Cancer Advisors are available to speak directly with patients in order to help them gather information that can be used to effectively and intelligently discuss their condition with their doctors.

- In addition to providing members with the latest information on all available treatments, ECPCP's advisors also supply members with the names and locations of the best doctors in the United States who specialize in specific prostate cancer treatments. These doctors have been identified as being the best by both patients and other physicians.

- ECPCP's Prostate Cancer Advisors are available to participate in conference calls with a member and his doctor. It is important to note that the advisors do not prescribe - or insist that a member undergo - any treatment. They only offer unbiased educational information so that a member can make an informed decision with his doctor.

- ECPCP operates a hotline for members to reach an advisor. ECPCP can be contacted by telephone at (516) 942-5000, by fax at (516) 942-5025, or by email at ecpcp@aol.com. You can also visit ECPCP's website at www.ecpcp.org.

- The Prostate Cancer Exchange, an informative newsletter, is filled with important and timely information from a variety of sources, including physicians, researchers, other health care professionals, and patients. Topics include: (1) the latest information on both conventional and alternative treatments and techniques, (2) information about ongoing clinical trials of new treatments, and (3) information on how nutrition can play a role in the prevention and treatment of prostate cancer. Also included are a calendar of noteworthy events, workshops, and seminars (held by both ECPCP and other organizations), book reviews, and a large Q&A section.

- ECPCP periodically holds national conferences to bring together patients, physicians, researchers, and others in the medical industry to discuss the latest information on the diagnosis and treatment of prostate cancer.

For more information, contact ECPCP at:

> Education Center for Prostate Cancer Patients
> 380 North Broadway – Ste. 304
> Jericho, NY 11753
> 516-942-5000

PCRI

A group that is not actually a support group but a valuable source for obtaining information about prostate cancer is the Prostate Cancer Research Institute (PCRI). PCRI not only advises patients with superior knowledge about various facets, but also publishes a four-color newsletter PCRI Insights, edited by Dr. Stephen Strum. Back issues of PCRI Insights can be reviewed or downloaded from the PCRI website, www.pcri.org.

Prostate Forum

Prostate Forum is an informal newsletter written by Dr. Charles E. Myers, one of the country's most knowledgeable medical oncologists. The newsletter can be ordered by calling 1-800-305-2432 or through Dr. Myers' website at www.prostateforum.com. Dr. Myers is a sought after physician who is also a prostate cancer survivor.

How to Use This Information

- Every person whose life has been affected by prostate cancer should join a support group. The best strategy may be to join a group that meets in your area, one or more of the top national support groups, and the Education Center for Prostate Cancer Patients. This will ensure that you have access to all of the different services available.
- Subscribe to the Prostate Forum.

Chapter 41

SUPPORTIVE THERAPY

Everyone at one time or another needs support. Men who have prostate cancer probably need such support more than most. Support groups and their own support team can play a vital role in their recovery. Many prostate cancer patients — as well as their families — go through an emotional shock when they are diagnosed with the disease, including apprehension, fear, anger, and then resolve to battle the illness. The psychological forces that come into play create a roller coaster of emotions for the patient and his family. Oftentimes, psychological support from outside sources such as friends, support group members, family members, and healthcare professionals becomes necessary.

Fighting Prostate Cancer with Nutrition

Nutrition, exercise, and dietary supplements - including lycopene, calcium, vitamin D (calcitriol), vitamin E, and selenium - are all important in the fight against prostate cancer, whether the patient is participating in watchful waiting or fighting advanced disease. Drugs are available to help fight the symptoms of lethargy, tiredness, shortness of breath, and headache that can develop, for example, as a result of anemia. It has been shown that pharmaceuticals such as Epogen, Procrit, and Aranesp improve the hemoglobin and hematocrit of patients who are undergoing both hormonal and chemotherapy for prostate cancer. These drugs have few side effects, and their potential benefit outweighs those effects. In the last several years, pharmaceutical research and development has advanced so that we can now mimic the body's ability to produce substances such as erythropoietin, which can therapeutically improve the red blood cell counts of patients undergoing treatment. This has been a dramatic breakthrough in that red blood cell transfusions are required in many fewer patients than in previous decades. The quality-of-life indicators and the ability to exercise and endure the daily rigors of life have, therefore, been markedly improved since the discovery of these agents.

Colony-Stimulating Agents

Similarly, colony-stimulating agents such as Leukine, Neupogen, and Neulasta increase patients' white blood cell counts - specifically cells

337

that fight infection – and can thus keep patients who are on chemotherapy out of the hospital and functioning without infections. These agents directly stimulate the bone marrow to produce more neutrophils, the cells that fight infection, as well as other cells that help bolster the immune system. Before the development of these agents, patients needed to undergo intravenous antibiotic therapy, frequently in a hospital, sacrificing days or weeks of their lives. This can now usually be avoided.

Better Antibiotics

The pharmaceutical industry has made great strides in producing better antibiotics. These are often given orally to those who have very low white-cell counts or who have infections, thereby avoiding hospitalizations that were once inevitable. These broad-spectrum oral agents are a positive addition to the therapeutic quiver of arrows needed to help keep patients ambulatory.

Chemotherapeutic agents (see Chapters 30 and 34) help many prostate cancer patients improve their quality of life as far as performance status and pain control are concerned. Hopefully, we are on the cusp of improving disease-free and overall survival with these agents as well (see Chapters 26 and 34). Sometimes, however, the side effects of these agents need to be overcome with pharmacological assistance. We now have good antinausea agents available. These drugs, such as Anzemet, Zofran, and Kytril, are 80 percent effective in controlling the nausea and vomiting caused by many of the chemotherapeutic drugs used to treat advanced prostate cancer patients. These drugs will also come into play if these chemotherapeutic agents are deemed worthy enough to be used in an adjuvant setting. Trials are ongoing.

Controlling Pain

The ability to control pain with pharmacological agents continues to improve as advances in analgesia are made (see Chapter 38, Managing Prostate Cancer Pain).

The various forms of radiation, including radiopharmaceuticals such as strontium and Quadramet, have been invaluable in controlling multifocal sites of pain in select groups of patients. These agents can be given with little toxicity and have about an 80 percent success rate. The major side effect that needs to be monitored with these agents is blood count suppression.

Furthermore, pharmaceutical agents such as Zometa (see Chapter 33) have improved the ability to decrease pain as well as prevent complications of progression of metastatic disease to bone. These include spinal cord compression and pathologic fractures. A simple 15-minute infusion on a monthly basis of Zometa has been shown to be quite effective in delaying the onset of pain as well as helping prevent bony complications.

Many prostate patients undergo hormonal manipulations, the side effects of which have been well documented. Now, a multitude of pharmacologic agents exists to prevent these undesirable symptoms. Antidepressant drugs such as Effexor, Zoloft, Prozac, and Wellbutin alleviate the hot flashes and sweats caused by orchiectomy or LHRH-A therapy. The use of agents such as Tamoxifen and Arimidex helps alleviate the breast swelling and tenderness that men who are on antiandrogens, either alone or with Proscar or Avodart, can have. Dostinex is another drug that can prevent similar effects from excess prolactin secretion.

Zometa has also been shown to be effective in reducing the osteoporosis frequently associated with the LHRH agonists.

Overall, there are now many valuable agents to help the prostate cancer patient deal both psychologically and physically with his disease. In addition, over the next several years more and more pharmaceutical agents will become available to further enhance the quality - and hopefully, quantity - of life available to patients with prostate cancer.

How to Use This Information

When diagnosed with prostate cancer, consider engaging in the following activities:
1. Join a local or national prostate cancer support group before undergoing treatment.
2. Exercise one-half to one hour daily.
3. Keep a log of all of your prostate cancer activities.
4. Get some spiritual guidance.
5. Ask your doctor what agents are available to treat the symptoms you have.
6. Know what services your medical insurance covers.
7. When making a treatment decision, consider getting a second opinion.
8. Accumulate a pertinent library.

Chapter 42

PSYCHOSOCIAL ASPECTS OF PROSTATE CANCER

"In the depth of winter, I finally learned that within me there lay an invincible summer." Albert Camus

Illness can be a terrifying experience. Acute anxiety and distress immediately after diagnosis can reach levels sufficiently high to impair the ability to process information and make responsible decisions. Today's health care professionals have become very sensitive to the psychological effects of prostate cancer on both the patient and his family members. Caring for the patient's emotional and social needs has become a recognized aspect of overall prostate cancer management.

Ten to 20 percent of men with prostate cancer are found to have clinically significant levels of psychological distress. _Distress_ is defined by the National Comprehensive Cancer Network as an unpleasant experience of an emotional, psychological, social, or spiritual nature that interferes with the ability to cope with cancer treatment. Symptoms vary from normal feelings of vulnerability, sadness, and fearfulness to disabling depression – for example, some cancer drugs, pain medications, steroids, etc., affect the mood center of the brain. Fatigue, a common result of treatment, and the debilitating effects of pain and physical discomfort, can also cause depression. Watchful waiting, surgery, radiation, chemotherapy, and hormonal treatment can all have significant psychological impacts. Feelings of helplessness and loss of control over one's physical health usually intensify at the beginning of treatment.

Side Effects of Treatment

The most debilitating side effects of prostate cancer treatment are usually incontinence and impotence. Incontinence can cause social embarrassment as well as physical discomfort. Sexual dysfunction, besides being emasculating and humiliating, can create difficulties in a relationship already stressed by a partner's cancer. Some men withdraw completely from physical and emotional intimacy to avoid dealing with their erectile dysfunction. Health care providers can help them adapt to these changes in functioning, aiding them in maintaining their sense of self.

Traditionally, men tend to withdraw into themselves and become isolated from the very people who can offer emotional and concrete support. Women dealing with serious illness usually find it much easier to reach out.

Assimilating Information

When diagnosed with prostate cancer, men tend to be overwhelmed. They find it difficult to assimilate the enormous amount of information about their diagnosis, treatment choices, financial and logistical details, and aftercare. They may be grappling with fears of changes in their lifestyle and possibly in their sexual functioning, anticipating pain and discomfort, and they may be confused about health insurance entitlements and concerned about a possible disruption of income. They often feel embarrassed about how family, friends, and coworkers will view their condition. They may experience a loss of self-esteem (i.e., perceived "sense of masculinity"), as well as an acute fear of death and dying, common to most people diagnosed with a life-threatening illness. It may be the first time they have been forced to confront their own mortality. A normal reaction to being diagnosed with a life-threatening illness such as prostate cancer is anger toward the physician. Because the physician is the one breaking the bad news and dishing out the disagreeable treatments, anger and blame are easily misdirected toward him or her. These initial feelings are not usually diminished by the reality that, with advances in medical treatment, men with prostate cancer are living longer and the quality of their lives is improving. For many, in the early stage, there is no "best" treatment, which adds to the anxiety often experienced in the early weeks after diagnosis.

Although the oncology team is the frontline in providing supportive therapy to patients, other resources — support groups, psychotherapy, and if indicated, psychopharmacology — can strengthen patient's adaptive capacities and improve his coping skills. Regardless of prognosis or uncertainty about the future course of their illness, all patients can benefit from psychosocial intervention. At the very least, their quality of life can be improved, and at best, the course of their illness may be positively affected.

Although men with cancer have been shown to be less interested in support groups than have women, support groups can be very beneficial in helping them to maintain past coping mechanisms and encouraging them to use their support systems. Patients learn from each other how to help friends and family help them, as well as how to ask for what they need. Many people don't understand cancer, and they may withdraw from prostate cancer patients because they are afraid of the illness or worry that they will upset them by saying the wrong thing. Whether a self-help group is run by a mental health professional (the ideal) or run by peers, patients in these groups are encouraged to verbalize their thoughts and concerns through the "we are all in the same boat" mindset and to feel understood on a gut level. Expressing fears, frustrations, anger, etc., is like removing a heavy burden – it is cathartic. Information and experiences are shared, creating a sense of normalcy toward one's own thoughts and feelings. Grieving the loss of a sense of wellness is appropriate, as is anger, regressive (childlike) behavior, and thoughts. Illness brings out the "small child" in all of us. This doesn't indicate a lack of courage or strength.

Individual psychotherapy can help in the form of "crisis management," with problem-solving and supportive techniques reinforced. Cognitive-behavioral methods, such as keeping a journal and learning the art of positive self-talk, are empowering and will assist patients in taking an active role in their care plan. According to Herbert Benson, M.D., at the Harvard Medical School, various forms of meditation – such as mindfulness meditation, visualization, guided imagery, abdominal breathing, repetitive mantras, progressive relaxation exercises, self-hypnosis, biofeedback, yoga, affirmations, and prayer - "decrease oxygen consumption, heart rate, respiratory rate, and blood pressure and increase the intensity of alpha, theta, and delta brain waves – the opposite of the physiological changes that occur during the stress response."

In dealing with serious illness, stress management is vital. A substantial body of evidence has shown the negative effects of stress on the immune system. There is also impressive proof that pain management techniques can actually alter the perception of pain, as any woman who has practiced Lamaze exercises during childbirth will tell you. Medical researchers are discovering that high determination and purpose can enhance the working of the immune system, allowing specific medical treatments to work optimally.

Psychology and the Immune System

The field of psychoneuroimmunology (PNI) - the interface between psychology and the immune system – has brought to light the theory that one's attitudes and actions at times of adversity can make a difference. And, the human brain may actually convert these attitudes and actions into specific immune-system changes. Psychobiologist Candace Pert, M.D., has shown that neuropeptides (which enhance the immune system by raising the T-cell level) are actually generated by positive thoughts and self-talk. The natural healing capacity of the body is very powerful.

Supportive psychotherapy can focus on impotence and intimacy issues and the discomfort of incontinence. It can also assist men in strengthening their adaptive capacities, helping them regain a sense of hope, control, comfort, and dignity, even in the face of physical uncertainty. A life-threatening illness can leave you forever changed, and most people need to reestablish their emotional equilibrium and reprioritize, which a skilled psychotherapist can facilitate. Also, with the patient's permission, healthy communication between the patient and his significant others can be enhanced by therapy sessions that include these people. A positive attitude is not a substitute for competent medical attention, but it can and does affect the quality of life, regardless of present circumstances. In his exploration of the "mind-body connection," Bernie Siegel, M.D., states, "In the absence of certainty, there is nothing wrong with hope."

People who think of themselves as survivors often respond significantly better than people who have a victim's mentality, according to Candace Pert, Ph.D. and other behaviorists. In recent years, based on scientific studies by David Spiegel, M.D., and others, new respect has developed for the importance of psychosocial factors in contributing not only to cancer patients' quality of life but also to their longevity. A total of 649 oncologists, reporting in a national survey undertaken at UCLA, ranked various psychosocial factors according to their importance in successful treatment outcomes. These factors, based on the treatment of more than 100,000 cancer patients, were:

1. a strong will to live
2. confidence in your physician and believing in treatment choices
3. ability to cope with stress
4. emotional support from friends and family

Psychotropic Medications

Psychotropic medications are being used increasingly in patients with cancer. Selective serotonin-reuptake inhibitors (SSRIs) can treat both depression and anxiety, allowing patients to tap into their own inner strengths to draw on past successes and coping skills. Low-dose antidepressants, particularly SSRIs and venlafaxine (Effexor), have been shown to alleviate hot flashes in many men, an uncomfortable side effect of prostate cancer treatment. For acute anxiety, short-term use of mild tranquilizers (i.e., benzodazepines or low-dose atypical neuroleptics) have proved effective.

Norman Cousins in his classic <u>Anatomy of an Illness</u> suggests that watching funny movies should be a part of every patient's treatment and that laughter helps the body heal because it lowers stress hormones, blood pressure, and pain. Cousins states that there is something about making a supreme effort in coping that gives meaning to life, even under the most trying and poignant circumstances. Living in the moment and deriving the most satisfaction out of every minute of every day is often the lesson learned when, through illness, human beings discover how tentative, fragile, and precious life can be. You can choose to live a rewarding and meaningful life amidst the challenges of a serious illness.

How to Use This Information

Remember:

1. Depression can be a side effect of some medicines.
2. Sexual problems from cancer can have physical or emotional causes, or both.
3. Reach out to other prostate cancer patients to socialize and to get as much information as you need.
4. Far too many prostate cancer patients struggle alone with their problems when there are patients in their communities able and willing to assist them.

Chapter 43

USING A NOMOGRAM TO MAKE A TREATMENT DECISION

Sooner or later, one out of five men in the United States will learn that he has prostate cancer. Of the men who are diagnosed with the disease, a large percentage will have a localized early-stage cancer. The dilemma they face is this; What should I do about eradicating my disease? Should I watchful-wait, undergo surgery, have seed implantation and/or external beam radiation, or have cryosurgery?

The more he understands the consequences of his decision, the more a man can make a decision he is comfortable with. A new and effective tool—a *prostate nomogram*—enables patients to better understand the outcomes of the various treatments for prostate cancer.

What Is a Nomogram?

The prostate nomogram is a graphic procedure that make forecasts about the outcome of medical treatment for prostate cancer. It does this by associating information about a prostate cancer patient with a database of information about hundreds or thousands of other patients.

Nomograms are available for prostate cancer patients who are considering radical prostatectomy, external beam radiotherapy, and seed implantation, as well as for patients who have already had these procedures.

Each nomogram is based on thousands of patients who had their prostate cancer treated at a major hospital. These data were compiled and then studied to determine their collective characteristics. As a result, an artificial neural network was produced to duplicate the data.

A number of disease factors appear in a treatment nomogram:

- PSA level
- Gleason score at biopsy
- clinical stage
- whether hormone therapy will be used
- If external beam radiation is used, what dose will be given?
  When inputting data in the treatment nomogram, the results may show the following:
- 5 years progression biochemical (using PSA–non-progression) free probability after radical prostatectomy

345

- 5 years biochemical progression-free probability after external beam radiation
- 5 years biochemical progression-free probability after brachytherapy

Not only can a nomogram be designed as a prognostic tool, it can also be designed to predict treatment failure among patients who already have undergone other therapies for the disease. Such a nomogram is called a *recurrence nomogram*. Figure 43-4 shows a typical recurrence nomogram for predicting a recurrence of prostate cancer based on 3D conformal radiation therapy. Input data consists of:

- pretreatment PSA level
- clinical stage
- Gleason score at biopsy
- dose of external beam radiation received
- whether the patient underwent hormone therapy

Data Required for the Nomogram

The prediction nomogram may require the following data depending on the nomogram used:

- pretreatment PSA level
- Gleason grade and score
- clinical stage
- capsular penetration
- surgical margin status
- seminal-vesicle invasion
- lymph-node status
- previous radiation therapy

For predicting survival in patients with hormone-refractory disease, other data needed include:

- visceral disease (i.e., organ involvement)
- performance status
- LDH level
- alkaline phosphatase level
- hemoglobin level

Prostate nomogram calculator from www.nomograms.org is needed. At the end of this chapter you will find the following nomograms:

1. preoperative nomogram for disease recurrence (Figure 43-1)
2. postoperative nomogram for disease recurrence after radical prostatectomy (Figure 43-2)
3. pretreatment nomogram for predicting freedom from recurrence after permanent prostate brachytherapy (Figure 43-3)
4. pretreatment nomogram for predicting recurrence after 3D conformal radiation therapy (Figure 43-4)
5. prognostic model for predicting survival in men with hormone-refractory prostate cancer (Figure 43-5)

Advantage of a Nomogram

A nomogram has the following advanges:

*   It improves the ability of the patient and physician to decide on a treatment that will yield the most beneficial results.
*   It gives prostate cancer patients a genuine feeling of hope.
*   It helps give the patient confidence that he made the most appropriate treatment decision.
*   It lessens the subjective basis and enhances the objective basis for the patient to choose a treatment.
*   It may improve the survival rate of prostate cancer patients with localized disease.
*   It enables the patient to explore the different options before deciding on a treatment.
*   It helps the patient to understand what the consequences of his decision will be.
*   It can help the patient to better understand his prognosis.
*   It challenges the patient to explore a number of treatments.

Disadvantages of a Nomogram

There are at least three disadvantages to a nomogram:

1. It may not predict well when applied to new patients if the predictor variables are irreproducible, unavailable, or conformed by other factors.
2. If the sample size or follow-up used to develop the nomogram is inadequate, the estimates may not optimal.

3. The statistical model of the nomogram may not match the nomogram. As a result, validation in one or several of the cohorts represents an important step before a nomogram can safely be implemented in routine clinical practice.

Nomogram Types

As stated earlier, nomograms can be developed for a number of reasons. These include:

*   to determine if the disease will return after radical prostatectomy.
*   to determine which treatment will yield the most beneficial results.
*   to determine if treatment with or without hormones or radiation will improve the effectiveness of the treatment.
*   to predict freedom from recurrence after brachytherapy.
*   to predict the outcome of 3D conformal radiation.
*   to predict survival in patients with hormone-refractory disease.

Actualizing Your Nomogram

There are four steps you can take to actualize your nomogram:

1. Get a reliable PSA level by avoiding factors that may affect it, such as the following:
    *   urinary retention
    *   sexual intercourse within 48 hours of the test
    *   acute or chronic prostatitis (If you have bacteria-induced prostatitis, have the PSA test after an appropriate course of antibiotics).
    *   use of Proscar or Avodart (If these drugs are being used, double the PSA level).
2. Obtain an accurate biopsy. The probability of getting an accurate diagnostic biopsy using the standard sextant method is 72.6 percent, compared to the 10-12 pattern biopsy, which is 99 percent accurate.
3. Obtain an accurate clinical stage (ask your physician what it is).
4. Use appropriate imaging technology. If it is necessary to determine lymph node invasion, have a ProstaScint scan with either an MRI or CT scan to increase its sensitivity.

The data you gather from the various nomograms may help you answer some of these questions:

- Should I undergo brachytherapy alone or with external beam radiation?
- Should I undergo external beam radiation alone or with hormonal therapy?
- Should I undergo hormonal therapy alone. If so how much?
- Should I undergo hormone therapy with other treatment?
- Should I try to predict whether I will experience a recurrence and within what period of time?
- Should I undergo a radical prostatectomy?
- Should I predict the probability of getting a recurrence?

To help determine a treatment decision, insert all of the factors describing your condition into the nomogram, and then tabulate your results. Once you have collected all your decision-making data, you will have a much better idea where you stand.

Validating A Nomogram

Validating a nomogram is accomplished by the networks with a set of cases that have not been seen by the networks. Based on the networks performance on this unseen case, the accuracy of the nomograms can be tested.

Limitations of Nomograms

Any patient with clinical variables outside the range of the variables used to develop the nomogram will not be able to use it. For instance the upper limit of the PSA level in patients who use the postoperative nomogram in the model is 100 ng/ml. Any patient whose pretreatment PSA is higher than 100 ng/ml would not be eligible to use this model.

Identifying Pertinent Information Regarding Treatment Nomograms

Table 43-1 illustrates the treatments, type of prognostic tool, design, and limitations of certain treatment nomograms.

E. Roy Berger, M.D., F.A.C.P. and James Lewis, Jr., Ph.D

Definitive Therapy	Prognostic Tool/Nomogram	Design	Limitations
Radical prostatectomy (preoperative nomogram for disease recurrence) Nomogram 43-1	Predictor variables: PSA, clinical stage, biopsy Gleason sum	Patient number: 1,055 (T1-3a NX, MO)	Single-institution study # All - Caucasian population
Radical prostatectomy (postoperative nomogram for disease recurrence) Nomogram 43-2	Kattan Predictor variables: preoperative PSA, specimen Gleason score, capsular invasion, surgical - margin status, seminal -vesicle invasion, lymph - node status	Patient number: 996 (T1a-T3c, NX, MO, majority of patients T2)	Single-institution study # All - Caucasian population
Brachytherapy Nomogram 43-3	Kattan Predictor variables: pretreatment PSA, clinical stage, biopsy Gleason score, adjuvant external beam radiotherapy Predicted outcome: 5-year biochemical risk of recurrence without neoadjuvant hormonal therapy	Patient number: 920 (T1c-T2b, majority of patients T1c) # 18% received external beam adjuvant radiation therapy	Single-institution study

Definitive Therapy	Prognostic Tool/Nomogram	Design	Limitations
External beam radiation therapy (3D conformal) Nomogram 43-4	Kattan Predictor variables: clinical stage, biopsy Gleason score, pretreatment PSA, radiation dose, administration of neoadjuvant hormonal therapy Predicted outcome: 5-year biochemical risk of recurrence	Patient number: 1,042 (T1c-T3c, NX, M0, majority of patients T2) # 62.9% did not receive neoadjuvant hormonal therapy	Single-institution study # Limited African-American population
Prognostic model for predicting survival in men with hormone = refractory metastatic prostate cancer # Nomogram 43-5	Kattan Predictor variables: visceral disease, Gleason sum, performance status, baseline PSA, LDH, alkaline phosphatase, hemoglobin	Patient number: 1,101	All - Caucasian population

Nomograms Studies

A retrospective study was conducted by F. A. Vicini and Colleagues of the Department of Radiation Oncology, William Beaumont Hospital, Royal Oak, Michigan, entitled *An Interinstitutional and Interspecialty Comparison of Treatment Outcome Data For Patients With Prostate Carcinoma* based on predefined prognostic categories. The study involved 6,877 men with prostate cancer treated between 1989 and 1998 at seven different institutions with six different types of therapy. Five-year actuarial rates of PSA failure were calculated based on predefined prognostic categories, combinations of pretreatment PSA level, tumor stage, and Gleason score. In addition, outcome was calculated using consistent biochemical failure definitions with a minimum, median length of follow-up.

Substantial differences in outcome were observed for the same type of treatment and at the same institution, depending on the number of prognostic variables used to define treatment groups. However, estimates of 5-year PSA outcomes for all forms of therapy for low-risk and intermediate-risk groups were remarkably similar (regardless of the type of treatment) when all three pretreatment variables were used to define prognostic categories. For patients in high-risk groups, the 5-year PSA outcomes were suboptimal, regardless of the treatment technique used. This is most likely due to the high likelihood of systemic disease.

The current data suggest that interinstitutional and interspecialty comparisons of treatment outcomes for prostate cancer patients are possible but that results must be based on all major prognostic variables to be meaningful. Analyzed in this fashion, 5-year PSA results were similar for patients in low-risk and intermediate-risk groups, regardless of the form of therapy. Finding from prospective, randomized trials using survival (cause specific and overall) as the end point for judging treatment efficacy require longer follow-up to validate the PSA findings and to identify the most appropriate management option for patients with all stages of disease.

A study conducted by Michael W. Kattan, Ph.D., and colleagues at Memorial Sloan- Kettering Cancer Center "*International Validation of a Preoperative Nomogram for Prostate Cancer Recurrence after Radical Prostatectomy,*" Journal of Clinical Oncology examined 6,232 prostate cancer patients. The nomogram was able to accurately predict recurrencein 75 percent. When the nomogram was used to predict the probability of freedom from recurrence (as measured by PSA) for different risk groups, it predicted probabilities of 87 percent (low-risk), 64 percent (intermediate low-risk), 39 percent (intermediate high-risk), and 14 percent (high-risk). Among these patients, the actual outcomes for remaining free from recurrence match these predictions closely: 86, 64, 42, and 17 percent, respectively.

Researchers tested the accuracy of the nomogram in two ways. First, they analyzed the ability of the nomogram to correctly identify higher-risk patients. Second, researchers retrospectively inserted patients' records into the nomogram program to obtain patients, disease -recurrence predictions and then compared these results to actual outcomes.

Researchers also found that the accuracy of the nomogram was not adversely affected for those patients who received neoadjuvant hormone therapy to treat their prostate cancer.

How to Use This Information

Use the prostate nomogram to predict your treatment results, Click on the Calculate box or choose Online Prostate Nomogram to download the prostate nomogram software available in Palm Pilot, Access 97, 2000, or Pocket PC format. Remember these are approximations, so do not pick one treatment over another based on small differences in predictions of PSA freedom from recurrence.

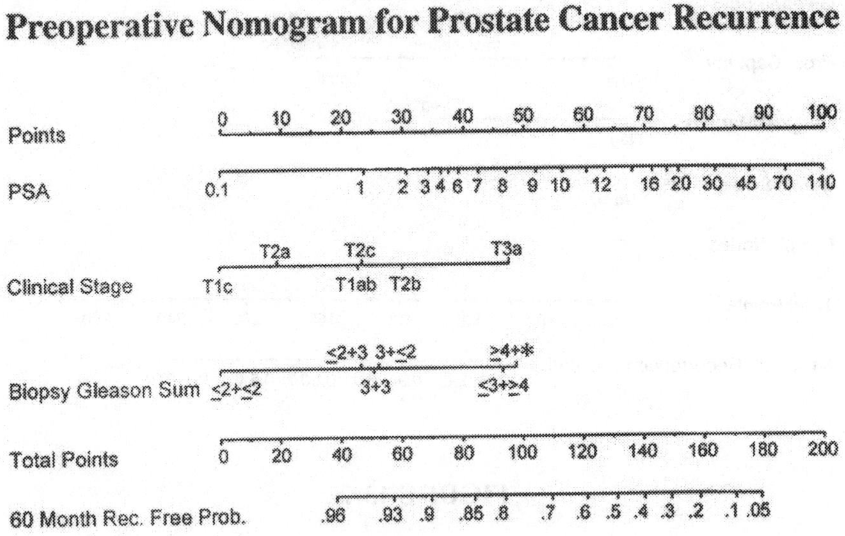

Preoperative Nomogram for Prostate Cancer Recurrence

Points	0 10 20 30 40 50 60 70 80 90 100
PSA	0.1 1 2 3 4 6 7 8 9 10 12 16 20 30 45 70 110
Clinical Stage	T2a T2c T3a / T1c T1ab T2b
Biopsy Gleason Sum ≤2+≤2	≤2+3 3+≤2 ≥4+* / 3+3 ≤3+≥4
Total Points	0 20 40 60 80 100 120 140 160 180 200
60 Month Rec. Free Prob.	.96 .93 .9 .85 .8 .7 .6 .5 .4 .3 .2 .1 .05

FIGURE 43-1

Instructions: Locate the patient's PSA on the PSA axis. Draw a line straight upward to the Points axis to determine how many points toward recurrence the patient receives for his PSA. Repeat this process for the other axes, each time drawing straight upward to the Points axis. Add the points achieved for each predictor, and locate this sum on the total points axis. Then draw a line straight down to find the patient's probability of remaining recurrence - free, assuming he does not die of another cause first.

E. Roy Berger, M.D., F.A.C.P. and James Lewis, Jr., Ph.D

Postoperative Nomogram for Prostate Cancer Recurrence

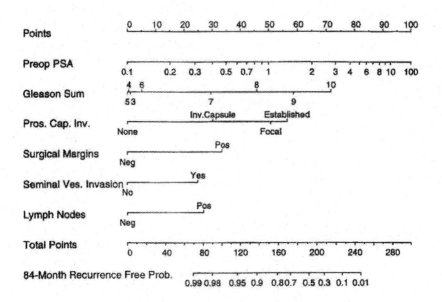

FIGURE 43-2

Instructions: Locate the patient's PSA on the PSA axis. Draw a line straight upward to the Points axis to determine how many points toward recurrence the patient receives for his PSA. Repeat this process for the other axes, each time drawing straight upward to the Points axis. Add the points achieved for each predictor, and locate this sum on the total points axis. Then draw a line straight down to find the patient's probability of remaining recurrence - free, assuming he does not die of another cause first.

Brachytherapy Nomogram

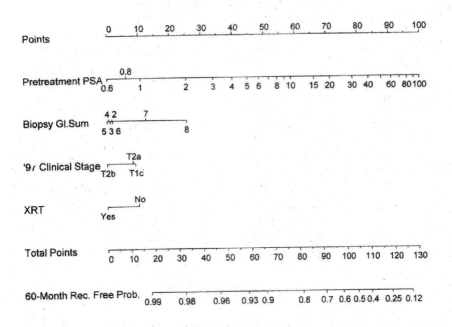

Figure 43-3

Instructions: Locate the patient's PSA on the PSA axis. Draw a line straight upward to the Points axis to determine how many points toward recurrencethe patient receives for his PSA. Repeat this process for the other axes, each time drawing straight upward to the Points axis. Add the points achieved for each predictor, and locate this sum on the total points axis. Then draw a line straight down to find the patient's probability of remaining recurrence - free, assuming he does not die of another cause first.

E. Roy Berger, M.D., F.A.C.P. and James Lewis, Jr., Ph.D

3D Conformal Radiation Therapy Nomogram

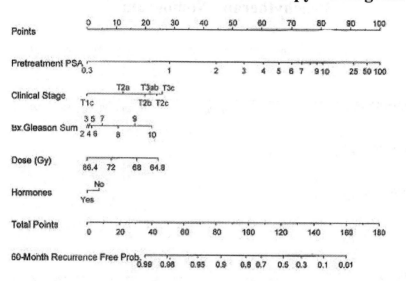

Figure 43-4

<u>Instructions</u>: Locate the patient's PSA on the PSA axis. Draw a line straight upward to the Points axis to determine how many points toward recurrence the patient receives for his PSA. Repeat this process for the other axes, each time drawing straight upward to the Points axis. Add the points achieved for each predictor, and locate this sum on the total points axis. Then draw a line straight down to find the patient's probability of remaining recurrence - free, assuming he does not die of another cause first.

Hormone-Refractory Nomogram

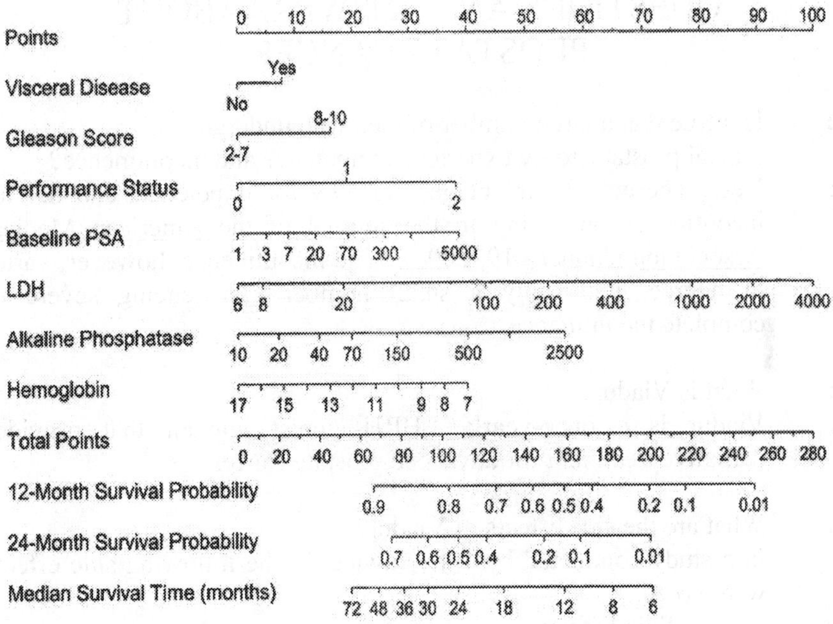

Figure 43 –5

Instructions: Locate the patient's PSA on the PSA axis. Draw a line straight upward to the Points axis to determine how many points toward recurrencethe patient receives for his PSA. Repeat this process for the other axes, each time drawing straight upward to the Points axis. Add the points achieved for each predictor, and locate this sum on the total points axis. Then draw a line straight down to find the patient's probability of remaining recurrence - free, assuming he does not die of another cause first. In the case of Figure 43-5, 12 months, 24 months, and median survival probability can be calculated.

357

Chapter 44

QUESTIONS AND ANSWERS ABOUT PROSTATE CANCER

Q: Is it true that a large number of men who undergo radical prostatectomy experience impotence and incontinence?

A: Yes. The actual percentages are 59.9 for impotence, and 8.4 for incontinence according to the <u>Journal of the American Medical Association</u> (January 19, 2000). The incontinence, however, varies in degree, with only a small number experiencing severe or complete incontinence.

Q: What is Viadur?

A: Viadur is a once-yearly LHRH-agonist implant that provides palliative treatment for advanced prostate cancer.

Q: What are the side effects of Viadur?

A: In a study conducted by J. E. Fowler, Jr. the following side effects were noted.

Side Effects	Percentage
Hot flashes	67.9%
Loss of strength	7.6%
Enlarged and tender breasts	6.9%
Depression	5.3%
Sweating	5.3%
Bruising	34.6%
Burning	5.6%

Q: How can a prostate cancer patient get relief from hot flashes due to hormone treatment?

A: Consider using gabapentin or estrogen patches. Low doses of Megace also can reduce or eliminate hot flashes. However, these treatments all have side effects and should be monitored.

Q: What is cachexia?

A: Cachexia is a physical condition in which a person's body wastes away.

Q: How can cachexia be prevented?

A: The patient should take omega-3 fatty acids, which are found in fish oil and flaxseed oil.

Q: What is Amrit?

A: Amrit is a combination of 40 herbs that reportedly help the liver filter toxins out of the body and make chemotherapy easier to tolerate.

Q: What is a PSA bounce?

A: A PSA bounce is a temporary rise in the PSA level that occurs sometime between 12 and 36 months after radioactive seed implantation and/or external beam radiation, and then returns to a lower level.

Q: What is a FastPack system?

A: The FastPack system enables a physician to provide PSA test results in about 10 minutes. It was developed by Qualigen, of Carlsbad, California.

Q: What percentage of prostate cancer patients die of the disease annually?

A: Two to three percent.

Q. What drug reduces the risk of acute urinary retention and the need for the "terrible TURP"?

A. The Food and Drug Administration approved a supplemental drug called Avodart (dutasteride) on October 9, 2002. Avodart reduces the risk of acute urinary retention and lessens the need for TURP surgery.

Q: What is Aredia?

A: Aredia is a bisphosphonate drug designed to prevent and reverse osteoporosis and to prevent the loss of calcium from bones of patients on combination hormonal therapy. It also reduces pain in patients with hormone-refractory disease as well as possibly lowering their PSA. It can be used if Zometa is not tolerated.

Q: Can Aredia be used with combination hormonal therapy (CHT)?

A: Yes. A total of 302 patients with microscopic cancer cells in their bones (but normal bone scan) were given CHT for 2 years. One-half of them were also given Aredia, and the other half were not. The results indicated that there were 3.5 times more deaths among the men not receiving Aredia. Aredia also reduced the metastases.

Q: What are the side effects of Aredia?
A: The most frequent side effects of Aredia are:
- low-grade fever
- chills
- body aches
- muscle aches, mostly during the first one to three cycles

Q: Are all patients eligible for intermittent combination hormonal therapy?
A: No. Only those patients who respond to CHT are eligible. We do not yet know the optimal group of prostate cancer patients to apply this treatment to, nor do we know the optimal timing of it. Many physicians who have extensive experience with intermittent therapy do it differently. There are guidelines but no hard-and-fast rules about the best way to use this treatment.

Q: Can heavy metals like lead and mercury damage the body?
A: Heavy metals and other toxins can depress body temperature, suppress activity of the endocrine system, and slow down the immune system, making the body susceptible to infections and yeast overgrowth, as well as cancer.

Q: My doctor performed a sextant biopsy on me and came up with nothing. Then he performed about eight or nine other biopsies and found nothing. Should I allow him to perform another biopsy on me?
A: No. Several medical textbooks indicate that a biopsy may seed the prostate cancer. Instead, you should go to a hospital that gives the AMARC test (see Resources at the back of this book). This test involves microscopic examination of the tissue of your biopsy for prostate cancer, and it is very effective.

Q: How can I prevent osteoporosis?
A: The following steps help to prevent osteoporosis:
- Avoid smoking, reduce alcohol intake, and increase your level of activity. Have a daily calcium intake of 1,000 mg if you are 65 or younger, and consume 1,500 mg if you are over age 65.

- Be sure to get enough vitamin D. Normally, sufficient vitamin D is made from exposure to as little as 10 minutes of sunlight a day. If your exposure to sunlight is inadequate, however, take at least 400 IU of vitamin D - but not more than 800 IU - per day. Four hundred IU is the amount found in a quart of fortified milk and in most multivitamins.
- Engage in a regular regimen of weight-bearing exercise where bones and muscles work against gravity. This includes walking, jogging, racket sports, climbing stairs, team sports, lifting weights, and using resistance machines. A doctor should evaluate the exercise program of anyone diagnosed with osteoporosis to determine if twisting motions and impact activities, such as those used in golf, tennis, and basketball, need to be curtailed.
- Discuss with your doctor the use of medications such as steroids and hormones that are known to cause bone loss.
- Recognize and treat any underlying medical conditions that affect bone health.
- Undergo a bone-density test and take bone-building medications when appropriate.

Q: Can a man under the age of 55 get prostate cancer?
A: Yes. Frequently these cases run in families. They are seen in up to 50 percent of men whose father and/or brother have prostate cancer.

Q: My radiation oncologist says she will use either iodine-125 or palladium-103 to treat me with seed implantation. Is one of these preferable?
A: Although palladium-103 is more expensive, it is considered more effective in irradiating high-grade tumors. Iodine-125 seems to be more effective with low-grade tumors. However, more data are needed to definitively answer the question.

Q: What type of patient should consider seed implantation?
A: Excellent candidates for seed implantation are men with low-volume, low-grade disease and a low incidence of extracapsular penetration. However, patients with stage B3, C1, or C2 tumors may also be candidates for the treatment if there is no lymph-node, seminal-vesicle, or neurovascular involvement. If there is extracapsular involvement, it may be necessary for the patient to be put on CHT for 6 months or longer. However, because such involvement is difficult to determine with the present diagnostic tools, we recommend CHT prior to seed implantation in most cases.

CHT usually decreases the size of the prostate and the cancerous tissue, and it is especially useful in men with large prostates. Furthermore, most radiation oncologists combine this treatment with 3D-conformal external beam radiation for patients who have stage B3, C, or C2 tumors.

Q: Which of the standard treatments for prostate cancer has the fewest side effects?

A: A study indicated that of the three standard treatments — radical prostatectomy, external beam radiation, and seed implantation — seed implantation has the fewest side effects. These include short-term incontinence (less than 5%), impotence for men under the age of 70 (less than 20%), urinary frequency and urgency%, and mild or self-limited radiation proctitis (1%).

Q: What should a man's PSA be after a radical prostatectomy?

A: According to most of the literature, when a patient's prostate has been removed, the PSA level should be less than 0.3 ng/ml. It is well established that if a man has undergone a prostatectomy and his PSA level is 0.3 ng/ml or more, then there is a high probability that some cancer remains in him. When a man has been treated with either seed implantation, external beam radiotherapy, or cryosurgery, the PSA level should be 1.0 ng/ml or less. However, if the PSA level is higher than 1.0 but less than 4.0 and the level is stabilized, there may not be a clinical recurrence of prostate cancer. A PSA level of more than 2.0 after external beam radiation may mean a clinical recurrence of prostate cancer.

Q: What options are available to the patient whose radical prostatectomy fails to "cure" him?

A: The following options are based on an early-stage and early-grade tumor.

- If treatment fails locally, you can opt for external beam radiation to the prostatic fossa, combination hormonal therapy, or both. You could also select orchiectomy with or without Eulexin, Casodex, or Nilandron. Because your prostate has been removed, you may not be eligible for either cryosurgery or seed implantation. However, Frank Critz, M.D., in Atlanta, Georgia, performs seed implantation on patients who have undergone radical prostatectomy and had a recurrence.
- If cryosurgery fails, you can opt for a repeat treatment. In rare instances, a third cryosurgical procedure can be done.

Q: What option is available if external beam radiation fails?
A: Combination hormonal therapy.

Q: What options are available if seed implantation fails?
A: If seed implantation fails, patients with early-stage and early-grade tumors may be eligible for cryosurgery, orchiectomy with Eulexin or Casodex, or CHT. They may also be eligible for a radical prostatectomy under certain conditions. Seed implantation can also be repeated, but experience with this is limited.

Q: Of radical prostatectomy, cryosurgery, and seed implantation, which treatment is best for stage C patients?
A: There is not enough data to give a definitive answer. Most patients with stage C tumors will eventually have to deal with systemic disease. Therefore, in our opinion, CHT must be the mainstay of their treatment. In order to give patients a chance to get off CHT, a form of therapy that is less invasive than radical prostatectomy — such as 3D-conformal radiation, with or without seed implantation — should be considered.

Q: How long can a patient with advanced metastatic prostate cancer survive?
A: Although the survival rate is usually 2 to 3 years, it varies widely. For example, Fernand Labrie, M.D., found the median survival time in men on CHT who had five or fewer metastatic D2 sites on a bone scan to be 6.5 years.

Q: Is it true that CHT is not a cure for prostate cancer but a palliative treatment?
A: CHT is almost certainly not a cure for patients with stage D2 disease. There are, however, some patients who have low PSA levels and normal bone scans after 10 years or more of CHT. These men are rare, and most of them will probably eventually relapse if they do not die of other causes first.

Q: When is CHT the best treatment for prostate cancer?
A: CHT has been shown to be an effective treatment for men with stage D2 disease. Because a group of men with minimal metastatic cancer have done better on CHT than have those treated with one-hormone therapy, we assume that CHT will be even more effective in stages C, D, and D1. There are significant data indicating that CHT is

effective in downsizing (reducing the volume of the cancer) or downstaging disease when used before other forms of treatment.

Dr. Labrie maintains that for men aged 70 years or more, or for men with a life expectancy of less than ten years, CHT alone may effectively control the disease and prevent death from prostate cancer.

Q: I asked my doctor if I should be treated with CHT to shrink my prostate before my operation. He said CHT would not be necessary because I have early-stage cancer. Is he right?

A: Not necessarily. In a study conducted by Dr. Labrie and colleagues, 40 to 50 percent of patients were found to have a more advanced stage of prostate cancer following pathologic analysis of their surgically removed prostates.

Two groups of patients were studied. One group received 3 months of CHT prior to radical prostatectomy, and the other group underwent radical prostatectomy without CHT. The first group was able to reduce its cancer-positive margin to 7.8 percent (10 of 72 men), while the second group had a positive-margin rate of 33.8 percent (25 of 65 men). Similar results were reported in two other studies (Soloway and Fair).

Based on the tremendous number of patients initially understaged, it may be better to be safe than sorry. Consider asking your physician to give you 6 months of CHT before surgery. We are eagerly waiting to see if such treatment will improve the survival figures for those with early-stage disease.

The optimal period of time that CHT should be used is unknown. One study from Vancouver, Canada, suggested that it took about 8 months of CHT for the PSA level to reach its lowest point when an ultrasensitive PSA test was used. Interestingly, no hormonal-insensitive cells were detected in the specimens taken during surgery.

Q: I have a local recurrence of prostate cancer. I would like to live as long as I can. Can you recommend a treatment plan that will enable me to live longer?

A: Your doctor should explain the various options available to you: radical prostatectomy, external beam radiation, cryosurgery, and seed implantation. Which treatment he or she recommends will depend on the primary treatment that you had. For example, seed implantation can be repeated once, and cryosurgery can be repeated twice. When the only option available is CHT or bilateral orchiectomy plus an antiandrogen, you and your doctor should consider intermittent CHT with Proscar. This will hopefully do several things:

1. It should reduce your PSA level to an almost undetectable level.
2. It will improve your quality of life by minimizing the side effects of the hormonal therapy, and it may restore your sexual function if it existed prior to hormonal therapy.
3. It may lengthen your stay on CHT and therefore delay chemotherapy.
4. Proscar may prevent or delay your PSA from increasing while you are off the hormonal therapy.

Q: I understand some doctors and researchers believe that prostate cancer, as well as other cancers, is a systemic disease. If so, why don't doctors use systemic rather than local therapy?

A: Not much research has been done in this area. However, CHT *is* a systemic treatment. Unfortunately, CHT can only arrest hormonally sensitive cells. We also need a systemic treatment for hormonally insensitive or independent cells.

Q: If Proscar has such a positive effect on prostate cancer, why don't more physicians use it as a preliminary treatment by more physicians?

A: To date, Proscar has not been shown to have a major effect on prostate cancer. Perhaps used in combination with an LHRH agonist and Eulexin, Casodex, or nilutamide, it may show an advantage. Studies of such therapies are under way. In the meantime, a few doctors are using it as a maintenance treatment for patients undergoing intermittent hormonal therapy, but there are few data on the efficacy of this treatment.

Q: A few years ago, I received external beam radiation for prostate cancer. Recently, a blood test indicated my PSA level is 2.1 ng/ml. However, there is no evidence of clinical progression of my disease. My doctor recommends that I take Proscar. I understand Proscar is prescribed for patients who have BPH. Can you explain why my doctor is making this recommendation? Should I see another doctor?

A: No, you do not need to see another doctor unless you want a second opinion. Proscar inhibits the conversion of testosterone to a more potent androgen known as dihydrotestosterone (DHT). By lowering DHT but not testosterone, Proscar may possibly suppress prostate cancer cell growth. Therefore, if it can significantly delay the PSA level from increasing, Proscar may have a role in the treatment of patients with low-volume disease after radical prostatectomy or external beam radiation. It is not yet clear whether Proscar has a suppressive effect on the growth of prostate cancer or that it prevents or even delays relapse. Before beginning this therapy, however, be sure that your increased PSA level is not just a PSA bounce.

Q: I have stage D2 prostate cancer. Because I have no pain, my doctor wants to wait before treating my disease. What should I do?

A: Speak to another doctor. Patients who have been staged D2 should receive CHT as an initial treatment because prostate cancer is rapidly and extremely well controlled at both the level of the prostate as well as systemically. When the disease progresses, it affects the bones 95 to 98 percent of the time, whereas progression at the level of the prostate is less than 5 percent. Early treatment with CHT for stage D2 patients is important. A study has shown the median survival time to be more than 8 years in patients with one to five bone lesions, whereas survival is drastically reduced to 3.5 years when the number of bone lesions increases from six to ten.

Q: What is the purpose of an antiandrogen withdrawal response?

A: There are several antiandrogenic drugs, such as flutamide, Casodex, and nilutamide, that block the androgen-reception sights in prostate cancer cells. However, when these cells are exposed to antiandrogens for a long period of time, it is thought that the androgen receptor mutates; then the cell can actually be stimulated by the very drug that originally inhibited its growth. By discontinuing the treatment at this time, the cells stop growing, and the PSA decreases accordingly.

Q: I am undergoing combination hormonal therapy. One of the side effects is Gynecomastia or breast enlargement. What can I do about it?

A: Take Arimidex or Dostinex.

Q: What are some side effects of radical prostatectomy?

A: There are many side effects, some more common or more dangerous than others:
- deep vein thrombosis or embolism (blood clot)
- episodes of nerve palsy

- incontinence
- impotence
- blood loss
- rectal injury
- transient lower back pain
- death
- lymph leak/prolonged drainage
- wound infection and hematoma
- myocardial infarction and cardiac arrhythmia

Q: After radical prostatectomy and pelvic lymphadenectomy proves that lymph-node metastases exist, is it better to undergo immediate hormonal therapy or wait until the PSA level rises above 30 ng/ml?

A: We recommend immediate hormonal therapy.

Patients with lymph-node metastases were randomly assigned to receive immediate antiandrogen therapy, with either an LHRH agonist or bilateral orchiectomy, or to receive no treatment until the PSA level rose to 30 ng/ml. The patients were assessed quarterly for a year and then semiannually.

After a median 7.1 years of follow-up, only 7 of the 47 men (15%) who received immediate antiandrogen treatment had died, compared with 18 of 51 men (35%) in the observation group. At the time of the last follow-up, 36 patients in the immediate-treatment group (77%) and 9 men in the observation group (18%) had no evidence of recurrent disease, including undetectable PSA level.

Q: What is the risk of getting prostate cancer from sexual encounters with prostitutes and failing to use condoms?

A: A study by R. B. Hayes and colleagues was carried out among 981 men (479 black, 502 white) with pathologically confirmed prostate cancer and among 1,315 controls (594 black, 721 white). In-person interviews elicited information about sexual behavior and other potential risk factors for prostate cancer. Blood was drawn for serologic studies in a subset of the cases (276) and controls (295). Prostate cancer risk was greater among men who reported a history of gonorrhea or syphilis (odds ratio = 1.6) (95% confidence intervals) or showed evidence of syphilis. Patterns of risk for gonorrhea and syphilis were similar for blacks and whites. Risks increased with increasing occurrences of gonorrhea, rising to an odds ratio = 3.3 (95% CI 1.4-7.8) among patients with three or more events.

367

Q: Why is the DNA ploidy analysis not in favor with some urologists?

A: It is misleading to assume that a tumor is entirely diploid when only a small fraction of it may be diploid. Cells normally found in the seminal vesicles are normally tetraploid and will yield a false positive unless these cells are first recognized as noncancerous.

Q: What drugs should be used with caution when taking Viagra?

A: There are at least three: Tagamet, erythromycin, and Nizoral.

Q: Which patients are most likely to respond to combination hormonal therapy? Which patients are not likely to respond to CHT?

A: Men with a well-differentiated and diploid tumor are most likely to respond to CHT. Those patients with (1) a Gleason score of 8 to 10 and (2) a cancer that produces very little or no PSA, or that has small cell characteristics, are unlikely to benefit from CHT.

Q: What is the drawback of watchful waiting?

A: The possibility that an enlarged prostate gland may block urine flow.

Q: Is watchful waiting as effective as conventional therapies?

A: Several studies have shown that in terms of survival, watchful waiting may be as effective as surgery or radiation, at least for the first 10 years following diagnosis. Its pros and cons need to be carefully considered by patient and physician.

Q: What is a low-risk patient? A high-risk patient?

A: Patients are considered low-risk if they have nonbulky disease (i.e., stage T1 to T2b and B2), a PSA less than 10 ng/ml, and a Gleason score less than 7. Intermediate-risk patients have one only of the above, and high-risk have two or more of the above. Patients classified as intermediate- or high-risk may be better treated with a combination of treatments, such as seed implant and external beam radiation, than either of the above.

Q: What does each category of the Gleason score mean?

A: A Gleason score of 2 to 4 means the cancer has low aggressiveness. A score of 5 to 6 indicates intermediate aggressiveness, and a score of 7 means an aggressive tumor. A Gleason score of 8 to 10 indicates that the tumor is very aggressive, and the chance of cure is usually much less than for patients with lower Gleason scores.

Q: What salvage treatment is appropriate following radiation?

A: There are three: combination hormonal therapy, cryotherapy, and in some cases, radical prostatectomy.

Q: What is the average age of a prostate cancer patient?

A: The average age of a prostate cancer patient is 71.

Q: What are some facts about prostatic intraepithelial neoplasia (PIN)?

- PIN is considered the most likely precursor of prostate cancer.
- PIN has three grades: 1, 2, and 3.
- PIN coexists with prostate cancer.
- PIN mimics prostate cancer, but within the ducts only.
- PIN may predict prostate cancer by more than 10 years.
- The frequency of PIN appears to increase with age.

Q: I had a bilateral orchiectomy. When I asked my doctor if I should take flutamide to counteract any testosterone from the adrenal glands, she said it was unnecessary because the adrenal glands are responsible for only a small percentage of testosterone. Is this true?

A: No. An orchiectomy eliminates androgen and reduces circulating testosterone by 95 percent. The remaining 5 percent is emitted by the adrenal glands. Although the concentration of testosterone in the blood falls to less than one-tenth of normal, the amount of androgen detectable in prostate cancer tissue may be as high as 30 to 40 percent of what it was prior to orchiectomy. Therefore, anyone who has had either surgical or medical castration should consider taking an antiandrogen such as Eulexin, Casodex, or Nilandron.

Q: The prostate gland is divided into three zones. Can prostate cancer be found in all three?

A: No. The central zone is immune to prostate cancer. Prostate cancer tends to invade the peripheral zone, which can sometimes be felt through a digital rectal examination. Prostate cancer also invades the transitional zone, the area responsible for producing benign prostatic hyperplasia.

Q: Is an extended stay on CHT a good idea?

A: A few doctors believe it is undesirable. Fred Lee, M.D., of Valley Sinai Hospital in Commerce, Michigan, believes that if a patient has undergone CHT before getting a baseline reading from a transrectal ultrasound analysis, he should not be treated with cryosurgery until the effects of CHT have diminished. Frank A. Critz, M.D., of Urological Clinics of Georgia in Decatur, requires that patients have at most a minimal stay on CHT because the reduced gland size of some patients hampers his ability to insert an adequate number of seeds. Therefore, it is wise to ask the physician who will treat you just how long you should remain on CHT, if at all.

Q: CHT is no longer effective in treating my disease. Will I live longer by undergoing chemotherapy?

A: There is scant evidence indicating that chemotherapy prolongs survival. Chemotherapy affects each prostate cancer patient differently. Some may live 6 months or less, while others may live 3 years or more. Prior to undergoing chemotherapy, learn as much as you can about the various drugs that are being used with some success.

Q: I had a transurethral resection to treat a urination problem. Now my doctor says I have stage C prostate cancer. What are my treatment options?

A: Most doctors will probably recommend that you undergo external beam radiation. However, if you decide to do this, delay treatment for at least two months in order to avoid urethral stricture. You should begin CHT during this time and continue it at least until the radiation treatments are completed. There are data to support the use of hormonal therapy for up to 3 years. You may also be a candidate for seed implantation. Seek the opinions of at least one specialist in each of these treatment approaches.

Q: I underwent external beam radiation about 2 years ago. My PSA level has risen from 4.6 to 5.7 within a month. Is this acceptable?

A: In 1989, Thomas Stamey, M.D., in a controversial study, used a cutoff PSA level of 1.0 ng/ml to predict a recurrence of prostate cancer for patients undergoing external beam radiation. However, a study conducted by researchers in the Department of Urology, University of Texas, M. D. Anderson Cancer Center, concluded a higher PSA level indicated a recurrence. They maintained that the most clinically useful model for predicting an identifiable recurrence of prostate cancer after external beam radiation was either (1) a PSA level above 2.0 ng/ml or (2) a PSA level of 2.0 ng/ml or less and an abnormal image (or images) on an ultrasound. More important is monitoring sized PSAs if bounce is not a clinical consideration. Prostatic biopsy, depending on when it is done, may be diagnostic.

Q: African-American men have a higher incidence of prostate cancer than do white American men. How does prostate cancer affect these two groups differently?

A: This has perplexed both doctors and researchers for years. However, we do know several things about the disparity between blacks and whites in regard to prostate cancer:

1. On average, African-American men have prostate cancer in two to three lobes of their prostate, whereas whites tend to have it in one lobe.
2. On average, African-American men have a level of testosterone 15 percent higher than that found in whites.
3. Black men are more reluctant than white men to undergo a physical examination or a digital rectal examination.
4. Blacks are more likely to undergo radiation and watchful waiting, while whites are more prone to undergo radical prostatectomy.
5. African Americans have tumors that are on average 1 to 2.5 times the size of tumors in white men.
6. Black men develop prostate cancer about 3 years earlier than do white men.
7. Blacks are diagnosed more often than whites with advanced prostate cancer.
8. African Americans tend to have higher PSA levels than whites have.
9. Some researchers suggest that African-American men may develop a particularly aggressive form of prostate cancer not usually found in white men.
10. The upper limits of the PSA blood test are lower for African-American men (2.0 to 5.5 ng/ml) than for white men (2.5 to 6.5 ng/ml).

Q: I have advanced prostate cancer, stage D2. How long will I be able to remain on CHT before it begins to fail? How long will I be able to remain on a second hormonal management therapy before it too begins to fail? And, finally, how long will I be able to survive under chemotherapy?

A: Hormone-refractory disease usually appears after a median of 18 months of CHT; however, it cannot be predicted how long any individual will respond. We have seen some men with a Gleason score of 8 respond to CHT for more than 8 years. You will most likely be able to remain under a second hormonal manipulation therapy for about 3 to 6 months before it begins to fail, but again there are many exceptions. The median time of survival under chemotherapy is 12 months. However, prostate cancer is an individualized disease and affects each man differently. Some men have survived under CHT for 10 years, and a few patients have been known to remain chemotherapy-responsive for 3 years.

Q: A friend who has prostate cancer told me that his doctor has prescribed Proscar to improve CHT. However, when I asked my doctor about adding Proscar to my own hormonal regimen, he said that it adds nothing to CHT. Is this true?

A: Not necessarily. The concept of adding Proscar to CHT is based on findings published in *European Urology* (1993) on the treatment of advanced prostate cancer with a combination of Proscar and flutamide, as well as in an abstract of the American Urology Association Meeting in May 1994. It is also based on the concept of additional blockade in the conversion of testosterone to dihydrotestosterone by interfering with the enzyme involved in the conversion - namely, 5-alpha reductase. Dr. Labrie, who developed CHT, maintains that "the additional androgen blockade achieved by the addition of a 5-alpha reductase inhibitor could improve combination hormonal therapy." Stephen Strum, M.D., and others believe that use of Proscar during the "off after" of intermittent androgen blockade prolongs the time off therapy.

Q: I had a radical prostatectomy 2 years ago. Within the last 9 months, my PSA has risen from 0.4 to 1.7 ng/ml. My doctor said I have a recurrence and suggested I be retreated with external beam radiation. Do I have any other options?

A: Yes, you do. You could opt for combination or intermittent hormonal therapy, an orchiectomy with or without an antiandrogen such as Eulexin or Casodex, and/or external beam radiation. Some physicians also implant seeds in the setting. The first three options are standard procedures; however, seed implantation is not routine after a failed prostatectomy. Frank A. Critz, M.D., has treated 33 patients whose cancer recurred after prostatectomy. He reported that after surgery two patients had elevated PSA level of 2.6 and 4.4 ng/ml and so underwent seed implantation and external beam radiation. Although Critz could not locate any clinical evidence of recurrence, he strategically seeded the bed of the removed prostate.

Three weeks after seed implantation, he applied external beam radiation to the bed and surrounding areas. Each patient had a subsequent PSA level of 0.2 ng/ml or below. The median follow-up age for the patients is at least 10 years as reported by his 10-year results.

Q: Is the survival of prostate cancer patients related to their age or race?

A: Survival of patients with prostate cancer is related to the extent of the tumor in the prostate and number of tumors and whether the disease has spread beyond the gland. When the cancer is confined to the prostate, the disease is frequently curable, and median survival in excess of 10 years can usually be anticipated. Patients with locally advanced cancer are not usually curable, and a substantial number will eventually die from it, although median survival may well be more than 5 years. If prostate cancer has spread to distant organs, current therapy will not cure it. Median survival in such cases is usually 1 to 3 years, and the majority of such patients will die. However, even in this group of patients, some may live 10 years or more.

Q: I recently underwent an orchiectomy. I am now having terrible hot flashes, from the bottom of my legs to the top of my head. My doctor said that very little could be done about this condition. Is this true?

A: Your doctor is not necessarily correct. Hot flashes usually affect a patient's face, neck, upper chest, and back. It is unusual for the legs to be affected. Triggers of hot flashes caused by LHRH agonists, such as Lupron and Zoladex, and by antiandrogens, such as Eulexin and Casodex, include the warmth from radiant heaters, eating hot foods, drinking alcohol, and taking certain medications.

Usually, hot flashes can be treated with 1 mg of estrogen (DES) per day or by using progesterone-based drugs such as Provera or Megace. Antidepressants such as Effexor or an SSRI (e.g., Prozac) can help alleviate these symptoms.

373

Q: Can you explain the staging classifications for prostate caner?

A: The current staging employed in the United States follows:

Stage	Criteria
A1	One to three foci of well-differentiated, tumor or less than 5 percent of specimen contains tumor that is well-differentiated with Gleason score of 2, 3, or 4. Some authors accept up to Gleason score 7.
A2	Fewer than 3 foci or less than 5 percent well-differentiated tumor for any moderate- or poorly differentiated tumor.
B1n	Nodule occupying 1.5 cm or less in one lobe with normal prostate on four sides.
B1	Nodule, 1 to 1.5 cm in size, surrounded on three sides by normal prostate.
B1	Nodule, confined to prostate, involving less than one lobe.
B2	Nodule, confined to prostate, involving one whole lobe, both lobes, or bilateral nodules.
B3*	One tumor involving both lobes or nodules in both lobes; both biopsies positive.
C	Local extension beyond prostate.
C1	Lateral extension.
C2	Seminal-vesicle extension.
C3	Both lateral extension and seminal-vesicle extension.
D0*	Local disease rectally, elevated serum enzymatic acid phosphatase.
D1	Local disease rectally; positive obturator; hypogastric, external, or common iliac lymph nodes.

Stage	Criteria
D2	Nodal disease, outside pelvis; bone metastases and/or soft-tissue metastases.
D3*	Metastatic disease that has failed initial hormone therapy

* Stages not totally accepted.

The TNM system is not widely used in the United States, but its relationship to the Jewett-Whitmore staging is listed. It is a clinical and pathological staging.

T0a	Focal tumor at prostatectomy
T0b	Diffuse tumor at prostatectomy
T1a	1-cm nodule, confined to prostate
T1b	1-cm nodule, confined to one lobe
T1c	Involves both lobes, confined
T2	Invades but does not penetrate capsule
T3	Penetrates capsule with or without seminal-vesicle invasion
T4	Fixed to periprostatic side wall or adjacent organs
N1	Single lymph node, homolateral
N2	Multiple or contralateral lymph nodes
N3	Bulky pelvic lymph nodes
N4	Juxtaregional lymph nodes involved
Mx	No metastases found of incomplete assessment
M0	No known metastases
M1	Metastases present

Q: Andy Grove, CEO of Intel, opted for the "smart bomb" protocol to treat his prostate cancer. Do you think this was a wise choice?

A: We really do not know. However, we will answer your question to the best of our knowledge based on the following summary of protocols:

1. *Radiotherapy Clinics of Georgia:* A radioactive implant is done first, and then, beginning 3 weeks after the implant, external beam radiation is given. Thus, the cancer cells are irradiated simultaneously, producing a probable synergistic effect. In

addition, the iodine seeds are used as targets for the conformal beam radiation.

2. *Northwest Tumor Institute:* External beam radiation is given initially, followed approximately 6 weeks later by seed implant. The seeds used are either iodine or palladium. The two forms of irradiation are given separately.

3. *Swedish Medical Center:* A prostate implant using an intermittently high dose of irradiation is done over a 2-day period. This is not a permanent implant. Several weeks after the treatment, external beam radiation is delivered. The seeds are not in place for a target. Both forms of irradiation are given separately.

Q: My doctor said I have a Gleason score of 8 and should undergo a prostatectomy immediately. Do you agree?

A: Although it would be helpful if we knew your PSA level, your stage, and your age, we don't necessarily think so. Your Gleason score indicates you have an aggressive disease and that it has most likely spread beyond your gland. In this case, prostatectomy is futile.

Types of Differentiated Cells

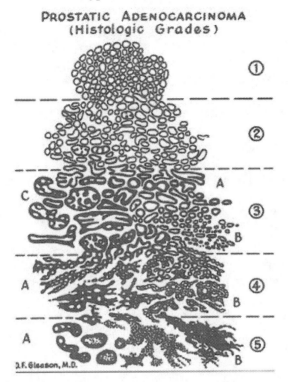

Fig 44-1 Gleason grading system of prostatic
adenocarcinoma.

Figure 44-1 shows the variations in shape, size, and arrangement of prostate cancer cells. Well-differentiated tumors (*top two panels*) — those that most resemble normal glandular tissue — are thought to behave less aggressively than the less organized, moderately differentiated (*middle panel*) or poorly differentiated tumors (*bottom two panels*). In the Gleason system, the degree of differentiation is indicated by a numerical value ranging from 1 to 5. The score for the predominant pattern is often added to that of the next most prevalent pattern to yield a final Gleason score ranging from 2 to 10.

We advise you to see another doctor, preferably a medical oncologist with a subspecialty in prostate cancer.

GLOSSARY

10-12 pattern biopsy: ten to twelve cores extracted from the prostate gland.

5-alpha reductase: enzyme in the prostate gland that converts testosterone to DHT (the active form of male hormone in the prostate).

5-region biopsy: tissue extracted from five regions of the prostate gland.

abdomen: the part of the body located below the ribs and above the pelvis.

acid phosphatase, total serum (ACP): enzyme that is present in the prostate gland, and in smaller amounts in blood cells, bones, and other body organs; elevated ACP levels may indicate extracapsular prostate cancer and other diseases.

adjuvant therapy: a treatment method used in addition to the primary therapy. Radiation therapy is often used as an adjuvant to surgery.

adrenal glands: two glands located above the kidneys (one above each kidney). They produce several kinds of hormones, including a small amount of sex hormones.

age-adjusted: statistical method used to adjust effects of age of an individual or group of individuals; for example, prostate cancer survival data and average normal PSA values may be adjusted according to the ages of groups of men.

alkaline phosphatase: an enzyme made by cells in the bone, liver, etc.

alprostadil: an FDA-approved drug to improve or restore potency in men.

alternative treatment: complementary therapy or alternative medicine, including homeopathy, holistic medicine, and Chinese medicine.

AMACR: a gene in which an overexpression indicates prostate cancer in tissues, thus nullifying the need for a repeat biopsy.

analog: a synthetic look-alike body chemical or drug.

androgen: male sex hormone produced by the testicles and, in small amounts, by the adrenal glands.

anesthesia: loss of feeling or sensation resulting from the use of certain drugs or gases.

aneuploid: a very aggressive prostate cancer tumor, which has more or less than the normal 46 chromosomes.

angiogenesis: formation of new blood vessels.

antiandrogen: a drug such as Casodex, Eulexin, and Nilandron used in hormone therapy to treat prostate cancer by blocking the impact of testosterone and DHT on prostate cancer cells by neutralizing their effects.

antiandrogen withdrawal response (AAWR): decrease in PSA caused by the withdrawal of an antiandrogen, such as bicalutamide or Eulexin, once combined hormonal therapy begins to fail; may occur when sensitized prostate cancer cells that have mutated feed on antiandrogens; the withdrawal destroys such sensitized cells.

antiangiogenesis: prevention of the development of new blood vessels.

anti-malignin antibody in serum (AMAS) test: a blood test that can be used to determine the presence of cancer in the body.

anus: opening at the lower end of the rectum through which solid waste is eliminated.

apoptosis: process by which cells create their own controlled death in response to intracellular or extracellular events; also called programmed cell death.

aspiration biopsy: biopsy that uses suction to remove fluid or cells from the body, usually through a fine needle.

atypia: a condition of being irregular or not standard.

autologous vaccine: preparation obtained from a process that combines the patient's own cancer cells with an agent that results in a significant immune response.

Befar: a topical cream for treating erectile dysfunction.

benign: a nonmalignant or noncancerous.

benign prostatic hyperplasia/benign prostatic hypertrophy (BPH): a noncancerous condition of the prostate; generally, an enlargement of the gland, sometimes obstructing urination, which can result in secondary complications.

bilateral orchiectomy: surgical removal of the testicles to halt production of testosterone.

biochemical failure: a process of ascertaining whether or not a treatment has failed by conducting a PSA blood test.

biopsy: the procedure used to obtain tissue, which is then examined by a pathologist to distinguish between cancerous and noncancerous conditions; for prostate cancer this may be a needle biopsy or transurethral resection of the prostate (TURP).

bladder: the hollow organ that stores urine.

blood chemistry profile: analysis of multiple components in the blood, including tests to evaluate function of the liver and kidneys, minerals, cholesterol, etc.; abnormal values can indicate spread of cancer or side effects of treatment(s).

blood count: analysis, primarily of red blood cells (which help transport oxygen in the body), white blood cells (which protect against infection), and platelets (necessary for clotting of blood); abnormal values can indicate cancerous involvement of the bone marrow, or side effects of treatment(s).

Bluestein table: a probability table for determining clinical stages.

bone scan: more sensitive technique than conventional X-rays; uses a radioactive agent injected into the bloodstream to identify abnormal or cancerous growths within or attached to bone. In the case of prostate cancer, a bone scan is used to identify metastases of cancer cells that have escaped from the prostate and set up house in a bony location; metastases appear as "hot spots" on the film; however, the absence of hot spots does not prove the absence of microscopic metastases; suspicious areas are often difficult to distinguish from arthritis.

brachytherapy: treatment with radioactive sources placed into or very near a tumor; includes surface application, body cavity application, and placement into the tissue. Sometimes used interchangeably with internal radiation therapy.

Calcitriol: a form of vitamin D.

cancer: a general term for more than 200 diseases in which abnormal cells multiply without control. Cancer cells can spread through the bloodstream and lymphatic system to the other parts of the body.

capsule: muscle-like tissue surrounding the prostate gland.

carcinoma: cancer cells that form in the lining of an organ or cavity.

Careseng: an extract from the herb ginseng capable of destroying prostate cells.

Casodex: antiandrogen used to block the uptake of testosterone at the receptors of the adrenal gland.

castration: elimination of testicular function, either by surgical removal of the testes (surgical castration) or by administration of an LHRH agonist (a class of drugs designed to inhibit testicular function).

catheterization: insertion of a catheter through the urethra into the bladder.

Caverject: see Alprostadil.

chemiluminescent assay: test to detect extremely minute amounts of PSA that may be secreted by tissue cells other than prostate cancer cells.

chemotherapy (chemo): use of pharmaceuticals or other chemicals to kill cancer cells; in many cases, chemotherapeutic agents kill not only cancer cells but also other cells in the body, which makes such agents potentially very dangerous; may be taken by mouth, or injected into a vein, artery, or muscle; considered a systemic treatment because, as the drugs travel through the body, they can kill cancer cells anywhere in the body.

clinical failure: a process for ascertaining by means other than a blood test whether a treatment has failed.

clinical trial: study conducted with cancer patients, usually to evaluate a promising new treatment. Each study is designed to answer scientific questions and find better ways to treat patients.

cobalt 60: a radioactive substance used as a radiation source to treat cancer.

combined hormonal therapy (CHT): use of more than one hormone in therapy; see ADT, monotherapy.

complementary treatment: see alternative treatment.

computed tomography: see CT scan.

conformal radiotherapy: therapy in which a radiation beam is shaped (conformed) to target the area that needs treatment.

contraindication: situation in which a medical treatment is not recommended because of undesirable side effects.

control group: in an experimental study, the group of subjects who do not receive the experimental treatment; the effects of treatment on the experimental group are compared to the effects of no treatment on the control group.

conventional treatment: a treatment falling into any one of three categories: surgery, radiation, and chemotherapy.

core biopsy: removal through a large needle of a piece of a tumor or lump, called a core; the core is then sent to the laboratory to determine if the tumor is benign or malignant.

corpora cavernosa: two cylindrical compartments situated alongside the penis.

cryoprobes: a chilled instrument used in cryosurgery to freeze tissue.

cryosurgery: use of liquid nitrogen probes to freeze a particular portion of an organ to extremely low temperatures to kill the tissue prior to surgery used to destroy cancerous tissue; when used to treat prostate cancer, the cryoprobes are guided by transrectal ultrasound.

CT scan: method of combining images from multiple X-rays under the control of a computer to produce cross-sectional or three-dimensional pictures of the internal organs; can be used to identify abnormalities; can identify prostate enlargement, but is not always effective for assessing the stage of prostate cancer; significantly more accurate for evaluating metastases to lymph nodes or distant soft-tissue sites.

cystoscope: a lighted instrument used to look at the inside of the urethra and bladder.

cytoluminescent Therapy (CLT): advanced form of photodynamic therapy that uses light to fight cancer.

dendritic cell therapy: immune therapy using specialized white blood cells that efficiently present antigen to other cells; such cells are removed from a patient's blood and pulsed in the lab to enhance their activity with prostate-specific membrane antigen (PSMA) peptides, then reinjected into the patient; plays a pivotal role in initiation of immune responses; under study.

deoxyribonucleic acid (DNA): basic biologically active chemical that maintains our genetic codes; may insure healthy cell division.

detoxifying: cleansing the body by eliminating toxins, waste materials, and dead cells.

DHT (dihydrotestosterone): active form of male hormone in the prostate gland that is made when testosterone is changed by an enzyme called 5-alpha reductase.

diagnosis: evaluation of symptoms and/or tests leading to a conclusion about a patient's medical condition.

digital rectal examination (DRE): examination by a physician in which a gloved and lubricated finger is inserted into the patient's rectum; used to screen for abnormalities of the prostate and rectum; the physician palpates (feels) the prostate gland through the rectal wall; the presence of lumps or hard areas indicate possible prostate cancer.

dihydrotestosterone: <u>see</u> DHT.

diploid: slow-growing prostate cancer cell that has the normal 46 chromosomes.

DNA ploidy analysis: study used to determine the growth characteristics of prostate cancer cells by determining the number of chromosomes.

DNA ploidy analysis through static cytometry: pathological analysis that may determine the ploidy patterns from a sample of tissue obtained from a fine-needle aspiration biopsy. This test compares the number of chromosomes and the DNA in a normal cell; may indicate whether the cell has the potential for fast or slow growth.

docetaxel: an anticancer chemotherapy drug sometimes referred to as Taxotere.

Doppler, power: highly sensitive form of color Doppler; shows blood flow and velocity in normal and abnormal blood vessels and detects the increased blood flow by growing prostate cancer.

double-blind study: form of clinical trial in which neither the physician nor the patient knows the actual treatment that any individual patient is receiving; double-blind trials minimize the influence of the placebo effect as well as the personal opinions of patients and physicians on the results of the trial.

doubling time: time that it takes a particular focus of cancer to double in size.

DR70: A test designed to detect at least 13 different tests.

DRE: see digital rectal examination.

dysplasia: abnormal growth or development, as of organs or cells.

ejaculation: release of semen through the penis during orgasm.

endorectal MRI: magnetic resonance imaging in which a long narrow tube containing radio-frequency coils is inserted into the rectum; this technique provides a clearer picture of the prostate gland than does the standard MRI; see magnetic resonance imaging.

erectile dysfunction (ED): consistent inability to achieve and/or maintain an erection sufficient for sexual activity: see impotence.

estrogen: a female sex hormone.

estrogen patch: female sex hormone, estrogen, which is absorbed through the skin.

external beam radiation therapy: treatment with high-energy radiation given from a source located outside the body.

extracapsular extension: condition in which a tumor has invaded and extended through and beyond the prostatic capsule, indicating a more advanced stage of the disease.

extracapsular prostate tissue: tissue that immediately surrounds the outside of the prostate; if the cancer has spread to this area or beyond, it is considered to be advanced.

EZH2 gene: a gene to express metastatic prostate cancer.

false negative: erroneous negative test results; for example, an imaging test that fails to show the presence of a tumor that is later found by biopsy to be present in the patient, is said to be a false negative result.

false positive: positive test result mistakenly identifying a state or condition that does not in fact exist.

flow cytometry: the process by which graphs or histograms are plotted based on the DNA content of the cancerous tissue cells.

Foley catheter: in terms of men, a tube that is inserted through the tip of the penis into the urethra until it enters the bladder.

ginseng: root found mainly in Asia; animal studies are under way to determine if Korean red ginseng saponins can modulate carcinogenic metabolism and impact the progression of established and developing cancerous lesions in the rat colon.

Gleason grading: system of describing the degree of aggressiveness of prostate cancer based on the appearance of the cancer cells.

Gleason score: widely used method for classifying the cellular differentiation of cancerous tissues; the less the cancerous cells appear like normal cells, the more malignant the cancer. Two numbers, each from 1 to

5, are assigned successively to the two predominant patterns of differentiation present in the examined tissue sample; added together, these produce the Gleason score. Low numbers of 2, 3, and 4 indicate a well-differentiated cancer; 5 and 6 indicate a moderately well differentiated cancer and grade 7 is considered significant. High numbers (8, 9, 10) indicate poor differentiation and a disease with a more aggressive clinical behavior.

Gray (Gy): 100 rads. The unit of radiation dosage; used in therapeutic cancer management usually vary from 45 to 65 gray; a <u>centigray</u> is 1/100 of a gray.

high-intensity focused ultrasound (HIFU): treatment for benign prostatic hyperplasia that uses heat from ultrasound energy to trim excess prostate tissue; <u>see</u> ablatherm.

hormonal (or hormonally) refractory: a condition in which hormonal therapy or medical castration is no longer controlling prostate cancer.

hormonally insensitive: prostate cancer cells that are no longer sensitive to hormonal therapy.

hormonally sensitive: prostate cancer cells that are sensitive to hormonal therapy.

hormone: a chemical substance that is formed in one part of the body, travels through the blood, and affects the function of cells elsewhere in the body.

hormone therapy (HT): use of hormones, hormone analogs, and certain surgical techniques to treat disease (e.g., advanced prostate cancer), either on their own or in combination with other hormones, or in combination with other methods of treatment. Because prostate cancer is usually dependent on male hormones to grow, hormonal therapy can be an effective means of alleviating symptoms and retarding the development of the disease.

hot spot: image on a bone scan that may indicate a site of prostate cancer that has spread to the bones.

hyperthermia: a treatment for cancer using heat produced by microwave radiation.

imaging: technique or method allowing a physician to see something in the body that would otherwise not be visible.

immune system: the human body's defense system, which fights disease, bacteria, and virus.

implant: device that is inserted into the body; for example, a tiny container of radioactive material inserted in or near a tumor. Also, a device to replace or substitute for an ability that has been lost; for example, an implant inserted into the penis to provide rigidity for intercourse.

impotence: partial or complete loss of erection, which may be associated with a loss of libido; may be a result of injury due to radiation therapy, surgical resection of the prostate, prostatectomy, hormone deprivation therapy, disease, or other cause.

IMRT: see intensity modulated radiation therapy.

incision: a cut into the body or an organ during surgery.

incontinence, urinary: partial or complete loss of bladder control; may be a result of injury due to radiation therapy, prostatectomy, or surgical resection of the prostate.

indium-111: radioactive material injected into a patient undergoing a ProstaScint scan; see ProstaScint.

infusion: technique for intravenous administration of drugs, or other treatments in liquid form, at a controlled rate.

intensity modulated radiation therapy (IMRT): sophisticated computer program that pinpoints the cancer for radiation treatment so that the surrounding healthy tissue of the bladder and rectum is spared.

intermittent combined hormone therapy (ICHT): hormonal treatment with LHRH agonists and an antiandrogen that is administered intermittently.

intermittent hormone therapy (IHT): hormone therapy administered periodically.

internal radiation: a type of therapy in which a radioactive substance is implanted into or close to the area needing treatment.

interstitial implant: a radioactive source placed directly into the tissue (not in a body cavity).

iodine-125: radioactive isotope implanted into the gland and used in brachytherapy.

iridium-192: radioactive isotope, with a prolonged half-life, used in brachytherapy.

laparoscopic prostatectomy: a radical prostatectomy using laparoscopy.

laparoscopic surgery: a minimally invasive form of abdominal surgery.

laparoscopy: technique that allows a physician to observe internal organs through optical
equipment inserted into the body through a small surgical incision.

linear accelerator: a machine that creates high-energy radiation to treat cancers by using electricity to form a stream of fast-moving subatomic particles.

local therapy: treatment that affects a tumor and the tissue near it.

luteinizing hormone-releasing hormone (LHRH) agonist: a substance that closely resembles LHRH, which controls the production of sex hormones. However, LHRH agonists affect the body differently than does LHRH. LHRH agonists keep the testicles from producing hormones.

lymph: the almost colorless fluid that travels through the lymphatic system and carries cells that help fight infection.

lymph-node involvement: presence of tumor cells in the lymph nodes of the pelvis.

lymph nodes: small, bean-shaped organs located along the channels of the lymphatic system. The lymph nodes store special cells that can trap bacteria or cancer cells traveling through the body.

lymphadenectomy: surgical removal of one or more lymph nodes for purposes of microscopic examination; may be performed as an <u>open pelvic lymphadenectomy</u> as the initial approach during radical prostatectomy, or as a separate procedure prior to radical prostatectomy by means of small incision(s) into the pelvic cavity (laparoscopic lymphadenectomy).

lymphatic system: the tissues and organs that produce, store, and carry cells that fight infection and disease. This system includes the bone marrow, spleen, thymus, lymph nodes, and channels that carry lymph.

magnetic resonance imaging (MRI): imaging process that uses magnetic resonance with atoms in body tissues to produce distinct cross-sectional and three-dimensional images of internal organs; MRI is useful in staging biopsy-proven prostate cancer.

magnetic resonance imaging scan (MRI): a sophisticated use of an electromagnet and sound waves to create a detailed X-ray - type image by measurement of signal intensity of a particular body part or region; in general, this may be the most effective means of detecting whether a tumor has penetrated through the capsule of the prostate gland, invaded the seminal vesicle(s), or both; can be used to evaluate whether pelvic lymph nodes are enlarged.

magnetic resonance spectroscope imaging (MRSI): imaging using a magnetic field and radio waves to obtain pictures based on the concentration of cellular chemicals; detects cellular metabolites, citrate, creatine, and choline.

malignant: cancerous; tending to become progressively worse and to result in death; having the invasive and metastatic properties of cancer.

metastasis (sing.), metastases (pl.): spread or transfer of a malignant tumor to another part of the body not directly connected to the original tumor location; all malignant tumors have the potential to metastasize (spread), while benign conditions do not.

metastasize: to spread to other parts of the body.

metastatic cancer: cancer that has spread to a site distant from the original site.

moderately differentiated: a classification of prostate cancer in which the cells are beginning to lose their shape; this corresponds to a Gleason score of 5, 6, or 7.

nanogram: a procedure that enables physicians and patients to render treatment decisions based on medical and personal data.

necrosis: the sum of the morphological (structure of animals and plants) changes indicative of cell death and caused by the progressive degradative action of enzymes; may affect groups of cells or part of a structure or an organ; <u>see</u> apoptosis.

neoadjuvant therapy: therapy given before the pharmacy treatment in order to shrink a cancerous tumor. At the present time, it is still not very accurate.

neutron beam radiation: a form of external beam radiation designed to kill prostate cancer cells.

neutron particles: supplement to photon beams of radiation to help improve the effectiveness of the therapy.

Nilandron: nilutamide (Hoechst Marion Roussel); a nonsteroidal antiandrogen used as add-on therapy after surgical or chemical castration due to prostate cancer; reduces bone pain in men with advanced prostate cancer; known in Canada as Anandron.

NMP 48: blood marker for detecting cancer.

oncologist: a doctor who specializes in treating cancer. Some oncologists specialize in a particular type of cancer treatment - for example, a radiation oncologist treats cancer with radiation.

orchiectomy: surgical removal of the testicles; certain drugs or radiation can result in a <u>nonsurgical orchiectomy</u>.

palladium-103: a seed used in seed implantation having a much shorter half-life than iodine-125, which is usually reserved for prostate cancer patients with moderate and poorly differentiated tumors.

palliate: to ease or relieve symptoms of prostate cancer to improve quality of life.

palliative therapy: a treatment that may relieve symptoms without curing the disease.

Papaverine: a drug approved by the FDA to restore potency in men through an injection.

Partin II tables: tables that use PSA growth after prostatectomy to distinguish local recurrence from distant metastases.

Partin tables: tables used to determine the probability that a prostate cancer patient's disease has spread to the lymph nodes, seminal vesicles, or beyond.

pathologist: a doctor who identifies disease by studying cells and tissues under a microscope.

pelvic: referring to the area of the body located below the waist and surrounded by the hip and pubic bones.

perineal prostatectomy: surgery to remove the prostate through an incision made between the scrotum and the anus.

perineum: in men, the area between the scrotum and anus.

PET scan: a diagnostic examination that involves the biologic images on the detection of subatomic particles.

pH: the controlling factor for hundreds of enzymes in the body involving digestion and assimilation of nutrients and the production of energy in the cells or potential hydrogen, which measures the number of hydroxl ions which are negative and alkaline-forming or opposed to the amount of hydrogen ions that are positive and acid-forming.

phase I: "first time in humans" trial to ascertain if a drug is safe and at what dose; the phase series usually starts after years of laboratory testing, followed by trials on animals; phase I trials usually involve fewer than a hundred participants.

phase II: small-scale trial of a drug's efficacy on human beings who are sick; usually involves a number of volunteers randomly selected as study and control groups.

phase III: large clinical trial using volunteers randomly selected and grouped for study and control to test the safety and efficacy of drug dosages; results are compared with the prevailing standard treatment, a placebo, or both.

phase IV: after approval of a drug, an ongoing study of its safety and efficacy; results are reported to the drug manufacturer, to the appropriate government regulatory agency, or both.

photon beam radiation: low-level laser therapy that transforms light of various frequencies into a very small and intense beam that produces very high heat and power.

phytotherapeutic agent: plant-delivered substance.

PIN (prostatic intraepithelial neoplasia): a pathologically identifiable finding believed to be a precursor of prostate cancer; also known as dysplasia; see atypia, dysplasia.

ploidy: number of sets of chromosomes in a cell; a human cell has 46 chromosomes in its nucleus: see diploid and aneuploid.

ploidy analysis: method used to tell the degree of abnormality of the DNA complement of cancer cells; abnormal ploidy is associated with a cancer's aggressiveness.

poorly differentiated: a classification of prostate cancer in which there is no definite shape of the cells; corresponds to a Gleason score from 8 to 10.

positron emission tomography (PET): type of X-ray that uses two radiotracer drugs to locate and determine tumor activity.

primary: refers to the organ or gland where a cancer begins, from which it may then spread (e.g., "primary" prostate cancer, which may "metastasize" to the bone).

prognosis: probable outcome or course of a disease; the chance of recovery.

progression: the continued growth of a cancer, or arecurrence of cancer after a previous response to treatment.

Proscar: finasteride (Merck); inhibitor of the enzyme 5-alpha reductase; often prescribed as part of a complete androgen blockade; used to treat complications of benign prostatic hyperplasia (BPH).

prostaScint: image in which a monoclonal antibody with great affinity for prostatic tissue - in particular, malignant tumor - is combined with a radioactive material (indium-111); the substance is injected intravenously and allowed to "settle" for 3 days; the radiolabeled antibody preferentially attaches itself to existing lesions. When the body is scanned, these lesions are detected by the radioactive emissions; used to help determine how far a tumor has spread.

prostate: a male sex gland that produces a fluid that forms part of semen.

prostatectomy: an operation to remove part or all of the prostate.

prostate-specific antigen (PSA): protein secreted by the epithelial cells of the prostate gland, including cancer cells; an elevated level in the blood indicates an abnormal condition of the prostate, either benign or malignant; used to detect potential problems in the prostate to follow the progress of prostate cancer therapy. It is recommended that the PSA blood sample be taken prior to a DRE, biopsy, or any other form of prostatic manipulation; see screening.

prostate specific antigen (PSA) test: blood test to measure a substance produced by prostate gland cells; used for screening (an elevated PSA level indicates an abnormal condition of the prostate, either benign or malignant, requiring further investigation); also used to monitor the progress of a patient undergoing treatment; it is the most sensitive "marker" of prostate cancer that is currently available.

prostate-specific antigen type II (free PSA, PSA II): the percentage of free PSA to total PSA (total PSA equals free PSA plus bound PSA); helpful for screening purposes when the PSA level is above the normal, but less than 10.

prostate-specific membrane antigen: a blood test used to determine the existence of prostate cancer by measuring the level of a substance called prostatic specific membrane antigen in the blood.

prostatic acid phosphatase (PAP): enzyme produced by the prostate; its level in the blood goes up in some men whose prostate cancer has reached the pelvic lymph nodes or gone beyond them.

prostatic acid phosphatase (PAP) assay: a blood test to measure a substance produced by prostate gland cells; also useful as a marker because the PAP is typically elevated if there is metastasis.

prostRcision: formerly known as <u>combined precision irradiation (CPI)</u>, a protocol for prostate cancer in which the patient receives iodine-125 followed by external beam radiation.

proton beam radiation: procedure that may use as many as 12 beams of radiation to treat tumors; proton subparticles are absorbed by the tumor instead of emerging through the lesion.

proton beam therapy: form of radiation using protons to treat cancer patients; the proton beam is focused on the site of the cancer; protons are elementary particles found in the nuclei of all atoms, rather than X-ray radiation.

Provenge: a prostate cancer vaccine.

PSA age-specific: suggested PSA level based on age.

PSA bump: an increase of 0.1 ng/ml or more above the preceding PSA level, followed by a subsequent decrease below that level.

PSA density (PSAD): formula in which the PSA is divided by the size or volume of the prostate.

PSA doubling time (PSADT): time it takes the PSA to double in value; an index of the aggressiveness of a tumor.

PSA II: the blood test used to determine if a patient has benign prostatic hyperplasia (BPH) by measuring the amount of free PSA.

PSA transitional zone: a method of determining prostate cancer by deciding the value of the transition zone of the prostate gland by the PSA level.

PSA velocity: the process of identifying the degree of change in the PSA level from year to year.

PSMA (prostate-specific membrane antigen): a diagnostic prostate marker.

Quadramet: samarium 153 (Cytogen); injectable radiotherapy treatment to minimize pain of bone metastases.

rad: short for <u>radiation absorbed dose</u>; a measurement of the amount of radiation absorbed by tissues (100 rad = 1 gray).

radiation: energy carried by waves or a stream of particles.

radiation oncologist: a doctor who specializes in using radiation to treat cancer.

radiation physicist: a person trained to ensure that the radiation machine delivers the right amount of radiation to the treatment site.

radiation therapy: treatment with high-energy rays from X-rays or other sources to damage cancer cells; the radiation may be from a machine (<u>external radiation therapy</u>) or from radioactive materials placed inside the body as close as possible to the cancer (<u>internal radiation therapy</u>).

radical prostatectomy: surgery to remove the entire prostate; the two types of radical prostatectomy are <u>retropubic</u> and <u>perineal</u>.

radiosensitizer: drug used to make tumors more sensitive to radiation.

rectal exam: a procedure in which a doctor inserts a gloved, lubricated finger into the rectum and feels the prostate through the wall of the rectum to check the prostate for hard or lumpy areas.

recurrence: reappearance of prostate cancer after the failure of an initial treatment.

refractory: resistant to therapy.

remission: real or apparent disappearance of some or all of the signs and symptoms of cancer; the period (temporary or permanent) during which a disease remains under control - that is, without clinical progression; complete remission does not necessarily indicate cure.

response: a decrease in the extent of a disease as evidenced by a reduction or disappearance of visible tumor and/or markers, which may be complete or partial; because untreated cancers are generally progressive, stability (no change) of disease is sometimes considered to be a positive response to treatment.

retropubic prostatectomy: surgical removal of the prostate through an incision in the abdomen.

retropubic: a surgical procedure in which the surgeon makes an incision in the lower abdomen.

RT-PCR PSA blood test: a test to determine if a patient's prostate cancer is in the bloodstream, which indicates that it has spread outside the capsule or beyond.

salvage therapy: treatment used to eradicate residual prostate cancer that may be outside the capsule and beyond.

scan: to systematically examine with a sensing device, such as a beam of radiation.

scrotum: pouch of skin that contains the testicles.

seed implantation: treatment for prostate cancer in which radioactive seeds are inserted in the prostate gland to kill malignant cells.

semen: the fluid that is released through the penis during orgasm; made up of sperm from the testicles and fluid from the prostate and other sex glands.

seminal-vesicle involvement: extension of prostate cancer into the seminal vesicles; indicates a more advanced stage of cancer.

sextant: having six parts; thus, a sextant biopsy takes six representative samples.

sextant biopsy: an attempt to get a comprehensive picture of the prostate by extracting six tiny samples of cells through the gland.

side effect: reaction to a medication or treatment; most commonly used to mean an undesirable effect.

simulation: a process involving special X-ray pictures that are used to plan radiation treatment so the areas to be treated are precisely located and marked.

smart bomb: drugs designed to seek out and destroy cancer cells while leaving normal cells unharmed.

Sonablate-200: a modified, high-intensity, focused ultrasound used to display sound to tumors for destruction.

specificity/sensitivity: a percentage ratio of disease versus nondisease states.

spectroscopic MRI: a combination of high-resolution anatomic (MRI) and metabolic (MRSI) imaging to improve the accuracy of staging prostate cancer.

spirulina: CLT (cytoluminescent therapy) sensitizer using medication to locate and kill cancer cells.

spot radiation: radiation specifically aimed at a specific spot on the human body.

stage: indication of the size of a tumor (or tumors), and the extent of the spread of the cancer.

Strontium 89: a radioactive isotope that seeks bone; designed to relieve a patient of severe pain, usually in two or more areas of painful bone metastasis.

support group: group of people on whom an individual can rely to provide emotional caring, concern, and reinforcement of a sense of personal value; may also provide practical or material aid, information, guidance, feedback, and validation of the individual's stressful experiences and coping choices.

Taxotere: docetaxel (Rhone-Poulenc Rorer); semisynthetic compound, belonging to the yew family, called <u>mitotic inhibitors</u>; approved for refractory breast cancer.

Ten-percenter: a man among the 10percent of prostate cancer patients who have a long-term survival of 10years or more while undergoing combination hormonal therapy.

tetraploid: an aggressive prostate cancer tumor, which has four times the normal number of chromosomes.

TGF-beta level: a predictor of biochemical progression after surgery.

total ablation: form of hormone therapy that treats prostate cancer by combining hormones or surgery to achieve a castrate level of testosterone.

total androgen blockade bf ablation: a form of hormonal therapy in which the production of testosterone is shut down, using either surgical castration plus an antiandrogen or chemical castration consisting of an LHRH agonist plus an antiandrogen.

toxic: poisonous.

toxin: a poison, usually from bacterial sources; may have negative effects on the body.

triple dose of Casodex: one hundred and fifty milligrams of Casodex.

triple therapy: a therapy using three types of hormones to treat prostate cancer.

triptorelin pamoate: a potent repressor of gonadotropin secretion when given continuously and in therapeutic doses.

TRUS: an ultrasound sometimes used to guide a biopsy.

tumor: excessive growth of cells caused by uncontrolled and disorderly cell proliferation; an abnormal tissue growth that can be either benign or malignant.

ultrasensitive PSA test: a test that can detect a recurrence much earlier than the routine PSA test.

ultrasonic power Doppler imaging: an image to denote blood flow signals in prostatic cancer using power Doppler imaging with a transrectal probe.

ultrasound: vibrations far beyond the hearing range.

ultrasound-guided biopsy in which a biopsy is obtained by ultrasound guidance.

ultrasound therapy: noninvasive therapy using sound waves of a particular frequency whose echoes are reflected from tissue; used to image internal organs or structures (e.g., tumor within a gland); may help to determine if a lump is solid tissue or cystic; also called <u>sonography</u>.

urologist: doctor who specializes in diseases of the urinary organs in females and the urinary and sex organs in males.

Viadur implant: osmotic tablets positioned at one end of the device that pushes a correct amount of medication out a small hole.

watchful waiting: a wait-and-see posture a prostate cancer patient takes to see how his disease progresses.

well-differentiated: a classification of prostate cancer in which the cells have definite shape; corresponds with a Gleason score of 2 to 4.

X-ray: high-energy radiation that can be used at low levels to diagnose disease or at high levels to treat cancer.

Zometa: a medication for bone metastases.

zone (there are three zones of the prostate gland): the central, peripheral, and transitional; the peripheral zone is most commonly affected by prostate cancer.

E. Roy Berger, M.D., F.A.C.P. and James Lewis, Jr., Ph.D

BIBLIOGRAPHY

Chapter 2
The Digital Rectal Exam

Association of Directors of Anatomic and Surgical Pathology: Recommendations for the reporting of resected prostate carcinomas. Hum Pathol 27:321-323, 1996.

Bostwick DG, Myers RP, Osterling JE: Staging of prostate cancer. Semin Surg Oncol 10:60-73, 1994.

Bova GS, Fox WM, Epstein JI: Methods of radical Prostatectomy specimen processing: A novel technique for harvesting fresh prostate cancer tissue and review of processing techniques. Mod Pathol 6:201-207, 1993.

Cohen MB, Soloway MS, Murphy WM: Sampling of radical prostatectomy specimens. How much is adequate? Am J Clin Pathol 101:250-252, 1994.

Donahue RE, Miller GJ: Adenocarcinoma of the prostate: Biopsy to whole mount. Denver VA experience. Urol Clin North Am 18:449-152, 1991.

Haggman M, Norberg M, de la Torre M, et al: Characterization of localized prostatic cancer: Distribution, grading and pT-staging in radical prostatectomy specimens. Scand J Urol Nephrol 27:7-13, 1993.

Hall GS, Kramer CE, Epstein JI: Evaluation of radical prostatectomy specimens: A comparative analysis of sampling methods. Am J Surg Pathol 16:315-324, 1992.

Henson DE, Hutter RVP, Farrow GM: Practice protocol for the examination of specimens removed from patients with carcinoma of the prostate gland. A publication of the Cancer Committee, College of American Pathologists. Arch Pathol Lab Med 118:779-783, 1994.

Litterup PJ, William CR, Egglin TK, et al: Determination of prostate volume with transrectal United States for cancer screening. Part II. Accuracy of in vitro and in vivo techniques. Radiology *179:49-53,* 1991.

Sakr W, Wheeler T, Blute M, et al: Staging and reporting of prostate cancer. Sampling of the radical prostatectomy specimens. Cancer 78:366-368, 1996.

Sakr WA, Grignon DJ, Visscher DW, et al: Evaluating the radical prostatectomy specimen, Part I. A protocol for establishing prognostic parameters and harvesting fresh tissue samples. J Urol Pathol 3:355-364, 1995.

Schmid H-P, McNeal JE: An abbreviated standard procedure for accurate tumor volume estimation in prostate cancer. Am J Surg Pathol 16:184-191, 1902.

Wheeler TM, Lebovitz RM: Fresh tissue harvest for research from prostatectomy specimens. Prostate 25:271-279, 1994.

Chapter 3

Transrectal Ultrasound

Benson MC, Whang IS, Pantuck A, et al.: Prostate specific antigen density: A means of distinguishing benign prostatic hypertrophy and prostate cancer. J Urol 147:815-816, 1992.

Cooner WH, Mosley BR, Rutherford CL, et al: prostate cancer detection in a clinical urological practice by ultrasonography, digital rectal examination and prostate-specific antigen. J Urol 143:1146-1154, 1990.

Lee F, Littru PJ, Loft—Christensen L, et al: Predicted prostate specific antigen results using transrectal ultrasound gland volume. Cancer 70:211-220, 1992.

Lee F, Littrup P, Torp-Pederson S, et al.: Prostate cancer: Comparison of transrectal ultrasound and digital rectal examination for screening. Radiology 168:389-394, 1988.

Mettlin C, Jones G, Averette H, et al: Defining and updating the American Cancer Society guidelines for cancer—related checkup: Prostate and endometrial cancers. CA Cancer J Clin 43:42-46, 1993.

Resnick M, Willard J, Boyce W: Recent progress in ultrasonography of the bladder and prostate. J Urol 117:444-446, 1977.

Rifken MD: Ultrasound of the Prostate, second edition. Philadelphia: Lippincott-Raven, 1997.

Rifkin M, Kurtz A, Choi H, Goldberg B: Endoscopic ultrasonic investigation of the prostate using a transrectal probe: Prospective evaluation and acoustic characterization. Radiology 149:265-271, 1983.

Rifkin MD: Transrectal prostatic ultrasonography: Comparison of linear array and radial scanners. J Ultrasound Med 4:1—5, 1985.

Watanabe H, Kaiho H, Tanaka M, Terasawa Y: Diagnostic applications of ultrasonotomography to the prostate. Invest Urol 8:548-599, 1971.

Watanabe H: History of transrectal sonography of the prostate. Urol Clin North AM 16:617-622, 1989.

Chapter 4

Biopsying the Prostate

Agatstein EH, Hernandez FJ, Layfield LJ, et al: Use of needle aspiration for detection of stage A prostatic carcinoma before transurethral resection of the prostate: A clinical trail. J Urol 138:551-553, 1987.

Bastacky SS, Silver SA, Epstein JI: Composite cytological smears of pelvic lymph nodes at the time of radical prostatectomy to identify nodal metastases. Hum Pathol 25:1352-1359, 1994.

Das DK, Hellund PO, Lowhagen T, et al: Squamous metaplasia in hormonally treated prostatic cancer. Significance during follow-up. Urology 38:70-75, 1991.

Esposti PL: Cytologic malignancy grading of prostatic carcinoma by transrectal aspiration biopsy A five-year follow-up study of 469 hormone-treated patients. Scand J Urol Nephrol 5:199-209, 1971.

Faul P, Schmidt E, Kern R: Prognostic significance of cytological differentiation grading in estrogen-treated prostatic carcinoma diagnosed by fine-needle aspiration biopsy (five-year follow-up of 496 patients) Int J Urol Nephrol 12:347-354, 1980.

Fox CH: Innovation in medical diagnosis-the Scandinavian curiosity. Lancet 1:1387, 1979.

Koss LG, Woyke S. Schreiber K, et al: Thin-needle aspiration biopsy of the prostate. Urol Clin North Am: 11:237—251, 1984.

Leistenschneider W, Nagel R: Atlas of Prostatic Cytology: Techniques and Diagnosis. New York: Springer Verlag, 1985.

Oyen RH, Van Poppel HP, Ameye FE, et al: Lymph node staging of localized prostatic carcinoma with CT and CT-guided fine-needle aspiration biopsy: Prospective study of 285 patients. Radiology 190:315-322, 1994.

Van Poppel H, Ameye F, Oyen R, et al: Accuracy of combined computerized tomogaphy and fine needle aspiration cytology in lymph node staging of localized prostatic carcinoma. J Urol 151:1324-1325, 1994.

Wolf JS, Cher M, Dall'era M, et al: The use and accuracy of cross—sectional imaging and fine-needle aspiration cytology for detection of pelvic lymph node metastases before radical prostatectomy. J Urol 153:993-999, 1995.

Chapter 5

A Gene for Metastatic Prostate Cancer

Chakravtri A, et al: Urology 55: 635-638, 2000.

Dhanasekaran SM, et al: Nature 412: 822-886, 2001.

Hanahan D, Weinberg, RA: Cell 100: 57-70, 2000.

Laible G, et al: Embo J 16: 3219-3232, 1997.

Latulippe E et al: Cancer Res 62: 4499-4506, 2002.

McMenamin ME, et al: Cancer Res 59: 4291-4296, 1999.

Nowell PC: Science 194: 23-28, 1976.

The polycomb group protein EZH2 is involved in progression of prostate cancer. Varambally S, et al: Nature 419: 624-629, 2002.

Van Kemenade FJ, et al: Blood 97: 3896-3901, 2001.

Chapters 6

The CT Scan

Hricak H, Dooms GC, Jeffrey RB et al: Prostatic carcinoma: Staging by clinical assessment, CT and MRI imaging. Radiology 162: 331-336, 1987.

Platt JF, Bree RL, Sdhwab RE: The accuracy of CT in the staging of carcinoma of the prostate. AJR 149:315—318, 1987.

Chapter 7

Monitoring Prostate Cancer with a Bone Scan

Chybowski FM, Larson Keller JJ, Bergstralh EJ, Oesterling JE: Predicting radio-nuclide bone scan findings in patients with newly diagnosed, untreated prostate cancer: prostate specific antigen is superior to all other clinical parameters. J Urol 145:313-318, 1991.

Corrie D, Timmons JH, Bauman JM, Thompson IM: Efficacy of follow-up bone scans in carcinoma of the prostate. Cancer 61:2453-2454, 1998.

Gerber G, Chodak CW: Assessment of value of routine bone scans in patients with newly diagnosed prostate cancer. Urology 37:418-422, 1991.

McGregor B, Tulloch AGS, Quinlan MF, Lovegrove F: The role of bone scanning in the assessment of prostatic carcinoma. Br J Urol 50:178-181, 1978.

The PET Scan and Lymph-Node Metastases

Cheng SS, Rifkin MD, Bajas MA, et al: Color Doppler imaging: an important adjunct to endorectal ultrasound in the diagnosis of prostate cancer. Radiology 201:338, 1996.

Chybowski FM, Larson Keller JJ, Bergstrahl EJ, et al: Predicting radionucleotide bone scan findings in patients with newly diagnosed untreated prostate cancer: Prostate specific antigen is superior to all other parameters. J Urol 145:313-318, 1991.

Danella JF, de Kernion JB, Smith RB, Steckel E: The contemporary incidence of lymph node metastases in prostate cancer: implications for laparoscopic lymph node dissection. J Urol 149:1488—1491, 1993.

Feneley MR, Chengazi VU, Kirby RS, et al: Prostatic radioimmunoscintigraphy preliminary results using technetium labeled monoclonal antibodies - CYT351. Br J Urol 77:373—381, 1996.

Gammelgaard J, Holm HH: Trans-urethral and trans-rectal ultrasound scanning in urology, J Urol. 124: 863—868, 1980.

Hricak H, Dooms GC, Jeffrey RB, et al: Prostatic carcinoma: Staging by clinical assessment, CT and MRI imaging. Radiology 162:331-336, 1987.

Jewett HJ: Significance of the palpable prostatic nodule. JAMA 160: 838—841, 1956.

Lantz EJ, Hattery RR: Diagnostic imaging of urothelial cancer. Urol Clin North Am 11:576—582, 1984.

Ohori M, Egawa S, Shinohara K, et al. Detection of microscopic extracapsular extension prior to radical prostatectomyfor clinically localized prostate cancer. Br J Urol 74:72—79, 1994.

Platt JF, Bree RL, Sdhwab RE: The accuracy of of carcinoma of the prostate. AJR 149:315—318, 1987.

Rifkin MD: Prostate cancer sonographic characteristics. In Ultrasound of the prostate. New York: Raven Press, 101, 1988.

Schnall MD, Imai Y, Tomaszewski J, et al: Prostate cancer: Local staging with endorectal surface coil MR imaging. Radiology 178:797—802, 1991.

Shreeve PD, Grossman HB, Gross MD, Wahl RL: Metastatic prostate cancer: initial findings of PET with 2-deoxy-2-[F-18]fluoro-D-glucose. Radiology 199:751—756, 1996.

Chapter 9

The ProstaScint Scan

Cheng S, Rifkin MD, Bajas MA, et al: Color Doppler imaging: an important adjunct to endorectal ultrasound in the diagnosis of prostate cancer. Radiology 201:338, 1996.

Gammelgaard J, Holm H: Trans-urethral and trans-rectal ultrasound scanning in urology. J Urol 124:863—868, 1980.

Kriby RS: Pretreatment staging of prostate cancer: Recent advances and future prospects. Prostate Cancer and Prostatic Diseases. London: Stockton Press, 1997, pp. 1-30.

Levran Z, Gonzalez JA, Diokno AC, et al: Are pelvic computed tomography, bone scan, and pelvic lymphadenectomy necessary in the staging of prostatic cancer? Br J Urol 75:778-781, 1995.

McCarthy P, Pollack HM: Imaging of patients with stage D prostate carcinoma. Urol Clin North Am 18:35-39, 1991.

Ohori M, Egawa S, Shinohara K, et al: Detection of microscopic extracapsular extension prior to radical prostatectomy for clinically localized prostate cancer. Br J Urol 74:72—79, 1994.

Petros JA, Catalona WJ: Lower incidence of unsuspected lymph node metastasis in 521 consecutive patients with clinically localized prostate cancer. J Urol 147:1574-1577, 1992.

Rifkin MD: Prostate cancer sonographic characteristics. In Ultrasound of the Prostate. New York: Raven Press, 1988, 101.

Schaffer DL, Pendergrass HP: Comparison of enzyme, clinical radiographic, and radionuclide methods of detecting bone metastases from carcinoma of the prostate. Radiology 121:431-5, 1976.

Wolfe JS, Shinohara K, Kerlikowski KM, et al: Selection of patients for laparoscopic pelvic lymphadenctomy prior to radical prostatectomy: a decision analysis. Urology 42:680-683, 1993.

Chapter 10

Using MRI and MRSI to Stage Prostate Cancer

Bartolozzi C, Menchi I, Lencioni R, Semi S, Lapini A, Barbanti G, Bozza A, Amorosi A, Manganelli A, Carim M. Local staging of prostate carcinoma with Endorectal Coil MRI: Correlation with whole-mount radical prostatectomy specimens. European Radiology 6:339-345, 1996.

Bessette A, Mueller-Lisse UG, Swanson M, Vigneron DV, Scheidler J, Srivastava A, Wood P, Hricak H, Caroll P, Nelson SJ, Kurhanewicz J: Localization of Prostate Cancer After Hormone Ablation by MRI and 3D 1H MRSI: Case-Control Study with Pathologic Correlation. Presented at Seventh Annual Meeting of the International Society for Magnetic Resonance in Medicine. 3:1519, 1999.

Byron PJ, Butler HE, Nelson AD, J.P. Lipuma JP: Magnetic resonance imaging of the prostate. American Journal Radiology 146:543-548, 1986.

Chen M, Hricak H, Kalbhen CL, Kurhanewicz J, Vigneron DB, Weiss JM, Carroll PR: Hormonal ablation of prostatic cancer: Effects on prostate morphology tumor detection, and staging by Endorectal Coil MR Imaging. American Journal Roentgenol 166:1157-1163, 1996.

Cohen JS: Phospholipid and energy metabolism of cancer cells monitored by 31P magnetic resonance spectroscopy: Possible clinical significance. Mayo Clinic Proceedings 63:1199-1207, 1988.

D'Amico AV, Whittington R, Malkowicz SB, Schultz D, Schnall M, Tomaszewski JE, Wein A: Critical analysis of the ability of the Endorectal Coil Magnetic Resonance Imaging Scan to predict pathologic stage, margin status, and postoperative prostate-specific antigen failure in patients with clinically organ-confined prostate cancer. Journal of Clinical Oncology 14:1770-1177, 1996.

D'Amico AV, Whittington R, Schnall M, Malkowicz SB, Tomaszewski JE, Schultz D, Wein A: The impact of the inclusion of endorectal coil magnetic resonance imaging in a multivariate analysis to predict clinically unsuspected extraprostatic cancer. Cancer 75:2368-2372, 1995.

Daly PF, Cohen JS: Magnetic resonance spectroscopy of tumors and potential in vivo clinical applications: A review. Cancer Research 49:770-779, 1989.

Heerschap A, Jager GJ, van der Graaf M, Barentsz JO, de la Rosette JJ, Oosterhof GO, Ruijter ET, Ruijs SH: In vivo proton MR 17 spectroscopy reveals altered metabolite content in malignant prostate tissue. Anticancer Research 17:1455-60, 1997.

Heerschap A, Jager GJ, van der Graaf M, Barentsz JO, Ruijs SH: Proton MR spectroscopy of the normal human prostate with an endorectal coil and a double spin-echo pulse sequence. Magn Reson Med 37:204-213, 1997.

Hricak, White HS, Vigneron D, Kurhanewicz J, Kosco A, Levin D, Weiss J, Narayan P, Carroll PR: Carcinoma of the prostate gland: MR imaging with pelvic phased-array coil versus integrated endorectal–pelvic phased-array coil. Radiology 193:703-709, 1994.

Kalbhen CL, Hricak H, Chen M, Shinohara K, Parivar F, Kurhanewicz J, Vigneron D: Prostate carcinoma: MR imaging findings after cryosurgery. Radiology 198:807-811, 1996.

Kayi, Kurhanewicz YJ, Hricak H, Sokolov D, Huang LR, Nelson S, Vigneron D: Localizing prostate cancer in the presence of postbiopsy changes on MR images: Role of proton MR spectroscopic imaging. Radiology 206: 785-790, 1998.

Kurhanewicz J, Dahiya R, MacDonald JM, Chang LH, James TL, Narayan P: Citrate alterations in primary and metastatic human prostatic adenocarcinomas: 1H magnetic resonance spectroscopy and biochemical study. Magn Reson Med 29:149-157, 1993.

Kurhanewicz J, Vigneron DB, Hricak H, Narayan P, Carroll P, Nelson SJ: Three-dimensional H-I MR spectroscopic imaging of the in situ human prostate with high (O.24-O.7-Cm3) spatial resolution. Radiology 198:795-805, 1996.

Kurhanewicz J, Vigneron DB, Hricak H, Parivar F, Nelson SJ, Shinohara K, Carroll PR: Prostate cancer: Metabolic response to cryosurgery as detected with 3D H-I MR spectroscopic imaging. Radiology 200:489-496, 1996.

Kurhanewicz J, Vigneron DB, Nelson SJ, Hricak H, MacDonald JM, Konety B, Narayan P: Citrate as an in vivo marker to discriminate prostate cancer from benign prostatic hyperplasia and normal prostate peripheral zone: Detection via localized proton spectroscopy." Urology 45:459-466, 1995.

Liney GP, Turnbull LW, Lowry M, Turnbull LS, Knowles AJ, Horsman A. In vivo quantification of citrate concentration and water T2 relaxation time of the pathologic gland using 1H MRS and MRI. Magnetic Resonance Imaging 15:1177-1186, 1997.

Ling D, Lee JKT, Heiken JP, Balfe DM, Glazer HS, McClennan GL: Prostatic carcinoma and benign prostatic hyperplasia: inability of MR imaging to distinguish between the two diseases. Radiology 158:103-107, 1986.

Lowry M, Liney, Turnbull LW, Manton DJ, Blackband SJ, Horsman A: Quantification of citrate concentration in the prostate by proton magnetic resonance spectroscopy: Zonal and age-related differences. Magnetic Resonance in Medicine 36:352-358, 1996.

Males R, Okumo W, Vigneron DB, Swanson M, Wood P, Nelson SJ, Roach M, Kurhanewicz J. Monitoring Effects of Prostate Cancer Brachytherapy Using Combined MRI/MRSI. Presented at Seventh Annual Meeting of the International Society for Magnetic Resonance in Medicine. 1:115, 1999.

McNeal JE, Kindrachuk RA, Freiha FS, Bostwick DG: Patterns of progression in prostate cancer. Lancet 1:60-63, 1986.

Moyher, SE, Vigneron DB, Nelson SJ. Surface coil MRI imaging of the human brain with an analytic reception profile correction. Journal Magn Reson Imaging 5:139-144, 1995.

Mueller-Lisse UG, Kurhanewicz J, Bessette A, Males R, SwansonM, Fang A, Nelson S, Hricak H, Barken I, Vigneron DB: Hormone Ablation of Localized Prostate Cancer: Effects of Duration of Therapy on Prostate Metabolism Demonstrated by 3D 1H MR Spectroscopy. Presented at

Seventh Annual Meeting of the International Society for Magnetic Resonance in Medicine. 3:1518, 1999.

Parivar F, Hricak H, Shinohara K, Kurhanewicz J, Vigneron DB, Nelson SJ, Carroll PR: Detection of Locally Recurrent Prostate Cancer after Cryosurgery: Evaluation by Transrectal Ultrasound, Magnetic Resonance Imaging, and Three-Dimensional Proton Magnetic Resonance Spectroscopy. 594-599, 1996.

Parivar F, Kurhanewicz J: Detection of Recurrent Prostate Cancer after Cryosurgery. Current Opinion in Urology 8:83-86, 1998.

Partin AW, Yoo J, Carter HB, et al: The use of prostate specific antigen, clinical stage and gleason score to predict pathological stage in men with localized prostate cancer. Journal of Urology 150:110-114, 1993.

Partin AW, Yoo J, Carter HB, Pearson JD, Chan DW, Epstein JI, Walsh PC: Partin AW. Kattan MW, Subong EN, Walsh PC, Wojno KJ, Oesterling JE, Scardino PT, Pearson JD: Combination of prostate-specific antigen, clinical stage, and gleason score to predict pathological stage of localized prostate cancer: A multi-institutional update. Journal of the American Medical Association 277:1445-1451, 1997.

Phillips ME, Kressel HY, Spritzer CE, Arger PH, Wein AJ, Marinelli D, Axel L, Gefter WB, Pollack HM: Prostatic disorders: MR imaging at 1 ST. Radiology 164:386-392, 1987.

Platt JE, Bree RL, Schwab RE: The accuracy of CT in the staging of carcinoma of the prostate. American Journal of Roentgenol 149:315-318, 1987.

Rifkin MD, Zerhouni EA, Gatsonis CA, Quint LE, Paushter DM, Epstein JI, Hamper U, Walsh PC, McNeil BJ: Comparison of magnetic resonance imaging and ultrasonography in staging early prostate cancer: Results of a multi-institutional cooperative trial. New England Journal of Medicine 323:621:626, 1990.

Scardino PT, Shinohara K, Wheeler TM, Carter SS: Staging of prostate cancer: Value of ultrasonography. Urol Clin North America 16:713-734, 1989.

Scharen-Guivek VLM, Males R, Nelson SJ, Mueller-Lisse UG, Vigneron DB, Kurhanewicz J: Evaluation of Local Prostate Recurrence after Radical Prostatectomy Using Magnetic Resonance Spectroscopic Imaging. Presented at Seventh Annual Meeting of the International Society for Magnetic Resonance in Medicine. 1:117, 1999.

Scheidler J, Hricak H, Vigneron DB, Yu KK, Sokolov DL, Huang RL, Zaloudek CJ, Nelson SJ, Carroll PR, Kurhanewicz J: 3D 11-I-MR spectroscopic imaging in localizing prostate cancer: Clinic-pathologic study. Radiology 1999 In Press.

Schick F, Bongers H, Kurz S, Jung WI, Pfeffer M, Lutz O: Localized proton MR spectroscopy of citrate in vitro and of the prostate in vivo at I.5T. Magn Reson Med 29:38-43, 1993.

Schnall MD, Imai Y, Tomaszewski J, Pollack HM, Lenkinski RE, Kressel FY: Prostate cancer: Local staging with endorectal surface coil MR imaging. Radiology 178:797-802, 1991.

Stamey TA: Cancer of the prostate: An analysis of some important contributions and dilemmas. Mono Urology 3:67-94, 1982.

Victor TA, Lawson CA, Wiebolt RC, Nussbaum S, Shattuch MC, Brodin AG, Degani H: Prediction of hormonal response of human breast carcinoma by spectroscopy. In Hasetine, ed. Magnetic Resonance of the Reproductive System. New Jersey: Slack, 67-80, 1987.

Vigneron D, Nelson S, Kurhanewicz J: Proton chemical shift imaging of cancer. In Hricak, Higgins and Helms, eds. Magnetic Resonance Imaging of the Body. New York: Raven Press, : 205-220, 1996.

Vigneron DB, Males R, Hricak H, Noworolski S, Carroll PR, Kurhanewicz J: Prostate Cancer: Correlation of 3D MRSI Metabolite Levels with Histologic Grade. Presented at RSNA. 209(P):181, 1998.

Vigneron DB, Nelson SJ, Moyher S, Kelley DAC, Kurhanewicz J, Hricak H: An Analytical Correction of MR Images Obtained with Endorectal or Surface Coils. Presented at Society of Magnetic Resonance Imaging Eleventh Annual Meeting. 3 (P):142, 1993.

Wice BM, Trugnan G, Pintom M, Rousset M, Chevalier G, Dussaulx E, Lacroix B, Zweibaum A: The Intracellular Accumulation of UDP=N-Acethylhexosamines.

Chapter 11

Balancing the Body's pH

Brewer AK, Clarke BJ, Greenberg M, Rothkopf N: The effects of rubidium on mammary tumor growth in C57L K/6J mice. Cytomios 24:99-101, 1979.

Brewer AK, Passwater R: Physics of the cell membrane. I. The role of the double bond energy states. Am Lab 6:49-72, 1974.

Brewer AK, Passwater R: Physics of the cell membrane. IV. Further comments on the role of the double-bond. Am Lab 6:49-62, 1975.

Brewer AK, Passwater R: Physics of the cell membrane. V. Mechanisms involved in cancer. Am Lab 8:7-45, 1976.

Brewer AK, Passwater R": Physics of the cell membrane. III. The mechanism of nerve action. Am Lab 6:49-62, 1974.

Brewer AK. Passwater R: Physics of the cell membrane. II. Fluorescence and phosphorescence in cell analysis. Am Lab 6:19-29, 1974.

Brewer AK: Cancer: Comments on the physics involved. Am Lab 5:12-23, 1973.

Brewer AK: The mechanism of carcinogenesis: Comments on therapy. J Int Acad Prev Med 5:29-53, 1979.

Brewer J: Abundance of the isotopes of potassium in mineral and plant sources. J Am Chem Soc 58:365-369, 1936.

Brewer J: Isotopes of potassium. Ind Chem Eng 30:893, 1938.

Chapter 12

Detoxifying the Body

Foster JS, et al. The Detox Boom Book 2002 E. Lyte, Millville, NJ.

Foster JS, et al. The Patient Detox Book 2002 E. Lyte, Millville, NJ.

Haas EM, The Detox Diet Celestia Ants, Buckley, CA, 1996.

Scrivner A. Detox Yourself Judy Paticus Publisher, London, England: 1990.

Chapter 14

Undergoing a Radical Prostatectomy

Beneventi PA, Cassebaum WH: Rectal flap repair of prostatorectal fistula Surg Gynecol Obstet 133:489, 1971.

Culp OS, Calhoon HW: A variety of recto-urethral fistulas: Experiences with 20 cases. J Urol 91:560, 1964.

Dahl DS, Howard PM, Middleton RG: The surgical management of rectourinary fistulas resulting from a prostatic operation: A report of 5 cases. J Urol 111:514, 1974.

Goodwin WE, Turner RD, Winter CC: Rectourinary fistula: Principles of management and a technique of surgical closure. J Urol 80:246, 1958.

Henderson DJ, Middleton RG, Dahl DS: Single stage repair of rectourinary fistula. J Urol 125:592, 1981.

Kilpatrick FR, York-Mason A: Post-operative recto-prostatic fistula. Br J Urol 41:649, 1969.

Middleton RG, Smith JA Jr, Melzer RB, et al: Patient survival and local recurrence rate following radical prostatectomy for prostatic carcinoma. J Urol 136:422, 1986.

Vose SN: A technique for the repair of recto-urethral fistula. J Urol 61:790, 1949.

Wood TW, Middleton RG: Single-stage transrectal transsphincteric (modified York-Mason) repair of rectourinary fistulas. Urology 35:27, 1990.

Zincke H, Oesterling JE, Blute ML, et al: Long-term (15 years) results after radical prostatectomy clinically localized (Stage T2c or lower) prostate cancer. J Urol 152:1850, 1994.

Chapter 15

IMRT: An Improved Version of External Beam Radiation

Dearnaley DP, Khoo VS, Norman AR, et al: Comparison of radiation side effects of conformal and conventional radiotherapy in prostate cancer: A randomized trial. Lancet. 353:267-271, 1999.

Hanks GE, Hanlon AL, Schultheiss TE, et al: Dose escalation with 3D conformal treatment five years outcomes, treatment optimization, and future directions. Int J Radiation Biol Phys 41:501-510, 1998.

Hanks GE, Schultheiss TE, Hanlon AL, et al: Optimization of conformal radiation treatment of prostate cancer: Report of a dose escalation study. Int J Radiation Oncol Biol Physics 37:543-550, 1997.

Kupelian PA, Mohan DS, Lyons J, et al: Higher than standard radiation doses with or without androgen deprivation in the treatment of localized prostate cancer. Int J Radiation Oncol Biol Phys 46:567-574, 2000.

Reinstein LE, McShan D, Webber B, et al: A computer assisted three-dimensional planning system. Radiology 127:259-264, 1978.

Smith AR, Ling CC: Implementation of three-dimensional conformal radiotherapy. Int J. Radiation Oncol Biol Physics 33:997-1995.

Smith AR, Purdy JA: Three-dimensional photon treatment planning report of the collaborative working group on the evaluation of treatment planning for external photon beam radiotherapy. Int J Radiation Oncol Biol Phys 21, 1991.

Sternick ES, The Theory and Practice for IMRT Advanced Medical Publishing, Madison, WI, 1997.

Zelefsky MJ, Leibel SA, Gaudin PB, et al: Dose escalation with three-dimensional conformal radiation therapy affects the outcome in prostate cancer. Int J Radiation Oncol Biol Phys 41:491-500, 1998.

Chapter 16

Cryosurgery

Boring CC, Squires TS, Tong T, et al: Cancer statistics. CA Cancer J Clin 44:7, 1994.

Chodak GW: Cryosurgery of the prostate revisited. CA 72:1145, 1993.

Epstein JI, Pizov G, Walsh PC: Correlation of pathologic findings with progression after radical retropubic prostatectomy. CA 72:1291, 1993.

Fowler FJ Jr, Barry MJ, Lu-Yao G, et al: Patient reported complications and follow-up treatment after radical prostatectomy. The national Medicare experience: 1988-1990. Urology 42:622, 1993.

Kabalin JN, Hodge KK, McNeal JE, et al: Identification of residual cancer in the prostate following radiation therapy: Role of transrectal ultrasound guided biopsy and prostate specific antigen J Urol 142:326, 1989.

Miller RJ, Cohen JK, Merlotti LA: Percutaneous transperineal cryosurgical ablation of the prostate for the primary treatment of clinical stage C adenocarcinoma of the prostate. Urology 44:170, 1994.

Murphy GP, Mettlin C, Menck H, et al: National patterns of prostate cancer treatment by radical prostatectomy: Results of a survey by the American College of Surgeons Commission on cancer. J Urol 132:1817, 1994.

Onik GM Cohen JK, Reyes GD, et al: Transrectal ultrasound-guided percutaneous radical cryosurgical ablation of the prostate. CA 72:1291, 1993.

Scardino PT: Early detection of prostate cancer. Urol Clin North Am 16:635, 1989.

Walsh PC, Partin AW, Epstein JI: Cancer control and quality of life following anatomical radical retropubic prostatectomy results at 10 years. J Urol 152:1831, 1994.

Zincke H, Oesterling JE. Blute ML, et al: Long-term (15 years) results after radical prostatectomy for clinically localized (stage T2c or lower) prostate cancer. J Urol 152:1850, 1994.

Chapter 17

High-Dose Radiation

Blasko J, Rade H, Luse R, Sylvester J, Cavanaugh W, Grimm P: Should brachytherapy be considered a therapeutic option in localized prostate cancer Urol Clin NA 23:633-650, 1996.

Fuks Z, Leibel SA, Walner KE: The effect of local control on metastatic dissemination in carcinoma of the prostate: Long-term results in patients treated with I-125 implantation. Int J Radiat Oncol Biol Phys 21:537-547, 1991.

Gottesman J, Tesh D, Weissman W: Failure of radioactive I-125 to control localized prostate cancer: A study of 41 patients. J Urol 146:1317-1320, 1991.

Holm HH, Juul N, Pedersen JF: Transperineal 125-iodine seed implantation in prostatic cancer guided by transrectal ultrasonography. J Urol 130: 283-286, 1983.

Koprowski CD, Berkenstock KG, Borofski AM: External beam irradiation versus I-125 implant in the definitive treatment of prostate cancer. Int J Radiat Oncol Biol Phys 21:955-960, 1991.

Kuban DA, El-Mahdi AM, Schellhammer PF: I-125 interstitial implantation I the definitive treatment of prostate cancer: what we have learned 10 years later? Cancer 63:2415-2420, 1989.

Mate T, Blasko J, Marshall S, Porter B, Schumaker D: Computed tomography-assisted permanent prostate implant dosimetry. Proceedings of the Twelfth Annual Mid-Winter Meeting of the American Endocurietherapy Society. 14, 1989.

McNeal JE, Redwine EA, Freiha FS, Stamey TA: Zonal distribution of prostatic adenocarcinoma: Correlation with histologic pattern and direction of spread. Am J Surg Pathol 12:897-906, 1988.

Russell K J, Blaski JC: Recent advances in interstitial brachytherapy for localized prostate cancer. In: Lange, P., ed. Problems in Urology. Vol. 7. No. 2. Philadelphia: Lippincott, 260-272, 1993.

Whitemore WF, Hilaris B, Grabstald H: Retropubic implantation of iodine–125 in the treatment of prostatic carcinoma. J Urol 108: 918-920,1972.

Chapter 18

Living with Hormone-Refractory Prostate Cancer

Meyer S, Nasti SC. Chicago, IL: University of Chicago Press, 124-135, 1994.

Prasad KN. Rochester, CT: Healing Arts Press, 1-81, 1993.

Buck CA. Prostate Cancer: Questions and Answers. Coral Springs, FL: Merit Publishing, 82-91, 1995.

McConnell JD. Physiologic basis of endocrine therapy for prostatic cancer. Urol Clin North Am 18(1):1-13, 1991.

Logothetis CJ, Samuels ML, von Eschenbach AC, et al: Doxorubicin, mitomycin-C, and 5-fluorouracil (DMF) in the treatment of metastatic hormonal refractory adenocarcinoma of the prostate, with a note on the staging of metastatic prostate cancer. J Clin Oncol 1:368-379, 1983.

Kelly WK, Scher HI, Mazumdar M, et al: Prostate-specific antigen as a measure of disease outcome in metastatic hormone-refractory prostate cancer. J Clin Oncol 11:507, 1993.

Seidman AD, Scher HI, Petrylak D, et al: Estramustine and vinblastine: Use of prostate specific antigen as a clinical trial end point for hormone refractory prostate cancer. J Urol 147:931, 1992.

Scher HI, Kelly WK; Flutamide withdrawal syndrome: Its impact on clinical trials in hormone-refractory prostate cancer. J Clin Oncol 11:1566-1572, 1993.

Dupont A, Gomez J-L, Cusan L, et al: Response to flutamide withdrawal in advanced prostate cancer in progression under combination therapy. J Urol 150:908-913, 1993.

Tong D, Gillick L, Hendrickson FR: The palliation of symptomatic osseous metastases: Final results of the study by the Radiation Therapy Oncology Group. Cancer 1985.

Chapter 19

Neutron Beam Radiation

Carlton E, Dawoud F, Hudgins P, et al. Irradiation treatment of carcinoma of the prostate: a preliminary report based on 8 years experience. J Urol 108:924-927, 1972.

Deming CL. Carcinoma of the prostate seminal vesicles treated with radium. Surg Gynecol Obstet 34:99-118, 1922.

Kuban D, Anas E, Schellhammer P. I-125 interstitial implantation for prostate cancer: What have we learned 10 years later? Cancer 63: 2413-2420, 1989.

Landis S, Murray T, Bolden S, et al. Cancer Statistics 1998. CA Cancer J Clin 48:6-29, 1998.

Mettlin C, Murphy G, Lee F, et al. Characteristics of prostate cancer detected in the American Cancer Society-National Prostate Cancer Detection Project. J Urol 152: 1737-1740, 1994.

Pasteau O. Traitment du cancer de la prostate par le radium (Treatment of prostate cancer with radium). Rev Malad Nutr 363-367, 1991.

Whitmore W, Hilaris B, Grabstald H. Retropubic implantation of iodine-125 in the treatment of prostate cancer. J Urol 108:918-920, 1972.

Chapter 20

Seed Implantation

Beyer DC, Priestly JB Jr. Biochemical disease-free survival following 125I prostate implantation. Int J Radiat Oncol Biol Phys 1997;37:559-563.

Chodak GW. Comparing treatment results in localized prostate cancer: Persisting uncertainty. JAMA 280:1008-1009, 1998.

D'Amico AV, Whittington R, Malkowicz SB, et al. Biochemical outcome after radical prostatectomy, external beam radiation therapy, or interstitial radiation therapy for clinically localized prostate cancer. <u>JAMA</u> 280:969-974, 1998.

Desai J, Stock RG, Stone NN, et al. Acute urinary morbidity following I-125 interstitial implantation of the prostate gland. <u>Radiat Oncol Invest</u> 6:135-141, 1998.

Hu K, Wallner K. Clinical course of rectal bleeding following I-125 prostate brachytherapy. <u>Int Radiat Oncol Biol Phys</u> 41:263-265, 1998.

Mantz CA, Song P, Farhangi E, et al. Potency probability following conformal megavoltage radiotherapy using conventional doses for localized prostate cancer. <u>Int J Radiat Oncol Biol Phy</u> 37:551-557, 1997.

Radge H, Blasko JC, Grimm PD, et al. Interstitial iodone-125 radiation without adjuvant therapy in the treatment of clinically localized prostate carcinoma. <u>Cancer</u> 80:442-453, 1997.

Robinson JW, Dufour MS, Fung TS. Erectile functioning of men treated for prostate carcinoma. <u>Cancer</u> 79:538-544, 1997.

Rousseau L, Dupont A, Labrie F, et al. Sexuality changes in prostate cancer patients receiving antihormonal therapy combining the antiandrogen flutamide with medical (LHRH agonist) or surgical castration. <u>Arch Sex Behav</u> 17:87-98, 1998.

Sharkey J, Chovnick SD, Behar RJ, et al. Outpatient ultrasound-guided palladium 103 brachytherapy for localized adenocarcinoma of the prostate: A preliminary report of 434 patients. <u>Urology</u> 51:796-803, 1998.

Stock RG, Stone NN, Iannuzzi C. Sexual potency following interactive ultrasound-guided brachytherapy for prostate cancer. <u>Int J Radiat Oncol Biol Phys</u> 35:267-272, 1996.

Wallner K, Roy J, Harrison L. Dosimetry guidelines to minimize urethral and rectal morbidity following transperineal I-125 prostate brachytherapy. <u>Int J Radiat Oncol Biol Phys</u> 32:465-471, 1995.

Wallner K, Roy J, Harrison L. Tumor control and morbidity following transperineal iodine-125 implantation for stage T1/T2 prostatic carcinoma. <u>J Clin Oncol</u> 14:449-453, 1996.

Chapter 22

Treating Cancers with Light Waves

Dougherty TJ. Photoradiation therapy: New approaches. Seminars in Surgical Oncology 5:6-16, 1989.

Hopper C. Photodynamic therapy: A clinical reality in the treatment of cancer. Lancet Oncol 1:212-9, 2000.

Liberman J. Light Medicine of the Future. Santa Fe: Bear and Co. 1991.

Perez C, Brady LW, eds. Principles and Practice of Radiation Oncology, 3rd ed. Philadelphia: Lippincott-Raven, 1998.

Chapter 25

Befar and Erectile Dysfunction

Feldman HA, Goldstein I, Hatzichristou DG, Krane RJ, McKinley JB. Impotence and its medical and psychological correlates: Results of Massachusetts Male Aging Study. J Urol 151:54-61, 1994.

Laumann EO, Paik A, Rosen RC. Sexual dysfunction in the United States. JAMA 281:6;537-544, 1999.

Chapter 30

Hormonal Therapy: A Definitive Treatment?

Byar DP. Proceedings: Veterans Administration Cooperative Urological Research Group's studies of cancer of the prostate. Cancer 32:1126-1130, 1973.

Fichtner J. The management of prostate cancer in patients with a rising prostate-specific antigen level [In Process Citation]. BJU Int 2000;86:II-III.

Iversen P, Madsen PO, Corle DK. Radical prostatectomy versus expectant treatment for early carcinoma of the prostate. Twenty-three-year follow-up of a prospective randomized study. Scand J Urol Nephrol Suppl 172:6572, 1995.

Melchior SW, Corey E, Elis WJ, et al. Early tumor cell dissemination in patients with clinically localized carcinoma of the prostate. Clin Cancer Res 3:249-256, 1997.

Middleton RG, Thompson IM, Austenfeld MS, et al. Prostate Cancer Clinical Guidelines Panel summary report on the management of clinically localized prostate cancer. American Urological Association. J Urol 154:2144-2148, 1995.

Moul JW. Prostate specific antigen only progression of prostate cancer. J Urol 163:1632-1642, 2000.

Oesterling JE, Fuks Z, Lee CT, et al. Cancer of the prostate. In: Devita VT, Hellman S, Rosenberg SA, eds. Cancer Principles and Practice of Oncology, 5th ed. Philadelphia: Lippincott-Raven, 1322-1386, 1997.

Pound Cr, Partin AW, Eisenberger MA, et al. Natural history of progression after PSA elevation following radical prostatectomy. JAMA 281:1591-1597, 1999.

Roach M, Weinberg V, McLaughlin P, et al. Does pretreatment PSA add to predicting long-term survival from prostate cancer? In: Perry MC, ed. Proceedings of the American Society of Clinical Oncology 36th Annual Meeting. New Orleans, LA, 1282, 2000.

Van den Ouden D, Hop WC, Schroder FH. Progression in and survival of patients with locally advanced prostate cancer (T3) treated with radical prostatectomy as monotherapy. J Urol 160:1392-1397, 1998.

Chapter 34

Treating Hormone-Refractory Prostate Cancer

Dupont A, Gomez J-L, Cusan L, et al: Response to flutamide withdrawal in advanced prostate cancer in progression under combination therapy. J. Urol 150:908-913, 1993.

Kelly WK, Scher HI, Mazumdar M, et al: Prostate-specific antigen as a measure of disease outcome in metastatic hormone refractory prostate cancer. J Clin Oncol 11:607, 1993.

Logothetis CJ, Samuels ML, Eschenbach AC, et al: Doxorubicin, mitomycin-C, and 5 fluorouracil (DMF) in the treatment of metastatic hormonal refractory adenocarcinoma of the prostate, with a note on the staging of metastatic prostate cancer. J Clin Oncol 1:368-379, 1983.

McConnell JD: Physiologic basis of endocrine therapy for prostatic cancer. Urol Clin North Am 189(1):1-13, 1991.

Scher HI, Kelly WK: Flutamide withdrawal syndrome: Its impact on clinical trials in hormone refractory prostate cancer. J Clin Oncol 11:1566-1572, 1993.

Seidman AD, Scher HI, Petrylak D, et al: Estramustine and vinblastine: Use of prostate specific antigen as a clinical trial end point for hormone refractory prostate cancer.

Tong D, Gillick L, Hendrickson FR: The palliation of symptomatic osseous metastases: final results of the study by the Radiation Therapy Oncology Group. Cancer 55:1468-1472, 1985.

Chapter 36

Intermittent Hormone Therapy

Albertson PC, Aronson NK, Muller MJ, et al. Health related quality of life among patients with metastatic prostate cancer. Urology 49:207-217, 1996.

Bolla M, Gonzalez D, Warde P, et al. Improved survival in patients with locally advanced prostate cancer treated with radiotherapy and goserlin. N Engl J Med 337:295-300, 1997.

Zelefsky MJ, Lyass O, Fuks Z, et al. Predictors for improved outcome for patients with localized prostate cancer treated with neoadjuvant androgen ablation therapy and three-dimensional conformal radiotherapy. J Clin Oncol 16:3380-3385, 1998.

Akakura K, Bruchovsky N, Glodenberg LS, et al. Effects of intermittent androgen suppression on androgen-dependent tumors. Apoptosis and serum prostate-specific antigen. Cancer 71:2782-2790, 1993.

Goldenberg LS, Bruchovsky N, Gleave ME, et al. Intermittent androgen suppression in the treatment of prostate cancer; a preliminary report. Urology 45:839-844, 1993.

Higano CS, Ellis W, Russell K, et al. Intermittent androgen suppression with leuprolide and flutamide for prostate cancer: A pilot study. Urology 48:800-880, 1996.

Strum SB, McDermed JE, Scholz MC, et al. Anaemia associated with androgen deprivation in patients with prostate cancer receiving combined hormone blockade. Br J Urol 79:933-941, 1997.

Asbell SO, Leon SA, Tester WJ, et al. Development of anemia and recovery in prostate cancer patients treated with combined androgen blockade and radiotherapy. Prostate 29:243-248, 1996.

Clarke NW, McClure J, George NJR, et al. The effects of orchiectomy on skeletal metabolism in metastatic prostate cancer. Scand J Urol Nephrol 27:475-483, 1993.

Chapter 37

PROSTATE CANCER AND HEART DISEASE

Gao X, et al. Elevated 12-lipoxygenase mRNA expression correlates with advanced stage and poor differentiation of human prostate cancer. Urology 46(2):227-237, 1995.

Liao S, et al. Growth inhibition and regression of human prostate and breast tumors in athymic mice by tea epigallocatechin gallate. Cancer Lett 96(2):239-243, 1995.

Clark LC, et al. Effects of selenium supplementation for cancer prevention in patients with carcinoma of the skin. A randomized controlled trial. Nutritional Prevention of Cancer Study Group [see comments] [published erratum appears in JAMA 1997, May 21;277(19):1520]. JAMA 276(24):1957-1963, 1996.

Ghosh J, Myers CE. Arachidonic acid stimulates prostate cancer cell growth: Critical role of 5-lipoxygenase. Biochem Biophys Res Commun 235(2):418-423, 1997.

Koide T, et al. Antitumor effect of anthocyanin fractions extracted from red soybeans and red beans in vitro and in vivo. Cancer Biother Radiopharm 12(4):277-280, 1997.

Clark LC, et al. Decreased incidence of prostate cancer with selenium supplementation: Results of a double-blind cancer prevention trial. Br J Urol 81(5):730-734, 1998.

Ghosh J, and Myers CE. Inhibition of arachidonate 5-lipoxygenase triggers massive apoptosis in human prostate cancer cells. Proc Natl Acad Sci USA 95(22):13182-13187. 1009.

Giovannucci E. Selenium and risk of prostate cancer. Lancet 352(9130):755-756, 1998.

Gross C, et al. Treatment of early recurrent prostate cancer with 1,25-dihydroxyvitamin D3 (calcitriol). J Urol 159(6):2035-9; discussion 2039-2040, 1998.

Heinonen OP, et al. Prostate cancer and supplementation with alpha-tocopherol and beta- carotene: Incidence and mortality in a controlled trial [see comments]. J Natl Cancer Inst 90(6):440-446, 1998.

Kamei H, et al. Anti-tumor effect of methanol extracts from red and white wines. Cancer Biother Radiopharm 13(6):447-452, 1998.

Nie D, et al. Platelet-type 12-lipoxygenase in a human prostate carcinoma stimulates angiogenesis and tumor growth. Cancer Res 58(18):4047-4051, 1998.

Pastori M, et al. Lycopene in association with alpha-tocopherol inhibits at physiological concentrations proliferation of prostate carcinoma cells. Biochem Biophys Res Commun 250(3):582-585, 1998.

Spiller GA, et al. Nuts and plasma lipids: An almond-based diet lowers LDL-C while preserving HDL-C. J Am Coll Nutr 17(3):285-290, 1998.

Yoshizawa K, et al. Study of prediagnostic selenium level in toenails and the risk of advanced prostate cancer [see comments]. J Natl Cancer Inst 90(16):1219-1224, 1998.

de la Puerta R, V Ruiz Gutierrez, and J.R. Hoult. Inhibition of leukocyte 5-lipoxygenase by phenolics from virgin olive oil. Biochem Pharmacol 57(4):445-449, 1999.

Fremont L, L Belguendouz, S Delpal. Antioxidant activity of resveratrol and alcohol-free wine polyphenols related to LDL oxidation and polyunsaturated fatty acids. Life Sci 64(26):2511-2521, 1999.

Gann PH, et al. Lower prostate cancer risk in men with elevated plasma lycopene levels: results of a prospective analysis. Cancer Res 59(6):1225-1230, 1999.

Ghosh J, CE Myers Central role of arachidonate 5-lipoxygenase in the regulation of cell growth and apoptosis in human prostate cancer cells. Adv Exp Med Biol 469:577-582, 1999.

Gupta S, et al. Prostate cancer chemoprevention by green tea: In vitro and in vivo inhibition of testosterone-mediated induction of ornithine decarboxylase. Cancer Res 59(9):2115-2120, 1999.

Hsieh TC, JM Wu. Differential effects on growth, cell cycle arrest, and induction of apoptosis by resveratrol in human prostate cancer cell lines. Exp Cell Res 249(1):109-115, 1999.

Kris-Etherton PM, et al. Nuts and their bioactive constituents: effects on serum lipids and other factors that affect disease risk. Am J Clin Nutr 70(3 Suppl):504S-511S, 1999.

Lagiou, P., et al. Diet and benign prostatic hyperplasia: A study in Greece. Urology 54(2):284-290, 1999.

Lyn-Cook BD, et al. Chemopreventive effects of tea extracts and various components on human pancreatic and prostate tumor cells in vitro. Nutr Cancer 35(1):80-86, 1999.

Mitchell SH, W. Zhu, CY Young. Resveratrol inhibits the expression and function of the androgen receptor in LNCaP prostate cancer cells. Cancer Res 59(23):5892-5895, 1999.

Norrish AE, et al. Prostate cancer risk and consumption of fish oils: A dietary biomarker- based case-control study. Br J Cancer 81(7):1238-1242, 1999.

Rao AV, N Fleshner, S Agarwal. Serum and tissue lycopene and biomarkers of oxidation in prostate cancer patients: A case-control study. Nutr Cancer 33(2):159-164, 1999.

Ripple MO, et al. Effect of antioxidants on androgen-induced AP-1 and NF-kappaB DNA-binding activity in prostate carcinoma cells. J Natl Cancer Inst 91(14):1227-1232, 1999.

Sabate J. Nut consumption, vegetarian diets, ischemic heart disease risk, and all-cause mortality: Evidence from epidemiologic studies. Am J Clin Nutr 70(3 Suppl):500S-503S, 1999.

Tzonou A, et al. Diet and cancer of the prostate: a case-control study in Greece. Int J Cancer 80(5):704-708, 1999.

Agarwal C, Y Sharma, Agarwal R. Anticarcinogenic effect of a polyphenolic fraction isolated from grape seeds in human prostate carcinoma DU145 cells: Modulation of mitogenic signaling and cell-cycle regulators and induction of G1 arrest and apoptosis. Mol Carcinog 28(3):129-138, 2000.

Attiga FA, et al. Inhibitors of prostaglandin synthesis inhibit human prostate tumor cell invasiveness and reduce the release of matrix metalloproteinases. Cancer Res 60(16):4629-4637, 2000.

Coni E, et al. Protective effect of oleuropein, an olive oil biophenol, on low density lipoprotein oxidizability in rabbits. Lipids 35(1):45-54, 2000.

Curb JD, et al. Serum lipid effects of a high-monounsaturated fat diet based on macadamia nuts. Arch Intern Med 160(8):1154-1158, 2000.

Gunawardena K, Murray DK, Meikle AW. Vitamin E and other antioxidants inhibit human prostate cancer cells through apoptosis. Prostate 44(4):287-295, 2000.

Gupta S, et al. Growth inhibition, cell-cycle dysregulation, and induction of apoptosis by green tea constituent epigallocatechin-3-gallate in androgen-sensitive and androgen-insensitive human prostate carcinoma cells. Toxicol Appl Pharmacol 164(1):82-90, 2000.

Israel K, et al. Vitamin E succinate induces apoptosis in human prostate cancer cells: Role for Fas in vitamin E succinate-triggered apoptosis. Nutr Cancer 36(1):90-100, 2000.

Kampa M, et al. Wine antioxidant polyphenols inhibit the proliferation of human prostate cancer cell lines. Nutr Cancer 37(2):223-233, 2000.

Knowles LM, et al. Flavonoids suppress androgen-independent human prostate tumor proliferation. Nutr Cancer 38(1):116-122, 2000.

Madaan S, et al. Cytoplasmic induction and overexpression of cyclooxygenase-2 in human prostate cancer: implications for prevention and treatment. BJU Int 86(6):736-741, 2000.

Nelson JE, and Harris RE. Inverse association of prostate cancer and non-steroidal antiinflammatory drugs (NSAIDs): results of a case-control study. Oncol Rep 7(1):169-170, 2000.

Norrish AE, et al. Men who consume vegetable oils rich in monounsaturated fat: Their dietary patterns and risk of prostate cancer (New Zealand). Cancer Causes Control 11(7):609-615, 2000.

Owen RW, et al. Phenolic compounds and squalene in olive oils: The concentration and antioxidant potential of total phenols, simple phenols, secoiridoids, lignans and squalene. Food Chem Toxicol 38(8):647-659, 2000.

Owen RW, et al. The antioxidant/anticancer potential of phenolic compounds isolated from olive oil. Eur J Cancer 36(10):1235-1247, 2000.

Rein D, et al. Epicatechin in human plasma: In vivo determination and effect of chocolate consumption on plasma oxidation status. J Nutr 130(8):2109S-2114S, 2000.

Rein D, et al. Cocoa and wine polyphenols modulate platelet activation and function. J Nutr 130(8):2120S-2126S, 2000.

Rotem R, Y Tzivony, Flescher E. Contrasting effects of aspirin on prostate cancer cells: suppression of proliferation and induction of drug resistance. Prostate 42(3):172-180, 2000.

Visioli F, et al. Olive oil phenolics are dose-dependently absorbed in humans. FEBS Lett 468(2-3):159-160, 2000.

Wang, JF, et al. A dose-response effect from chocolate consumption on plasma epicatechin and oxidative damage. J Nutr 130(8):2115S-2119S, 2000.

Yamagishi M, et al. Antimutagenic activity of cacao: Inhibitory effect of cacao liquor polyphenols on the mutagenic action of heterocyclic amines. J Agric Food Chem 48(10):5074-5078, 2000.

Aronson WJ, et al. Modulation of omega-3/omega-6 polyunsaturated ratios with dietary fish oils in men with prostate cancer. Urology 58(2):283-288, 2001.

Chung BH, et al. Effects of docosahexaenoic acid and eicosapentaenoic acid on androgen-mediated cell growth and gene expression in LNCaP prostate cancer cells. Carcinogenesis 22(8):1201-1206, 2001.

Davis PA, Iwahashi CK. Whole almonds and almond fractions reduce aberrant crypt foci in a rat model of colon carcinogenesis. Cancer Lett 165(1):27-33, 2001.

Hughes-Fulford M, Chen Y, Tjandrawinata RR. Fatty acid regulates gene expression and growth of human prostate cancer PC-3 cells. Carcinogenesis 22(5):701-707, 2000.

Ioku K, et al. Various cooking methods and the flavonoid content in onion. J Nutr Sci Vitaminol (Tokyo) 47(1):78-83, 2001.

Jiang Q, et al. Gamma-tocopherol, the major form of vitamin E in the US diet, deserves more attention. Am J Clin Nutr 74(6):714-722, 2001.

Myers C, et al. Proapoptotic anti-inflammatory drugs. Urology 57(4 Suppl 1):73-76, 2001.

Nikolic D, van Breemen RB. DNA oxidation induced by cyclooxygenase-2. Chem Res Toxicol 14(4):351-354, 2001.

Ornish DM, et al. Dietary trial in prostate cancer: Early experience and implications for clinical trial design. Urology 57(4 Suppl 1):200-201, 2001.

Saxe GA, et al. Can diet in conjunction with stress reduction affect the rate of increase in prostate specific antigen after biochemical recurrence of prostate cancer? J Urol 166(6):2202-2207, 2001.

Uotila P, et al. Increased expression of cyclooxygenase-2 and nitric oxide synthase-2 in human prostate cancer. Urol Res 29(1):23-28, 2001.

Xing N, et al. Quercetin inhibits the expression and function of the androgen receptor in LNCaP prostate cancer cells. <u>Carcinogenesis</u> 22(3):409-414, 2001.

Heber D. Prostate enlargement: The canary in the coal mine? <u>Am J Clin Nutr</u> 75(4):605-606.

John JH, et al. Effects of fruit and vegetable consumption on plasma antioxidant concentrations and blood pressure: A randomized controlled trial. <u>Lancet</u> 359(9322):1969-1974, 2001.

Liu M, et al. Mixed tocopherols have a stronger inhibitory effect on lipid peroxidation than alpha-tocopherol alone. <u>J Cardiovasc Pharmacol</u> 39(5):714-721, 2002.

Chapter 42

Psychosocial Aspects of Prostate Cancer

Borysenko J. <u>Minding the Body, Ending the Mind</u>. Massachusetts: Addison-Wesley, 1987.

Collinge W. Mind/body medicine: Separating the hope from the hype. <u>Coping: Living with Cancer</u> Winter, 1992.

Cousins N. <u>Anatomy of an Illness</u>. New York: Norton, 1979.

Cousins N. <u>Head First: The Biology of Hope</u>. New York: Dutton, 1989.

Kabat-Zinn J. <u>Full Catastrophe Living</u>. New York: Delta, 1991.

Passik SD, Dugan W, McDonald MV, et al. Oncologists recognition of depression in their patients with cancer. <u>J Clin Oncol</u> 16:1594-1600, 1998.

Pert C. <u>Molecules of Emotion: The Science Behind the Mind-Body Medicine</u>. New York: Touchstone, 1999.

Pirl WF, Mello, J. Psychological complications of prostate cancer. <u>Oncology</u> 16:1448-1467, 2002.

Pirl WF, Roth AJ. The diagnosis and treatment of depression in cancer patients. <u>Oncology</u> 13:1293-1301, 1999.

E. Roy Berger, M.D., F.A.C.P. and James Lewis, Jr., Ph.D

Rossman ML. <u>Healing Yourself</u>. New York: Walker, 1987.

Siegel B. <u>Love, Medicine, and Miracles</u>. New York: Harper & Row, 1986.

Spiegel D. <u>Living beyond Limits</u>. New York: Random House, 1993.

Walsh PC, Worthington JF. <u>Dr. Patrick Walsh's Guide to Surviving Prostate Cancer</u>, New York, Warner, 2001.

RESOURCES

BRACHYTHERAPY/BEFORE OR AFTER IMRT SITES

Alabama

U. Alabama, Birmingham Medical Center
Birmingham, AL
205-934-1747

Arizona

Arizona Oncology Services, Scottsdale Radiation Oncology
Scottsdale, AZ
602-274-4484

Mayo Clinic for Medical Education & Research
Scottsdale, AZ
480-301-1735

California

Beverly Oncology and Imaging Center
Montebello, CA
323-724-8780

City of Hope Medical Center
Durate, CA
626-301-8247

Redding Cancer Treatment Center
Redding, CA
530-245-5900

Sharp Chula Vista Medical Center
Chula Vista, CA
619-482-5851

Sharp Grossmont Hospital
La Mesa, CA
619-644-4500

Santa Monica Cancer Treatment Center
Santa Monica, CA
310-828-0061

St. Vincent Medical Center
Los Angeles, CA
213-484-7111

U. California, Irvine
Orange, CA
714-456-5508

U. California, San Francisco
San Francisco, CA
415-353-7174

Florida

Dattoli Cancer Center
Dr. Michael Dattoli
2803 Fruitville Road
Sarasota, FL
941-957-4926

Tenet St. Mary's Medical Center
Kaplan Radiation Ctr.
West Palm Beach, FL
561-881-2815

Georgia

Radiotherapy Clinics of Georgia
Dr. Frank A. Critz
2349 Lawrenceville Hwy
Decatur, GA 30033
770-289-2652

Columbus Regional Healthcare System
Amos Cancer Center
Columbus, GA
706-571-1911

Regional Radiation Oncology Center
Rome, GA
706-234-1400

Kansas

Wesley Medical Center
Wichita, KS
316-688-2920

Louisiana

Northeast Louisiana Cancer Institute
West Monroe, LA
318-329-4800

West Jefferson Medical Center
Marrero, LA
504-349-1480

Massachusetts

Tufts-New England Medical Center
Boston, MA
617-636-6161

Minnesota

Abbott Northwestern Hospital
Minneapolis, MN
612-863-5171

Missouri

Mallinckrodt/Barnes Jewish Hospital
St. Louis, MO
314-747-1230

Mississippi

Baptist Medical Center
Jackson, MS
601.968.1416

North Dakota

Altru Health System
Grand Forks, ND
701-780-5860

Bismarck Cancer Center
Bismarck, ND
701-222-6100

New Jersey

Hackensack U. Medical Center
Hackensack, NJ
201-996-2210

New York

**Advanced Radiation Oncology
of Nyack**
Nyack, NY
845-727-0628

**Long Island Jewish Medical
Center**
New Hyde Park, NY
718-470-7190

**North Shore Radiation
Oncology**
Dr. Martin Silverstein
Dr. Joseph Cirrone
181 Belle Mead Road
East Setauket, NY 11733
631-689-6776

Staten Island U. Hospital
Staten Island, NY
718-226-8862

Ohio

Cleveland Clinic Foundation
Cleveland, OH
216-444-1938

Pennsylvania
**Cancer Center of Wyoming
Valley**
Wilkes-Barre, PA
570-822-9822

Fox Chase Cancer Center
Philadelphia, PA
215-728-2996

**Sacred Heart Hospital Center
for Cancer Care**
Allentown, PA
610.776.4674

**Radiation Medicine Specialists
of NE PA, PC,** Forty Fort, PA
570-714-8686

South Dakota

**Prairie Lakes Healthcare
System**
Watertown, SD
605-882-6800

Tennessee

Centennial Medical Systems
Nashville, TN
615-342-4850

Texas
**CTRC/Grossman Cancer
Center**
San Antonio, TX
210-616-5500

Southwest Cancer Center
Lubbock, TX
806-743-1900

Houston Methodist Hospital
Houston, TX
713-790-2091

Tomball Regional Hospital and
Cancer Center
Tomball, TX
281-351-3914

Moncrief/UT Southwestern
Ft. Worth, TX
817-923-7393

VA-Houston
VA Medical Center
Houston, TX
713-794-7190

<u>**West Virginia**</u>

Princeton Radiation Oncology
Center
Greenbrier, WV
304-425-3514

CYTOLUMINESCENT THERAPY (CLT) SITES

Charles Knouse, D.O.
Oncologist
Aidan Clinic
621 South 48th St.
Ste. 111
Tempe, AZ 85281
Tel: 480-446-8181
Toll-free: 1-877-585-7684
Fax: 480-446-8858
aidan@aidan-az.com

William Porter, M.D.
Pascal Paschal Carmody, M.D.
East Clinic in Killaloe
PO Box 618
Killaloe, County Clare
Ireland
Tel: +353-0-61-375815

Wolfgang Woeppel, M.D.
Hufeland Clinic for Holistic
Immunotherapy
D-97980 Bad Mergen Tehern
Germany
Tel: +49-7931-6192

EXTERNAL BEAM RADIATION SITES USING IMRT ALONE

Arizona

East Valley Oncology
Mesa, AZ
602-274-4484

Good Samaritan Medical Center
Phoenix, AZ
602-239-3400

St. Joseph's Hospital
Phoenix, AZ
602-406-3170

Thunderbird Samaritan Medical Center
Glendale, AZ
602-588-5555

California

Beverly Hills Radiation Oncology
Beverly Hills, CA
310-659-6770

Daniel Freeman Hospital
Inglewood, CA
310-674-7050

East Bay Radiation Oncology Center
Castro Valley, CA
510-581-0556

Glendale Adventist Medical Center
Glendale, CA
818-409-8198

Glendale Memorial Hospital
Glendale, CA
818-502-2380

Good Samaritan Hospital
Los Angeles, CA
213-977-2360

Mercy San Juan Radiation Oncology Center
Carmichael, CA
916-537-5470

Sharp Memorial Hospital
San Diego, CA
858-541-5500

St. Agnes Medical Center
Fresno, CA
559-449-3156

St. Francis Medical Center
Lynwood, CA
310-900-2760

St. Jude's Medical Center
Fullerton, CA
714-446-5632

St. John's Health Center
Santa Monica, CA
310-829-8913

Stanford Hospital and Clinics
Stanford, CA
650-725-8060

Colorado

Porter Adventist Hospital
Denver, CO
303-778-5714

Connecticut

**University of Connecticut
Health Center**
John Dempsey Hospital
Farmington, CT
860-679-3225

Danbury Hospital
Danbury, CT
203-797-7190

Yale-New Haven Hospital
New Haven, CT
203-688-2951

Florida

VA-Tampa/VA Hospital
Tampa, FL
813-972-7667

**M.D. Anderson Cancer Center,
Orlando**
Winter Park, FL
407-628-0991

St. Vincent Medical Center
Jacksonville, FL
904-308-7300

U. Miami School of Medicine
Sylvester Comprehensive Cancer
Center
Miami, FL
305-243-4255

Georgia

**Southeast GA Regional Medical
Center**
Brunswick, GA
912-466-5200

Hawaii

Hawaii Pacific Cancer Center
Hilo, HI
808-933-0625

Iowa

U. Iowa Hospital and Clinic
Iowa City, IA
319-356-7592

Illinois

American Cancer Center
Elgin, IL
847-695-3555

Loyola U. Medical Center
Maywood, IL
708-216-9017

**Northwestern Memorial
Hospital**
Chicago, IL
312-926-4634

Berwyn Nuclear Oncology
Berwyn, IL
708-484-0011

U. Chicago Medical Center
Chicago, IL
773-702-3309

Louisiana

Willis-Knighton Medical Center
Shreveport, LA
318-632-4939

Maryland

National Naval Medical Center
Bethesda, MD
301-295-5000

U. Maryland Medical Center
Baltimore, MD
410-328-0324

Michigan

Harper U. Kamanos Cancer Institute
Detroit, MI
313-745-8376

Huron Valley Sinai Hospital
Commerce Township, MI
248-937-3605

McLaren Regional Medical Center
Flint, MI
810-342-1032

Oakwood Medical Center
Dearborn, MI
313-593-7335

Radiation Therapy Associates
Garden City, MI
734-522-8540

St. Mary's Mercy Medical Center
Grand Rapids, MI
616-752-6218

Seton Cancer Institute
Saginaw, MI
517-776-8115

Weisberg Cancer Center
Farmington Hills, MI
248-538-6624

North Dakota

Dakota Cancer Clinic
Fargo, ND
701-280-8910

Trinity Health-St. Joseph's
Minot, ND
701-857-2299

Nebraska

Clarkson Hospital
Nebraska Health System
Omaha, NE
402-552-3844

New Hampshire

Elliot Regional Cancer Center
Optima Healthcare
Manchester, NH
603-628-2363

New Jersey

Christ Hospital
Jersey City, NJ
201-795-5282

Clara Maass Medical Center
Belleville, NJ
973-450-2270

Community Medical Center
Toms River, NJ
732-557-8148

Shore Memorial Hospital
Somers Point, NJ
609-652-3409

**Monmouth/St. Barnabas
Healthcare**
Long Branch, NJ
732-923-6894

St. Barnabas Medical Center
Livingston, NJ
973-322-5634

**St. Joseph's Hospital and
Medical Center**
Patterson, NJ
973-754-2181

Valley Hospital
Ridgewood, NJ
201-447-8220

New York

Batavia Radiation Oncology
Batavia, NY
716-344-3050

**Finger Lakes Radiation
Oncology**
Clifton Springs, NY
315-462-5711

**North Shore Radiation
Oncology**
E. Setauket, NY 11733
631-689-6776

Radiotherapy of Syracuse
Syracuse, NY
315-472-7500

University Hospital Brooklyn
Brooklyn, NY
718-270-1591

**VA-Albany/Veteran's
Administration**
Medical Center, Albany, NY
518-462-4512

VA Hospital Bronx
Bronx, NY
732-363-2699

Ohio

Flower Hospital
Sylvania, OH
419-824-1855

Medcentral Health Systems
Mansfield, OH
419-526-8883

Oklahoma

Southwestern Regional Medical Center
Tulsa, OK
918-496-5121

Mercy Health Center
Oklahoma City, OK
405-752-3381

Oregon

Bay Area Hospital
Coos Bay, OR
541-269-8520

Pennsylvania

Allegheny General Hospital/West Penn
Allegheny Health System
Pittsburgh, PA
412-359-3400

Apple Hill Medical Center
York, PA
717-741-8126

Guthrie Healthcare System
Sayre, PA
570-882-4048

Jefferson Radiation Oncology
Pittsburgh, PA
412-653-8944

Hershey/Pennsylvania State University
Hershey, PA
717-531-8210

Thomas Jefferson U. Hospital
Philadelphia, PA
215-955-6702

Westmoreland Regional Hospital
Greensburg, PA
724-832-4267

Rhode Island

Rhode Island Hospital
Providence, RI
401-444-8546

Tennessee

St. Jude Children's Research Hospital
Memphis, TN
901-495-3604

Texas

Christus Spohn Hospital Shoreline
Corpus Christi, TX
361-887-4521

Joe Arrington Cancer Research and Treatment Center
Lubbock, TX
806-725-7924

MD Anderson Cancer Center
Houston, TX
713-745-4502

Paris Regional Cancer Center
Paris, TX
903-785-0066

Virginia

Danville Regional Medical Center
Danville, VA
804-799-4592

U. Virginia Medical Center
Charlottesville, VA
434-924-5191

Washington

Swedish Tumor Institute
Seattle, WA
206-386-2323

Wisconsin

Appleton Medical Center
Appleton, WI
920-738-6340

Froedtert Memorial Lutheran Hospital
Milwaukee, WI
414-805-4400

West Virginia

Greenbrier Valley Cancer Center
Lewisburg, WV
304-647-3500

Canada

Jewish General Hospital
Montreal, Quebec
514-934-8052

Toronto-Sunnybrook Hospital
Toronto, Ontario
416-480-5853
514-340-8288

HIGH-DOSE RADIATION (HDR) SITES

Douglas A. Kelly, M.D.
Oncologist, Brachytherapy
Specialist
Southwestern Regional Medical
Center
2408 East 81 St., Ste. 100
Tulsa, OK 74137-4210
Tel: 918-496-5121
Fax: 918-496-5146
dak@ctcoftulsa.com

**Chicago Prostate Cancer
Center**
One Oak Hill Center
Ste. 100
Westmont, IL 60559
Tel: 630-654-2515
Fax: 630-654-2516
www.prostateimplant.com

Jeffrey Demanes, M.D.
California Endocurietherapy
Cancer Center
3012 Summit St., Ste. 2675
Oakland, CA 94609
Tel: 510-986-0690
www.info@cetmc.com

**Southwestern Regional Medical
Center**
2408 E. 81st St., Ste. 100
Tulsa, OK 74137
Tel: 800-615-3055
Fax: 918-496-5052
www.brachytherapy.com

Loma Linda U. Medical Center
Dept. of Radiology
11234 Anderson St.
Loma Linda, CA 92354
Tel: 909-558-4356
Fax: 909-558-0147
www.llu.edu/llumc

Latrobe Area Hospital
121 W. Second Ave.
Latrobe, PA 15650-1096
Tel: 724-537-1000
Fax: 724-537-1935
www.lah.com

Timothy Mate, M.D.
Swedish Cancer Radiation
Oncology Group
1221 Madison, 1st Floor
Seattle, WA 98104
Tel: 206-386-2323
Fax: 206-215-6150

INTENSITY MODULATED RADIATION THERAPY (IMRT) SITES

University of Alabama
Birmingham Medical Center
Birmingham, AL
205-934-1747

Arizona Oncology Service
Scottsdale Radiation Oncology
Scottsdale, AZ
602-274-4484

Mayo Clinic for Medical Education & Research
Scottsdale, AZ
480-301-1735

Beverly Oncology and Imaging Center
Montebello, CA
323-724-8780

City of Hope Medical Center
Duarte, CA
626-301-8247

Redding Cancer Treatment Center
Redding, CA
530-245-5900

Sharp Chula Vista Medical Center
Chula Vista, CA
619-482-5851

Sharp Grossmont Hospital
La Mesa, CA
619-644-4500

Santa Monica Cancer Treatment Center
Santa Monica, CA
310-828-0061

St. Vincent Medical Center
Los Angeles, CA
213-484-7111

University of California, Irvine
Orange, CA
714-456-5508

University of California, San Francisco
San Francisco, CA
415-353-7174

Dattoli Cancer Center
Sarasota, FL
941-957-4926

Tenet St. Mary's Medical Center
Kaplan Radiation Center
West Palm Beach, FL
561-881-2815

Frank A. Critz, MD
Radiotherapy Clinics of Georgia
2349 Lawrenceville Highway
Decatur, GA 30033
404-320-1550

Columbus Regional Healthcare System
Amos Cancer Center
Columbus, GA
706-571-1911

Regional Radiation Oncology Center
Rome, GA
706-234-1400

Wesley Medical Center
Wichita, KS
316-688-2920

West Jefferson Medical Center
Marrero, LA
504-349-1480

Tufts-New England Medical Center
Boston, MA
617-636-6161

Abbott Northwestern Hospital
Minneapolis, MN
612-863-5171

Mallinckrodt/Barnes Jewish Hospital
St. Louis, MO
314-747-1230

Altru Health System
Grand Forks, ND
701-780-5860

Bismarck Cancer Center
Bismarck, ND
701-222-6100

Hackensack University Medical Center
Hackensack, NJ
201-996-2210

Advanced Radiation Oncology of Nyack
Nyack, NY
845-727-0628

North Shore Radiation Oncology
Martin Silverstein, MD
Joseph Cirrone, M.D.
181 Belle Meade Road
East Setauket, NY 11733
631-689-6776

Long Island Jewish Medical Center
New Hyde Park, NY
718-470-7190

Mt Sinai Medical Center
Mt Sinai, NY
212-241-7502

Staten Island University Hospital
Staten Island, NY
718-226-8862

Cleveland Clinic Foundation
Cleveland, OH
216-444-1938

Fox Chase Cancer Center
Philadelphia, PA
215-728-2996

Cancer Center of Wyoming Valley
Wilkes Barre, PA
570-822-9822

Sacred Heart Hospital Center for Cancer Care
Allentown, PA
610-776-4674

Radiation Medicine Specialist of Northeast PA, PC
Forty Fort, PA
570-714-8686

Prairie Lakes Healthcare System
Watertown, SD
605-882-6800

Centennial Medical Systems
Nashville, TN
615-342-4850

CTRC/Grossman Cancer Center
San Antonio, TX
210-616-5500

Southwest Cancer Center
Lubbock, TX
806-743-1900

Houston Methodist Hospital
Houston, TX
713-790-2091

Tomball Regional Hospital and Cancer Center
Tomball, TX
281-351-3914

Moncrief/UT Southwestern
FT. Worth, TX
817-923-7393

VA-Houston, VA Medical Center
Houston, TX
713-794-7190

Princeton Radiation Oncology Center
Greenbrier, WV
304-425-3514

LAPARASCOPIC PROSTATECTOMY SITES

Mani Menon, M.D., Urologist
Vatt, Kut, Urology Institute
Henry Ford Hospital
2799 W. Grand Blvd.
Detroit, MI 48202
Tel: 800-653-6568

Garth A. Ballantyne, M.D., Urologist
Hackensack University Medical Center
20 Prospect Ave., Ste. 901
Hackensack, NJ 07601
Tel: 201-996-2959

Bertrand D. Guillonneau, M.D., Urologist
Memorial Sloan-Kettering Cancer Center
1275 York Ave.
New York, NY 10021
Tel: 646-422-4387

Inderbir Gill, M.D.
Craig D. Zippe, M.D., Urologists
Cleveland Clinic Foundation
Urological Institute
9500 Euclid Ave., Desk A100
Cleveland, OH 44195
Tel: 216-445-1530

Jamil Rehman, M.D., Urologist
Stony Brook U. Hospital
Stony Brook Medical Park
Dept. of Urology
2500 R.347, Bldg. 23
Stony Brook, NY 11794

Benjamin R. Lee, M.D.
Arthur D. Smith, M.D.
Urologists
Long Island Jewish Medical Center
270-05 76th Ave.
New Hyde Park, NY 11040
Tel: 718-470-7220

Michael Fabrizio, M.D.
Win Robey, M.D., Urologists
Devine Tidewater Urology
400 West Brambleton Ave.
Ste. 100
Norfolk, VA 23510
Tel: 757-457-5128

Li-Ming Su, M.D.
Louis R. Kavoussi, M.D., Urologists
John Hopkins Bayview Medical Center
Dept. of Urology, A3East
4940 Eastern Ave.
Baltimore, MD 21224
Tel: 410-550-3506

Robert Mordkin, Urologist
Georgetown U. Hospital
Division of Urology
3800 Reservoir Rd. NW
Bldg. PHC, 4th Fl.
Washington, DC 20007
Tel: 202-687-4922

Douglas M. Dahl, M.D.
Urologist
Laparascopic Urologic Surgery
Massachusetts General Hospital
55 Fruit St.
GRB1102
Boston, MA 02114
Tel: 617-726-0875

Ingolf Tuerk, M.D., Ph.D.
Urologist
Chairman of Dept. of Urology
Lehey Medical Center
41 Mall Rd.
Burlington, MA 01805
Tel: 781-744-2503

MAGNETIC RESONANCE SPECTROSCOPIC IMAGING (MRSI)
SITES

Hedvig Hricak, M.D.
Chairman of Radiology
Memorial Sloan-Kettering Cancer
Center
1275 York Ave.
New York, NY 10021
Tel: 212-639-2000

Arlene Lennox, M.D.
Clinical Physicist
Fermi National Accelerator
Laboratory
PO Box 500, Mailstop 301
Batavia, IL 60510
Tel: 630-840-4850
www.fnal.gov

John Kurhanewicz, Ph.D.
Asst. Professor
Radiology, Bioengineering,
Pharmaceutical Chemistry
U. California at San Francisco
Dept. of Radiology
Box 1290
San Francisco, CA 94143
Tel: 415-479-9023

NEUTRON BEAM RADIATION SITES

Jeffery Foreman, M.D.
Radiation Oncologist
Gershenson Radiation
Oncology Center
399 John R St.
Detroit, MI 48201
Tel: 313-745-9191
www.roc.wayne.edu

Harold Kim, M.D.
Radiation Oncologist
Harper Hospital
Dept. of Radiation Oncology
3990 John R St.
Detroit, MI 48201
Tel: 313-745-8040
Fax: 313-993-0036
www.harperhospital.org

Arlene J. Lennox, M.D.
Geoffrey Smoron, M.D.
Jeffrey Shafer, M.D.
Clinical Physicist/Radiation
Oncologists
Midwest Institute for Neutron
Therapy at Fermilab
PO Box 500, Mailstop 301
Batavia, IL 60510
Tel: 630-840-3865
Fax: 630-840-8766
www.neutrontherapy.org

PATHOLOGY LABORATORY PERFORMING GENE TEST SITES

Arul M. Chinnalyan, MD, PhD
Department of Pathology
University of Michigan Medical School
1301 Catherine Road
Ann Arbor, MI 48109-0602
Tel: 734-936-1889
arul@umich.edu

PROSE MRI SITES

University of California, San Francisco
UCSF Comprehensive Cancer Center
Box 1290, UCSF
San Francisco, CA 94143-1290
Tel: 415-476-0312

National Institute of Health
9000 Rockville Pike
Bethesda, MD 20892
Tel: 301-496-2535

Edison Imaging Associates
60 James St.
Edison, NJ 08820
Tel: 732-632-1650

Hackensack Radiology Group
Imaging Center at Newman Street
30 S Newman St.
Hackensack, NJ 07601
Tel: 201-488-1188

MD Anderson Cancer Center
1515 Holcombe Blvd.
Houston, TX 77030
Tel: 800-392-1611 (USA)
Tel: 713-792-6161

STUDY SITES USING PROVENGE

California

City of Hope Medical Center
Medical Oncology
Mortensen Hall R. 138
1500 East Duarte Rd.
Duarte, CA 91010
Study coordinator: Dorie Garcia
Tel: 626-359-8111 ext. 3021
Principal investigator:
Kim Margolin, M.D.

Cancer and Blood Institute of the Desert
39-700 Bob Hope Dr., Ste. 110
Rancho Mirage, CA 92270
Study coordinator: Susan Sagle, RN, OCN
Tel: 760-568-4461 ext. 124
susan@cbirm.com
Principal investigator: Robert Lemon, M.D.

Sutter Cancer Center
2800 L Street, Ste. 410
Sacramento, CA 95810
Study coordinator: Kirsten Babski
Tel: 916-454-6931
Fax: 916-454-6596
babskik@sutterhealth.org
Principal investigator: Vincent Caggiano, M.D.

Neil M. Barth, MD, Inc.
4000 W Pacific Coast Hwy, Ste. 3C
Newport Beach, CA 92663
Study coordinator: Kelly Ditmore
Tel: 714-536-4640
Fax: 714-536-2382
Kelly-rn@pacbell.net
Prinicpal investigator: Neil M. Barth, M.D.

South Orange County Urological
24301 Paseo de Valencia, Ste. 100
Laguna Woods, CA 92653
Study coordinator: Erika Pirtle
Tel: 949-215-9515 ext. 236
Fax: 949-215-9510
Erika.pirtle@urologymedical.com
Principal investigator: Jay Young, M.D.

UCSF Cancer Center
Urologic Oncology, 1600 Divisadero St.
3rd Floor Bosx 1711
San Francisco, CA 94115
Study coordinator: Wilma Batiste, CRC
Tel: 415-885-7329
Fax: 415-353-9566
wbatiste@medicine.ucsf.edu
Principal investigator: Eric Small, M.D.

LLUMC for Molecular Biology and Gene Therapy
Dept. of Sponsors Research
11085 Campus St., Room 142
Loma Linda, CA 92354
Study coordinator: Richard
Gurrola, M.D.
Tel: 909-558-1000 ext.(1)81397
Principal investigator: Michael
Lilly, M.D.

Sharp Health Care
Clinical Oncology Research
7901 Frost St.
San Diego, CA 92123
Study coordinator: Cathy Wood
Tel: 858-541-3839
Principal investigator: Charles
Redfern, M.D.

Colorado

Rocky Mountain Cancer Centers
1800 Williams St.
Denver, CO 80218
Study coordinator: Joni Newman
Tel: 303-285-5011
Joni.Newman2@usoncology.com
Principal investigator: Robert
Rifkin, M.D.

Urology Associates, PC
850 East Harvard, Ste. 525
Denver, CO 80210
Study coordinator: Tanya Frazier
Tel: 303-733-8873 ext. 1262
Fax: 303-733-3107
T.Frazier@uradenver.com
Principal investigator: Barrett
Cowan, M.D.

Florida

Hematology/Oncology Associates of the Treasure Coast
1801 SE Hillmoor Dr., Ste. B108
Port St. Lucie, FL 34952
Study coordinator: Christine
Baker
Tel: 772-335-5666 ext. 244
Fax: 772-335-0102
cbaker@hemoncfl.com
Principal investigator: Michael
Wertheim, M.D.

Moffitt Cancer Center & Research Institute
12902 Magnolia Drive
Tampa, FL 33612-9497
Study coordinator: Kathy
McCollister, R.N.
Tel: 813-972-8395
Principal investigator: John D.
Seigne, M.D.

Georgia

Georgia Urology, P.A.
5445 Meridan Mark Rd., Ste. 430
Atlanta, GA 30342
Study coordinator: Patti Huebner,
RN BSN OCN CCRC
Tel: 404-943-1957
Fax: 404-493-1958
Principal investigator: Vahan
Kassabian, M.D.

Maryland

Urology Associates
7500 Hanover Pkwy., Ste 206
Greenbelt, MD 20770
Study coordinator: Liz D'Antonio
Tel: 301-441-8900 ext. 104
Principal investigator: Myron
Murdock, M.D.

New Jersey

Hackensack University Medical Center
Institute for Biomedical Research
20 Prospect Ave., Ste. 400
Hackensack, NJ 07601
Study coordinator: Laura
Kudlacik
Tel: 201-996-5917
Principal investigator: Richard J.
Rosenbluth, M.D.

Associates in Urology, LLC
741 Northfield Ave., Ste. 206
West Orange, NJ 07052
Study coordinator: Kathleen
Murtha
Tel: 973-325-6100
Principal investigator: Jeffrey
Katz, M.D.

New York

North Shore Hematology/Oncology Associates
235 North Belle Mead Rd.
East Setauket, NY 11733
Study coordinator: Sharon
Goldberg
Tel: 631-751-3000 ext. 170
Fax: 631-689-5813
Principal investigator: E. Roy
Berger, M.D., F.A.C.P.

Staten Island Urological Research, PC
242 Mason Ave., Ste. 5
Staten Island, NY 10305
Study coordinator: Nicole
Zampordi
Tel: 718-226-6460
Principal investigator: Ron
Israeli, M.D.

Ohio

AKSM Clinical Research Corporation
797 Thomas La.
Columbus, OH 43214
Study coordinator: Anne Berkal
Tel: 614-447-0281
Fax: 614-447-9374
aberkal@aksm.com
Principal investigator: Wayne
Poll, M.D.

Oregon

Oregon Urology Specialists
1200 Hilyard St., Ste. S150
Eugene, OR 97401
Study coordinator: Tamara
Whittle
Tel: 541-284-5508
twhittle@peacehealth.org
Principal investigator: Peter
Bergreen, M.D.

Pennsylvania

Bryn Mawr Urology
101 S. Bryn Mawr Ave.
Ste. 220
Bryn Mawr, PA 19010
Study coordinator: Carol Wenger
Tel: 610-520-0137
Principal investigator: James
Squadrito, M.D.

Office of Guy Bernstein
245 Bryn Mawr Ave.
Bryn Mawr, PA 19010
Study coordinator: Joan Brown
Tel: 610-525-2515
Principal investigator: Guy T.
Bernstein, M.D.

Rhode Island

**Univ. Urological Research
Institute**
100 Highland Ave., Ste. 106
Providence, RI 02906
Study coordinator: Betsy Parrott
Tel: 401-331-9242
Fax: 331-7429
Staff0029@americasdoctor.com
Principal investigator: Barry Stein,
M.D.

Texas

US Oncology
American Oncology Resources
3535 Worth St., Collins Building,
5th Fl.
Dallas, TX 75246
Study coordinator: Amy Morris-
Bosley
Tel: 214-370-1845
Fax: 214-370-1886
Ami.Bosley@usoncology.com
Principal investigator: John
Nemunaitis, M.D.

**Urology Associates of North
Texas**
1325 Pennsylvania Ave., Ste. 540
Fort Worth, TX 76104
Study coordinator: Nancy
Resmini
Tel: 817-332-8595 ext. 61
Fax: 817-332-8599
nresmini@uant.com
Princinpal investigator: David
Shepherd, M.D.

Utah

University of Utah
School of Medicine
30 North 1900 East
Salt Lake City, UT 84132
Study coordinator: Elizabeth
Lignell
Tel: 801-581-3739
Fax: 801-585-2891
Elizabeth.lignell@hscu.utah.edu
Principal investigator: Robert
Stephenson, M.D.

Cancer Care Northwest
605 E Holland St., Ste. 100
Spokane, WA 99218
Study coordinator: Rose Miller
Tel: 509-228-6951
Fax: 509-228-6952
Rosalee.miller@usoncology.com
Prinicipal investigator: Stephen
Anthony, M.D.

Virginia

Devine Tidewater Urology
600 Gresham Dr., Ste. 203
Norfolk, VA 23507
Study coordinators: Lenny
Strickland
Tel: 757-457-5163
Cindy Cutter
Tel: 757-459-9219
Principal investigator:
Paul Schellhammer, M.D.

Washington

Virginia Mason Medical Center
1100 9th Ave., MS C7-URO
Seattle, WA 98101
Study coordinator: Kathryn Dahl,
R.N.
Tel: 206-341-0578
Kathryn.dahl@vmmc.org
Principal investigator: John
Corman, M.D

INDEX

About the Authors

E. Roy Berger, M.D., F.A.C.P.

E. Roy Berger, M.D., a medical oncologist, is one of a small number of physicians in the United States whose subspecialty is in prostatic malignancies. He has participated in numerous research studies that have led to U.S. Food and Drug Administration (FDA) approval of such drugs as strontium. One of his most important achievements is participation in research that ultimately led to FDA approval of flutamide, an antiandrogenic drug used in combination hormonal therapy for treating prostate cancer.

In addition to lecturing, making presentations at conferences and hospitals around the nation, and publishing a multitude of professional articles, Dr. Berger is in private practice with a well-known and highly regarded group of physicians, the North Shore Hematology-Oncology Associates on Long Island, New York.

Dr. Berger has served as a consultant and as a clinical affiliate at Memorial Sloan-Kettering Cancer Center, where he was trained as a medical oncologist. He has also served on the Prostate Cancer Education Council, a group that has sponsored free prostate cancer screenings nationwide and has been instrumental in heightening prostate cancer awareness. Dr. Berger holds staff positions at Mather Memorial Hospital and St. Charles Hospital in Port Jefferson, New York, and at St. Catherine of Siena Medical Center in Smithtown, New York. He serves on the faculty at both SUNY at Stony Brook and New York Medical College. He also serves on the Medical Advisory Boards of PAACT and US TOO International. Dr. Berger has been cited in the book *How to Find the Best Doctor for Your Family and Top Doctors New York Metro Area* (Castle, Connolly). He is also the author, with Linda A. Mittiga, of *Common Bonds: Reflections of a Cancer Doctor* (1st Books Library, Publisher, 2001), a book about the intimate cancer patient—doctor relationship.

James Lewis, Jr., Ph.D.

James Lewis, Jr., is a survivor of both colon and prostate cancer.

Dr. Lewis received a B.S. from Hampton University, an M.S. from Columbia University, and a Ph.D. from Union Graduate School. In 1970, he was identified as one of the promising educators in the United States and received the prestigious Alfred North Whitehead fellowship at Harvard

University. He also attended the Massachusetts Institute of Technology. He was later superintendent of schools in Wyandanch, New York and in the Central Berkshire School District in Dalton, Massachusetts. He served as associate professor of education and full professor of education at Villanova University and the City University New York, respectively, and taught on the undergraduate and graduate levels. As a noted education consultant, he conducted training tours at numerous universities and school districts throughout the United States. During his public education career he wrote the best-seller, *Achieving Excellence in Our Schools...By Taking Lessons from the Best Run Companies in America* (1986) and 29 other books on a variety of education and school administration subjects.

As an educator, Dr. Lewis was quick to realize that prostate cancer patients were dying not because of the disease itself, but because of their lack of timely and meaningful information. To remedy this situation, he cofounded the Education Center for Prostate Cancer Patients to realize a vision of "enabling men to live longer than they hoped possible." As executive director of ECPCP, he now pursues his mission to save or lengthen the lives of prostate cancer patients, to improve their quality of life, and to enable them to make effective diagnostic and treatment decisions through education, advice, counseling, and research. As a prostate cancer advisor, Dr. Lewis has advised and guided approximately 65,000 prostate cancer patients throughout the United States and several foreign countries.

Dr. Lewis is also the author of *How I Survived Prostate Cancer...And So Can You* (1994) *Guidelines for Surviving Prostate Cancer* (1997), *Best Options for Diagnosing and Treating Prostate Cancer* (1999), and *The Herbal Remedy for Prostate Cancer* (1999).